OUT OF OTHERNESS:

Characters and Narrators in the Dutch Venereal Disease Debates 1850–1990

THE WELLCOME INSTITUTE SERIES IN
THE HISTORY OF MEDICINE

Forthcoming Titles

Constructing Paris Medicine
Edited by Caroline Hannaway and Ann Le Berge

Cultures of Psychiatry:
Postwar British and Dutch Mental Health Care
Edited by Marijke Gijswijt-Hofstra and Roy Porter

Mathematical and Statistical Developments
in the History of Medicine
Eileen Magnello

Academic enquiries regarding the series should be addressed
to the editors W. F. Bynum, V. Nutton and Roy Porter at
the Wellcome Institute for the History of Medicine,
183 Euston Road, London NW1 2BE, UK

OUT OF OTHERNESS:
Characters and Narrators in the Dutch Venereal Disease Debates 1850–1990

Annet Mooij

Translated from the Dutch by Beverley Jackson

Amsterdam – Atlanta, GA 1998

First published in Dutch, under the title *Geslachtsziekten en besmettingsangst*, 1993.

This English translation first published in 1998
by Editions Rodopi B. V., Amsterdam – Atlanta, GA 1998.

© 1998 Annet Mooij

Design by Christine Buckley, typesetting by Alex Mayor,
the Wellcome Trust.
Printed and bound in The Netherlands by Editions Rodopi B. V.,
Amsterdam – Atlanta, GA 1998.

British Library Cataloguing in Publication Data
A catalogue record for this book is available from the British Library
ISBN 90-420-0257-3 (Paper)
ISBN 90-420-0267-0 (Bound)

Annet Mooij
Out of Otherness – Amsterdam – Atlanta, GA:
Rodopi.
(Clio Medica 47 / ISSN 0045-7183;
The Wellcome Institute Series in the History of Medicine)

Front cover:

Illustration from a poster distributed by the Dutch Anti-Venereal
Disease Society as a warning to seamen, c.1920,
Universiteitsmuseum De Agnietenkapel, Amsterdam

© Editions Rodopi B. V., Amsterdam – Atlanta, GA 1998

Printed in The Netherlands

The translation of this book was funded by the Netherlands
Organization for Scientific Research (NWO)

Contents

Introduction

In the Dutch novel *De Klop op de Deur* (*The Knock on the Door*, 1930) by Ina Boudier-Bakker, the character Otto de Block finds himself increasingly troubled by severe fits of giddiness, that gradually turn his boyish, buoyant gait into an uncertain, creeping pace, and change his fresh features into a yellow countenance in which the dull eyes are sunk in deep hollow cavities. These alarming changes have set in only a few months after his marriage. And as if all the cares wrought upon Otto and his wife Stance by this baffling deterioration of the young man's health were not enough, other calamities follow in their train. Their first child dies quite unexpectedly when only a few years old, and the little boy born shortly afterwards, as soon becomes clear, is far from normal. His curious, angular head and his slow, aimless movements would immediately arouse suspicion in any experienced mother's eye. As he grows older, his retarded development is obvious to everyone; the fits to which he is prey, his unseeing stare and the raw cries he is apt to emit leave no room for doubt. While the origins of this misfortune are apparent to some of the better-informed persons in the neighbourhood, the hapless parents themselves are completely unaware of the cause. And then finally, each of them separately is made aware of the truth. Otto decides to seek another medical opinion about his condition, from a doctor whose questions 'suddenly brought into focus a period from before his marriage, a time his memory had elected to suppress'.

> He was thunderstruck.
> 'That? That?'
> He had sat there, pale, ashen, his dry,
> stammering lips scarcely able to form the words.

1

'Surely it couldn't be that? After so many years?'

'I'm afraid it's quite possible.'

'You mean it never went away?'

'Apparently not.'

His life collapsed in an instant. A flood of memories – acquaintances, men he had seen cut down in the prime of life – and then the shock of realization that split his head: 'His child. That child ...'.[1]

Otto cannot bring himself to break the terrible news to Stance. But meanwhile, she is conducting an investigation of her own. In a little book about feeble-mindedness, she learns something she has never heard of before. 'A child like Dolfje could be the result of a sickness of the father.'[2] Stance's love for Otto is shaken by this discovery, but it eventually triumphs over her resentment and sense of disillusionment. This generosity, however, can do nothing to avert the inexorable course of the disease: soon afterwards, on the same day, both father and son are laid to rest.

The author does not name the ailment that destroys her characters' lives, but readers will have understood what was meant: here was the tragic aftermath of an old syphilis infection. This minor episode in Boudier-Bakker's novel is set towards the end of the 19th century, and is typical of some people's rude confrontation, at the time, with the realities of venereal disease. Certain things in particular about this story will pull the present-day reader up short. In the first place, we are struck by the drastic consequences of a syphilis infection a hundred years ago. Otto believes himself completely cured when he is suddenly felled without the remotest chance of recovery. And not only is he himself quickly transformed from an apparently healthy man in the prime of life to a helpless wreck, he also infects those dearest to him. The telltale symptoms that the novelist describes, as terrifying as they are fascinating, were typical of the largely inscrutable course followed by syphilis at the time. Physicians, victims and the well-informed public were all equally gripped by the visible and often repulsive symptoms during the first stages, and even more so by the protracted periods of apparent cure, which could nevertheless be followed, years later, by physical or mental collapse.

Another aspect that dates this story is the veil of secrecy in which venereal diseases were shrouded, making it possible for so many people to remain ignorant of the truth. Conventions and rules of decorum kept women and young people from being properly informed about the dangers of syphilis and gonorrhoea.[3] This approach did not always produce the desired result: the whispers, the half-information and charged atmosphere rather served to focus attention on the 'secret diseases'. Nevertheless, shame was the prevailing emotion. In the novel, Stance is the most obvious victim of the conspiracy of silence, but Otto too sees himself in this light. 'Who had ever warned him? What did a boy know of such matters? Nothing. Later you heard things from friends. But who had told him, inexperienced as he was, of the possible consequences for his future life as a man? No one.'[4] And it is his own sense of shame that prevents him, too, as an adult, from speaking to his wife.

One further detail of this episode that will strike the present-day reader is the symbolic meaning accorded the story of Otto and Stance de Block. In tune with late 19th-century reality, it is linked almost directly to the imbalance in power between the sexes. Annette Craets, the novel's protagonist, has often wondered to herself why her own family life, in contrast to that of her childhood friend Stance, is a pattern of health and happiness. At one point she exclaims in near-indignation to her husband Frederik:

'However did Stance come by such a wretched child?'
'Well, that's not hard to see. It must be Otto.'
'What do you mean, it must be Otto?'
'Well ... his trouble ...'
'But there are other men who are not healthy – and they don't all have children like that, do they?'
'No, but this thing ... what he had before his marriage.'
Annette's eyes got bigger and bigger.
'Frederik! Do you mean that a woman can suffer *that* because of what a man has done?'
She stood before him, deathly pale and appalled, her eyes full of revulsion. [...] 'Oh, that we should just get married without knowing anything! And then *something like that* can happen. We are at your mercy! [...].'

Later, alone, she had thought to herself: she had reached the age of thirty-six, and had not known life. She had thought she knew, because she had borne children – was married – and yet she had lived in a box, had not suspected anything of the terrible things that may exist within a marriage. She had been a woman [...] like all the men in her circle wanted women to be: ignorant. [...] She also thought of Truida Leedebour, who had said: there will be no beauty, while women are doomed to give birth to sickly children through

the fault of men. For the first time she understood the indignation,
the struggle waged by all those angry, fierce, hating women.

Thus the fate of Stance and Otto de Block reflects social problems as
well as medical ones.

All this combines, in *De Klop op de Deur*, to produce a useful
impression of the late 19th-century concept of venereal disease, an
image of the problem as it was then understood. But we can also infer
from these features certain more general observations. They constitute
what is, as it were, the typical late 19th-century interpretation of
three determinants of this problem that retain their significance
when stripped of their timebound context. For the purposes of
simplification, these determinants are somewhat artificially separated
here, whereas in reality they are not entirely unrelated.

The mysterious clinical picture, the apparent cure, the insidious
spread of the disease, the infection of offspring, all these are bound
up with the medical knowledge and the available treatment of the
day. These constitute the first element that determines the form that
the problem of venereal diseases takes on at a certain moment.
Secondly, there are the views concerning – and the social valuation
of – sexuality, in other words, the prevailing sexual mores. The wall
of silence, the shame, the threat of scandal and the notions of
punishment and atonement that emerge from *De Klop op de Deur*
are timebound examples of the impact of sexual mores on the
concept of venereal disease and on common perceptions of the
problem. The third and final element is the connection seen
between venereal disease and social issues, which in this case means
relations between men and women. This connection shows that the
balance of power in society also helps determine the way in which
the presence of venereal diseases and the actual danger of venereal
infection are viewed at a given point in time.

These determinants make it plain that the problem of venereal
disease is shaped by the wide range of responses that its presence and
the danger of infection tend to provoke. These responses in turn are
born of a specific constellation of medical knowledge and available
treatment, sexual mores and relationships within society. It follows
from this that the problems thus constituted are neither clear-cut
nor constant in nature. They are not clear-cut because the
constellation of knowledge, sexual mores and relationships in society
from which they derive constantly generates new symbolic
meanings. This means that the problem of venereal disease always
has a wider frame of reference than that of infectious diseases alone:

it is linked to sinfulness and vice, to moral degeneracy or to relations between the sexes, to class distinctions, the quality of family life, the health of the nation or other social issues. And as for constancy, the growth of knowledge, the shifts in sexual mores and changes in relationships within society also have repercussions on the way people react to venereal diseases, thus changing the nature and form of the problem.

This book deals with the different forms that the problem of venereal disease has assumed in the Netherlands over the past hundred years.[5] To put it differently, it examines the diverse social responses that have been prompted by the presence of venereal diseases and the danger of infection, and tries to explain them.

Infectious diseases

The history of a disease can be written in a variety of ways. If we start from the premise that the meaning attached to a disease is not clear-cut, but dependent on historical and social circumstances, a purely medical history will obviously not do. Various studies have already shown that biomedical factors are of only limited usefulness in clarifying the epidemiology of, and fight against, infectious diseases. William McNeill, in particular, has demonstrated convincingly that the way in which infectious diseases are classified among and within societies is determined neither by chance factors nor by autonomous biological processes that are more or less amenable to targeted medical intervention. In his book *Plagues and Peoples*, he shows the extent to which the history of diseases is bound up with that of human societies. Manipulations of the ecological environment in which people live, changes in modes of living together and new contacts among peoples have always been accompanied by new patterns of disease. Historically, with the establishment of larger communities and cities, outbreaks of disease became an ever-present threat. Clearly, such concentrations of people, animals and crops also meant concentrations of food for micro-organisms, thus creating favourable conditions for potential epidemics. Since then, wars, migration, trade and tourism have all contributed, over the centuries, to forming a homogeneous and comprehensive pattern of disease, what McNeill refers to as a 'common disease pool'. The current balance between men and microbes is based to a significant extent on the close-knit and extensive network of relations linking the different parts of the world, and it is in the light of changes in this network that the rise and spread of infectious diseases should be viewed.

McNeill's study encompasses many centuries and adopts a global perspective. It is interesting to focus on one particular society, within a fairly recent period, which allows the impact of social and historical circumstances on the epidemiology of infectious diseases to be studied in greater detail. The work of Thomas McKeown, which is based largely on data from England and Wales, has demonstrated that – well into the 20th century – the important breakthroughs in medical science in the realm of immunization and treatment scarcely contributed at all to the decline in mortality rates from infectious diseases.[6] The general improvements in health that became noticeable around the turn of the century cannot be explained, therefore, as the result of effective and successful techniques of treatment developed by the medical profession. Of greater importance was the broad improvement in standards of living: better nutrition and the expansion of sanitary facilities such as the water supply and sewers. For the Netherlands, Verdoorn's study of public health in Amsterdam in the previous century has likewise shown that it was mainly social developments – in his terms, a structural change in the dominant culture – that suddenly caused more, improved sanitary facilities to be perceived as a matter of some urgency, and that ultimately provided the motor for the improvements in public health after 1880.[7]

The differences in the spread of disease across the various population groups likewise underscore the importance of an approach based on social epidemiology. This is just as true for today's ailments as for 19th-century epidemics. Some groups are systematically more prone to disease than others. Although women in the Western world have a longer average life expectancy than men, they report illness more frequently, and are over-represented among users of the health service.[8] The most striking discrepancy between the sexes is in the field of psychiatric disorders.[9] The distribution of diseases among social classes likewise exhibits systematic discrepancies: the vast majority of diseases are more prevalent among the poor. Countless studies have demonstrated afresh this connection between socio-economic position and state of health, and over the years a variety of hypotheses has been aired in explanation.[10] The prevailing trend in the mid-19th century was to assume that poverty and sickness were natural bedfellows, the emphasis being on the unsanitary conditions in poor neighbourhoods and what was believed to be a natural preference among the indigent for a dissolute lifestyle. More recent research has focused on class-bound differences in the accessibility and use of medical facilities, and on the more hazardous living and working conditions in which people from the lower classes tend to find themselves. The obdurate nature of the differences, which have persisted in spite of the successful onslaught on infectious diseases, and in spite of the general decline in mortality rates from disease, has also focused attention on factors of the social environment such as mobility, stress and the functioning of social networks, which may affect susceptibility to disease.[11]

All this justifies the conclusion that if we want to understand the history of an infectious disease, it will not do simply to chart the steady progress of medical control. The spread of diseases is intimately bound up with changes in the way people live together: with social trends such as urbanization and migration, with shifts in social practices and the changes in mentality that accompany them. I shall accordingly place the development and spread of infectious diseases in what has been called a 'socio-genetic' perspective.

This said, my research focuses most explicitly on the *responses* that diseases and their sufferers have provoked among various population groups. A socio-genetic framework is every bit as essential to understanding these responses as it is to understanding the spread of the disease itself. If we want to identify the meanings that are attached to diseases, as well as the people or population groups who are held responsible for distributing them and the kind of images that certain categories of patients acquire in the public eye, it is not enough to study the most obvious data on prevalence and seriousness of the disease in question; it is essential to come to grips with the historical circumstances and social structure within which specific responses come about.

Many studies – some empirical, others reflective – can be cited in justification of a sociological approach to the responses prompted by the presence of the sick and the danger of infection. Several researchers have investigated the process whereby collective images are formed of patients and the experience of sickness. The work of Claudine Herzlich and Janine Pierret falls into this category, as does a well-known study by Susan Sontag. In their book *Illness and Self in Society*, Herzlich and Pierret show that the image of the prototypical sickness that dominates a society at a given point in time and the associated individual experience of sickness vary according to their historical and social framework. They conclude:

> The sick person is a social figure in at least two respects. [...] Illness
> is related to society by its nature and its distribution, which vary
> according to the period and the society. Moreover, the condition

7

and the identity of the sick – the place that is assigned to them in the social space and in the collective consciousness – fit into the value system of each society, the body of knowledge it develops and the caretaking institutions it puts into place.[12]

In her famous book *Illness as Metaphor*, Susan Sontag discusses the tendency to ascribe to a disease meanings that help generate collective fantasies about its victims. Ignorance about a disease and its mode of transmission stimulate this process. Focusing on popular images and cultural representations of TB sufferers in the past, and of cancer patients in our own time, Sontag shows that the mysterious natures of the two diseases have spawned a whole range of moralistic reflections and speculative psychologizing about their victims.

Alongside the literature on the representation of sickness and the sick, countless studies have chronicled the history of and fight against specific diseases such as cholera, bubonic plague and tuberculosis.[13] All demonstrate to some extent that the way the medical profession, local and national authorities or the population at large react to a given disease cannot be separated from larger social trends.

Some authors – the Dutch sociologists Johan Goudsblom and Abram de Swaan among others – accord the historical and sociological framework an even more prominent role. Goudsblom, for instance, explains the dramatic sanitary reforms that were implemented in the 19th century largely as a result of changes in the sensitivities of the upper middle classes, which rendered the proximity of filth and evil-smelling slums intolerable to them. The campaigns for hygiene reform stemmed primarily from the need to make the unavoidable presence of the burgeoning working classes less distasteful and less hazardous. Furthermore, the development of the mutual dependency of factory-owners and workers had the effect of increasing the desire among the middle classes to combat disease and ignorance among the working classes, and to reduce the number of paupers. The sudden rage for hygiene therefore went hand-in-hand with the wide-ranging 'civilization offensive' that was waged in the 19th century with the aim of elevating the working classes.[14] Like Goudsblom, De Swaan sees the menacing proximity of a swelling proletariat in combination with an increased awareness of mutual interdependency as providing the main motive for the well-to-do citizenry to take collective action to install a water supply and sewers.[15] It was cholera, above all, that served as a metaphor for the dangers lurking within the new interdependency between the urban rich and their uncomfortably close poor neighbours.

Venereal diseases provide an even more fertile field than cholera for exploring a sociological view of illness. Whereas responses to cholera were bound up with the relations between rich and poor, the problems associated with venereal disease are a good deal more complex, with issues of sex and sexuality as well as class coming into play. This is what distinguishes venereal diseases from all other types of illness. There is another important distinction besides this. Whereas cholera reared its head, in the Netherlands, in sporadic short-lived epidemics, venereal diseases were, and are, an ever-present fact of life. This continuous presence is not without its usefulness for the researcher. It makes it possible to follow these infections and the responses they provoked in society over a long period, and to explore the relationships between social trends and changes in the significance of the problem of venereal disease.

The permanent presence of venereal disease – unlike sudden epidemics – raises the question of how we should explain the changing responses to it and fluctuations in the amount of attention it receives. The literature discussed above demonstrates convincingly that social responses to a disease also have social origins. They cannot be explained simply in terms of objective risk factors. Neither the seriousness of a disease nor its incidence can fully account for the intensity or nature of the responses it provokes.

Theoretical considerations aside, many empirical studies have shown quite clearly the disjunction between objective factors and society's response: the most extreme responses, in the form of sanitary measures or dogged efforts to fight a disease, often took place when the disease was past its highest point, with the number of victims falling. History also reveals that we cannot trace a simple parallel between the incidence of venereal disease and the degree of repugnance it provoked. Moreover, we can nearly always find other ailments that either claimed more victims or were increasing in incidence at the same time, without provoking a comparable public response.

Venereal diseases

Venereal diseases belong to the category of infectious diseases, and up to this point they have been discussed as such. Yet they stand out in certain respects from other infectious diseases. For instance, in general the control of infectious diseases in the Netherlands has improved dramatically in the course of the 20th century. Cholera, smallpox, typhoid fever, tuberculosis and diphtheria, which still assumed epidemic form in the 19th century, have been almost eradicated here over the past hundred years, and measles and scarlet fever, as endemic childhood diseases, have become increasingly mild. But the battle to contain infectious disease is not an unmitigated success story: venereal disease displays a striking deviation from the general pattern. Not only have the age-old afflictions of syphilis and gonorrhoea proved tenaciously resistant to effective individual treatment, but the list of known sexually transmitted diseases has actually lengthened over the past few decades. The most tragic development in this area, of course, is the advent and rapid spread, since the 1980s, of the new and deadly disease of Acquired Immuno-Deficiency Syndrome, or AIDS.

There is another respect in which venereal diseases have retained a somewhat anomalous position. Although they are no longer the unfathomable evils of a hundred years ago, improved medical knowledge and treatment have changed their nature without having completely dispelled the atmosphere of revulsion and fascination that they inhabit. The wall of silence may have been dismantled, but venereal diseases remain too intimate and emotionally charged an issue for them to be regarded as 'ordinary' illnesses. While they are no longer linked to the same problems as in the previous century, their connection with social friction has endured.

The specific nature of venereal diseases, of course, has to do with the fact that they are transmitted sexually. This partly explains why they constitute an intractable health problem, as people's sexual behaviour is not easy to regulate. The classic instruments of public health care, such as sanitary measures, protecting the drinking water supply and the inspection of foodstuffs, which proved useful weapons in the fight against other diseases, are ineffectual here. And the link with sexuality has not only fascinated countless contemporary observers over the course of time,[16] it also makes venereal diseases particularly interesting to historians and social scientists.

Most of the resulting studies have focused on syphilis, which – once identified as a specific disease – with its protracted insidious course, its eventual emergence into terrifying symptoms that were visible to all, and its congenital variants, made a strong appeal to the imagination.[17] Others, such as the entertaining, if heavily anecdotal, *Microbes and Morals* (1971) by Theodor Rosebury, discuss the problem of venereal disease in general. A more serious general study is Allan Brandt's *No Magic Bullet* (1987),[18] about the history of venereal diseases in the United States. Brandt places the link between venereal disease and sexuality centre stage; the book explores ways in which sexual mores and prevailing ideas about sex have influenced the fight against venereal disease over the past hundred years. Brandt highlights the exploitation of the problem of venereal disease as a rhetorical vehicle to propagate ideas about sexual mores and family life, and to a lesser extent about class and race. Brandt believes that this use of venereal disease as a means of regulating the sexual and social order has impeded the search for prevention and cure: 'In its transformation from a biological entity to a social symbol, venereal disease has defied control.'[19] Brandt argues convincingly that many of those involved in the fight against venereal disease have been motivated by a good deal more than the simple desire to seek an effective solution to this health problem.

Brandt's book is interesting from many points of view, but the choice of sexual mores as an organizing principle has certain limitations. The main weakness is a dearth of explanations for the phenomena he describes, as the entire history of venereal disease is squeezed into a perpetual opposition that Brandt perceives as existing between a medical, pragmatic approach focusing on practical information and treatment on the one hand and a traditional moralistic approach on the other, in which venereal disease is seen as the just deserts of the debauched, and which emphasizes individual responsibility, moral upbringing and behavioural change. Brandt classifies every involvement with the problem according to these two approaches. Depending on the situation, one of the two approaches triumphs over the other, although the unbiased, medical approach seldom gains ascendancy for very long. And depending on which side wins, the nature of the problem is defined differently, with different persons being held culpable and different solutions sought. Whatever the undoubted interest of these shifts of approach, as Brandt consistently places them within a single continuum his history of venereal disease and the efforts to combat it reads like a series of variations on the same theme; he describes trends in a supposedly eternal conflict. The intensity of the conflict may wax and wane, but the underlying contrast is completely separate from specific developments in society. It is only the *outcome* of the conflict that Brandt sees as depending on such developments: in wartime, the pragmatists tend to be in the ascendancy, but once life returns to normal, the moralists triumph again. However, the *content* of the conflict is always the same. The medical versus moralist opposition has never, according to Brandt, changed in character or lost its significance in the course of time. Right up to the present day, it dominates the debate in the same way as it always has, with hypocrisy and cant still obstructing our efforts to devise adequate methods of tackling venereal diseases.

By focusing so strongly on attitudes and value judgements relating to sexuality, Brandt has painted a picture in which the significance of venereal diseases and the fight against them is overwhelmingly dominated by conflicts in this area. The third and last book on the subject that I would mention here adopts a different perspective. In *The Secret Plague* (1987), historian Jay Cassel provides material that qualifies Brandt's assertion that preachers and moralists are most to blame for blocking the effective onslaught on venereal disease. His research into the history of the fight against venereal disease in Canada shows that much of what Brandt says should have been done in the realm of medical and social care has in fact been done in Canada. Cassel's detailed historical account (which spans the period 1838–1939) is organized around developments in medical research and treatment. According to Cassel, these developments are what mainly determine the significance of venereal diseases and the battle to eliminate them. While not losing sight of other aspects altogether, he does build his story on a basic structure of medical history, with social issues being brought in as additional factors complicating the work to be done.

At the beginning of this introductory chapter, I noted that the meaning attached to venereal diseases changes, and derives from the specific constellation of medical knowledge and available treatment, sexual mores and relationships within society that apply at a given moment in time. Cassel and Brandt, respectively, each focus on the first of these elements. In my own research into changing definitions of the problem of venereal disease in the Netherlands, I have adopted a somewhat different approach. A historical account of medical research and treatment is included, but is not the main aim of my research. And an overly monolithic interpretation of the issues in terms of a struggle between pragmatists and moralists can be avoided by looking at the different social groups that have been involved. The shifts in the nexus of social relations will thus be a major focus of attention in these pages.

Narrators and characters

This study looks at the past hundred years in the Netherlands, and attempts to answer the following questions: how have public responses to the problem of venereal disease changed in the course of time, and how may they be explained in sociological terms? In addition to syphilis and gonorrhoea, the book will also deal with the new scourges of the 20th century, genital herpes and AIDS, although the classification of AIDS as a venereal disease is controversial.[20] The responses will be explored in terms of three separate parameters.

The first of these parameters is intensity. Even the most cursory of glances at Dutch history reveals a pattern of gathering public furore followed by a relative lull in public interest in the problem of venereal disease. What causes this rise and fall in public concern? Under what circumstances does widespread alarm tend to peak? The scale of the actual problem, as already observed, does not hold the answer. It will prove helpful to look at social problems from the vantage-point of sociological theory.[21] Why is venereal disease labelled an urgent social problem at some times and not at others? To answer this, we need to know what groups in society focus attention on the issue, and when they do so. We must also identify the arguments they use, and the interests they serve.[22]

The second parameter is the *social function* of an increase in public concern. Brandt, among others, has already shown that the fear of infection has frequently been exploited to help regulate sexual activity, but is that all there is to it? And has this function remained the same in the course of time?

Inasmuch as any historical changes can be identified in this area, they must be considered in the light of the third parameter that will be investigated here – the *nature* of the concern with venereal disease. This will be formulated as a historical comparison: how and why do the current responses to sexually transmitted diseases differ, in qualitative terms, from those to the 'secret diseases' of the late 19th century?

To answer these questions, I have endeavoured to chart the public debate surrounding venereal diseases using periodicals, pamphlets and the occasional document from public records.[23] The next step was to identify the main groups that conducted this debate, their anxieties, the people they held responsible for the spread of infection, and the remedies they proposed. I stripped the key questions to their bare essentials when studying the printed sources, so that they became 'who says that who is being infected, and by whom, with what disease, and what should be done?'

The first part, 'who says that who is being infected by whom?', provides a basis for classification that will be important in the next few chapters, in the distinction between the various actors involved, whom I have chosen to label narrators and characters. The narrators are writers or speakers, expressing their views of the problem of venereal disease, thereby representing a certain group of interested parties. The story they have to tell introduces others, persons they use as graphic examples to back up their theories. These latter persons – culprits and victims alike – are the groups I have labelled the characters. Narrators single out specific characters to illustrate their view of venereal disease and the danger of infection. These characters thus embody a particular view of one or more aspects of infection, but more importantly, they reflect the unease and insecurity of the narrators themselves. The following chapters will identify the most prominent narrators and characters in the debate on venereal disease. It will become clear that while the persons cast in these parts change in the course of time, the changing relations between the two groups consistently express aspects of a few more wide-ranging power relations.

Much of the material presented in this book will thus amount to a dramatization of the debate on venereal disease.[24] The stories told by the narrators evoke spectacles varying from one-act plays to *tableaux vivants*, but each one is essentially a tragedy. The debate might therefore aptly be described as an ongoing drama series, or equally well as a series of dramas.

The theatrical metaphors should not be taken to imply a foregone conclusion that we are dealing with fiction. While the narrators' script and accompanying stage directions do not necessarily correspond to reality, they may well reflect parts of it with varying degrees of accuracy, and the narrators themselves, of course, hotly defend the realism encapsulated in their tales. It will certainly be necessary, therefore, to discuss the genre of these pieces; we shall have to decide whether they are to be considered largely as social realism, or whether they rather merit classification as morality plays or pageants. I shall endeavour as far as is possible to assess the accuracy of the narrators' casting, and to weigh their claims of veracity. The difficulty of evaluating the evidence for these claims will often dog our progress in the following pages, but this is no justification for abandoning the enterprise altogether.

Some comment is in order at this point concerning the available statistics. They constitute a major stumbling-block. We scarcely have at our disposal the neat rows of figures that we would wish for – and certainly not before the Second World War – that would enable us simply to read off incidence and the differential spread of infection. What figures we do have are often limited in scope or distorted.

I can now return to the second part of the question I have used to structure my examination of the material. 'With what disease are victims being infected, and what should be done about it?' Identifying the disease is of particular significance in helping us recall that venereal diseases are passed on not only in the narrators' stories but also in 'real life'. In other words, in gathering information about the history of venereal diseases and the groups affected, we cannot rely totally on the content of the debate. The advent of new types of infection and the changes in patterns of disease also tell us a great deal, albeit in other ways. For they can provide insight into the spread of new social and sexual practices, and into the formation of new patterns of contact between particular groups or communities, which may be taking place beyond the field of vision of the narrators who are active at that moment in time.

Finally, answers to the question of how best to curb the danger of infection are significant – just like the question of 'who says that who is being infected by whom?' – in helping us to follow the shifting contours of the problem of venereal disease in the course of time. After all, the measures propounded by narrators reveal a large part of their diagnosis. Furthermore, looking at these two questions in conjunction makes it easier to relate a solution that is advanced at a particular moment to the groups involved in the problem of venereal disease at that time.

The book follows a chronological course. Chapter 1 focuses on the controversy that developed in the late 19th century surrounding the twin problems of prostitution and venereal disease. For a long time, the regulation of prostitution was the main ingredient of the fight against venereal disease, but the 1880s witnessed a change of approach. A broad-based coalition that set out to dismantle the regulatory apparatus achieved a whirlwind success, and in 1911 procuring became a statutory offence. This chapter discusses the diverse parties involved in the prostitution debate, and looks at their arguments and strategies. It also endeavours to find an explanation for the determined efforts in the 1890s to stamp out prostitution and scrap its regulation.

The first section of chapter 2 looks at the way in which the two vacuums left by the new legislation were filled. Firstly, what took the place of regulation? And secondly, since physicians no longer had an obvious role to play, who stepped into the breach? At the beginning of the century, the establishment of health centres and dispensaries, the introduction of Salvarsan (arsphenamine) and the advent of a largely Protestant association to combat venereal disease proved successful replacements. The second part of this chapter deals with two separate circuits of venereal infection that became visible in the post-regulatory era, each with its own narrators, characters and solutions: the circuit of wives and children, and that of soldiers and sailors. In the 1920s, a new trend started to manifest itself, distinct from these two circuits, surrounding the rising complaints about licentiousness, particularly in young women.

During the 1930s, this third trend became the dominant one in the debate on venereal disease: the prostitute, previously the central character, was gradually supplanted by the promiscuous young woman. This change is described and explained in chapter 3, which also discusses a related practical development in the fight against venereal disease – the rise of social work. During the second wave of concern, in the wake of the Second World War, social work underwent rapid expansion as the issue of venereal disease was increasingly separated from that of prostitution. Immediately after the liberation of the Netherlands there was a short-lived panic about the perceived decay of moral standards in Dutch society. Once it had abated, the fight against venereal diseases was continued largely as part of the larger effort to reverse the trend towards antisocial behaviour.

During the 1950s, interest in venereal disease flagged. An important factor here, though not in itself sufficient to explain the new mood, was the success of penicillin. Chapter 4 focuses on this unique intermezzo in the history of venereal infection – the period in which all the (known) infections concerned were easily curable. Viewed in combination with other social developments occurring at the same time, namely the advent of what Paul Robinson has called 'sexual enthusiasm' and the definite shift of balance between moral and medical considerations in favour of the latter, this ushered in a period of unprecedentedly carefree attitudes to venereal disease. The increase in incidence of infection and the appearance of new diseases did little to alter this.

This blissful mood of unconcern was first shattered by the publicity surrounding herpes genitalis; then, with the arrival on the scene of AIDS, sexually transmitted diseases moved back to centre stage. Chapter 5 looks at the events of the 1980s against the backdrop provided by the rest of the book. In conclusion, it sets out to place the shifts in public attitudes to venereal disease in the Netherlands in the period 1850–1990 within the perspective of historical sociology.

Introduction

Notes

1. Boudier-Bakker 1930:270.
2. Boudier-Bakker 1930:284.
3. Boudier-Bakker 1930:272.
4. Boudier-Bakker 1930:330-32.
5. I shall use the term 'venereal disease' throughout this book, supplementing it for the recent period with 'sexually transmitted disease', which gained currency only in the late 20th century.
6. McKeown 1976a:Chap. 5; McKeown 1976b. Cf. also Dubos 1959; Kass 1971.
7. Verdoorn 1965:Chaps. IX-XII.
8. Nathanson 1975.
9. Standing 1980.
10. See Antonovsky 1967 for a survey of 30 studies that demonstrate, almost without exception, a significant correlation between social class and incidence of disease. The victory over infectious diseases has changed this to some extent, but not fundamentally.
11. Cf. Syme & Berkman 1976; Berkman 1981.
12. Herzlich & Pierret 1987 [1984]:237.
13. See e.g. Rosenberg 1982 on the three cholera epidemics that swept the United States during the 19th century; Brandt 1987 on venereal diseases in the United States; Bryder 1988 on the fight against tuberculosis in England. In the Netherlands, Sickenga 1980 deals with the fight against tuberculosis, Noordegraaf & Valk 1988 discusses the consequences of bubonic plague in the late middle ages and Renaissance periods, and Verkaik 1991 deals with 20th-century measures to combat rheumatic fever.
14. The term 'civilization offensive' is coined in De Rooy 1979:9.
15. De Swaan 1988:Chap. IV.
16. Witness the huge mass of literature on the subject that has appeared over the centuries. At the end of the 19th century, Proksch compiled a bibliography that ran to three volumes and included thousands of publications; Proksch 1889-1891. We could also point to the myriad of allusions to venereal disease – syphilis in particular – in works of art and literature through the ages; see Rosebury 1971:Chaps. 9-13; Böumler 1976.
17. For the history of syphilis, see e.g. Temkin 1927; Voorhoeve 1951; Quétel [1986]; and specifically in relation to the Netherlands Van der Valk 1910 and Van Lieburg 1982.
18. The book first appeared in 1985, but a second edition was published in 1987 including a new chapter on AIDS.
19. Brandt 1987:6.
20. Some of the arguments against this classification are unconvincing. Tielman & Van Griensven (1985:416) question it on extremely

formalistic grounds, reasoning that the crucial factor is not whether there has been sexual contact, but whether there has been any 'blood-blood' or 'sperm-blood' contact. Watney (1987:126-127) is particularly concerned about the stigmatizing implications of this classification. He argues that while AIDS is largely transmitted sexually, this is not the only mode of transmission; if we were to classify all diseases that can be passed on sexually as venereal diseases, he continues, we would be forced to include the common cold. This, of course, is a fallacious argument. The opposite is true: were we not to classify diseases that are passed on chiefly by sexual contact as venereal diseases, we would be left without any at all. This said, there is some justification for treating AIDS as 'less' of a venereal disease than syphilis or gonorrhoea, but as far as the situation in the Netherlands is concerned, where sexual contact is by far the most important mode of transmission of AIDS, there is insufficient reason to consider rejecting this classification (see Chapter 5 below).

21. See Spector & Kitsuse 1973:146, where the subject-matter of this branch of sociology is defined as 'the process by which members of groups or societies define a putative condition as a problem'. Spector and Kitsuse go on to define social problems as 'the activities of groups making assertions of grievances and claims to organizations, agencies, and institutions about some putative conditions'. Whether it is true to say that social problems exist solely by virtue of the efforts made by certain groups to have their grievances acknowledged and their claims upheld is disputed. This issue need not be resolved here. In order to explain the waves of intensity of public interest in the problem of venereal disease, conclusions borrowed from this school of sociology, one based on social constructivism, are of largely heuristic value, as they focus on questions similar to those I formulate in these paragraphs.

22. For studies already conducted in this area, see Pfohl 1977; Schneider & Kitsuse (eds.) 1984; Best 1987.

23. I made a thorough study of several periodicals: medical journals and those bordering on medical terrain, journals of military medicine, and the publications of Dutch organizations for the combating of venereal disease. The Bibliography includes a list of these publications.

24. This type of dramatization has been largely developed, in the social sciences, by Erving Goffman. Gusfeld (1981) is among those to have used it in analysing social problems. Applied to this area, dramatic analysis serves to describe the development of social problems as a public performance in which the various interested parties act out their parts, complete with the accompanying ceremony and ritual. Their aim is to attract public attention and to retain it (cf. Hilgartner & Bosk 1988). My own dramatization derives from written sources, however, and is presented in the form of a script.

1

Prostitution and Venereal Disease (1850–1911)

In his article 'On the history of morality and syphilis', the medical historian Owsei Temkin surveys historical changes in the significance attached to syphilis. He distinguishes four periods. During the first, from the arrival of syphilis in Europe in the 1490s until around 1520, the sexual transmission of syphilis was unknown or disputed.[1] In this period, which witnessed the rapid spread of a virulent form of syphilis throughout Europe, the new pestilence was viewed in much the same light as others that had afflicted humanity: it was universally thought to be a punishment for the sinfulness and godlessness of mankind. Although the treatment meted out to syphilitics – which ran to confinement, ostracism and even banishment – seems cruel to us today, there was no question of moral condemnation of the victims. They were not held personally responsible for their disease.

The second period stretches from the early 16th-century general recognition of syphilis as a venereal disease until the rise to dominance of the middle classes in the late 18th century. The connection with sexual intercourse had by then become incontrovertible, and syphilis started to be associated with transgressions against marital and sexual morality. Yet a clear, class-bound double standard prevailed in the moral judgements made of syphilitics and in their treatment. When commoners contracted the disease, received wisdom had it that they were being punished for their sins. And they were dealt with accordingly: surgeons and barbers prescribed dangerous mercury cures, aggressive sweat and saliva treatment that could be seen to some extent as part of the penitence that was required of any lowly mortal smitten with the 'vile pox'. Where the aristocracy was concerned, on the other hand, syphilis was generously labelled the 'cavalier's disease' – it was an acceptable risk run by the frivolous. These more elevated personages were treated by physicians, who used the far milder guaiacum, a tropical wood whose resin was endowed with medicinal properties.

In the third period, this double standard ceased to apply. The middle-class ethos attached morality more firmly to the family, and concepts of virtue and respectability gained the upper hand. Syphilis, now closely tied to extra-marital sexual relations, was no longer viewed as a scourge of God aimed at humanity in general, nor merely as a punishment for carnal knowledge, but increasingly as a sign of moral turpitude, a debasement of the infected man or woman, regardless of social class.

Finally, in the late 19th century, the wind of change and newly formed interest groups ushered in a fourth period, in which government concerned itself with a widening range of subject-matter that included venereal disease. Syphilis was now no longer – or not exclusively – seen as a violation of the prevailing family morality and as a stain on a person's moral standing. Where the emphasis had been on the defilement of one individual, there was now an increasing tendency to view the problem as a menace to society. Against the pernicious impact of this infection on the armed forces, the family and the new generation – in short, on the health of the nation – the state must arm itself. Hence in most European countries, national organizations were established to fight venereal disease. Some countries went so far as to create a statutory obligation to seek treatment for it. This brings us up to the early 20th century.

Temkin's four periods, whatever the inevitable limitations of any schematic classification, are very useful as a rough guide. The events of this chapter took place in the last of the four periods; they marked the gradual transition from the view of venereal disease as a personal disgrace to a preoccupation with social and political aspects of the problem.[2] Accompanying this shift of focus was an intensification in the public debate.

Two things complicated this debate. Firstly, around the turn of the century venereal diseases were inextricably linked to the fierce controversy surrounding prostitution. This chapter will accordingly discuss prostitution at some length. Secondly, the process whereby this dual problem of prostitution and venereal disease was brought into the open and defined as a social issue was itself a long and complex development; it resulted from the efforts of two successive, mutually antagonistic groups.

Initially, the delicate problems of prostitution and venereal disease were put on the public agenda by people who favoured a system of *regulated* prostitution. Then, many years later, they acquired still more emphasis as a social issue thanks to the exertions of a mixed lobby that took completely the opposite view – people committed to dismantling this very system. The 'abolitionist' lobby opposed the recognition of prostitution that was implicit in its regulation; its supporters wanted prostitution banned altogether, and they fixed on the dismantling of the regulatory apparatus as their first practical objective.

The regulation of prostitution[3]

The regulatory system was based on the organizing of prostitution along certain specified lines. It grew from a single assumption about what was a true and at the same time a desirable state of affairs – that prostitution was concentrated in certain special establishments, brothels. The whole thrust of the regulatory system was hence to subject brothels to supervision by a combination of medical and police authorities. All such establishments had to be registered with the police, as did the prostitutes working there, and the latter were required to submit to regular medical examinations in which they were screened for venereal disease. These physical examinations sometimes took place in the brothel itself, but more often they were performed in the physician's surgery. They varied in frequency, but weekly check-ups were the most common. Women who failed the medical examination would be forbidden to work for a period of time depending on the seriousness of their complaint. In the meantime they would be given a prescription, or admitted to hospital – forcibly, if need be – for medical treatment. If possible they would be treated in special infirmaries or closed hospital wards.[4] Any woman who defied a prohibition to work or who failed to appear for her check-up could expect any one of several possible sanctions, depending on the specific regulations in force: these ranged from a fine to a prison sentence, or temporary confinement to a reformatory. In some cases, the brothel itself would be closed down.

The Dutch regulatory system had its roots in France, where the combination of police and medical supervision was introduced at the beginning of the 19th century. This supervision was then primarily a military scheme designed to protect the French armies from venereal infections. But these military and political beginnings soon lost their relevance.[5] The French regulations functioned during most of the 19th century as a measure to shield the general public, based on the principles expounded by A.J.B. Parent-Duchatelet, a respected hygienist and expert in urban sewer systems, in his influential study *De la Prostitution dans la Ville de Paris* (1836). Alain Corbin was the first to subject the workings of the regulatory regime in French society to a detailed analysis, in his *Les Filles de Noce* (1978). One thing to emerge clearly from this book is that the medical function of regulation was not initially the most important. Corbin shows that the supervision in France was first and foremost a public order measure, a rigorous effort designed both to confine prostitution to certain neighbourhoods and to channel extra-marital sexual relations as much as possible into registered brothels. It was only later, with a new generation of regulators, that the dimension of medical justification was added, and that the salutary effects on health that were claimed for regulation acquired a dominant role.

The project of regulation was pursued in France with dogged determination and the rules were applied with unflinching rigour. The supervisory apparatus that was developed in the Netherlands is worlds apart from this. The Dutch system was never more than a shadow of its counterpart in France, and what rules did exist were often applied half-heartedly.[6] Yet here too, regulation was long believed to hold the solution to the problem of prostitution.

The first experience with regulation was under French rule. When Napoleon annexed the Netherlands in 1810, the French ordinances on prostitution entered into force, and they remained in force until the end of French rule three years later. Yet some municipalities retained these ordinances after the French had left. The statutory requirement to retain them had lapsed, but the Dutch government repeatedly urged municipal authorities – in 1818, 1828, 1846 and again in 1860 – to introduce a supervisory system for prostitution.[7] In 1860 the Ministry of the Interior's memorandum called for 'the medical and police supervision of women who are engaged in public or clandestine prostitution to be improved where necessary ... and the combating of syphilis to be made an object of special concern'.[8] All these exhortations to pass local ordinances on prostitution were prompted by the same disquieting figures – the rising incidence of venereal disease in the armed forces. In explanation of his 1860 memorandum, for instance, the Minister of the Interior observed that 'information received concerning the vast numbers of soldiers afflicted by venereal disease, which according to a five-year table of statistics averages 2,665 annually, has impelled His Excellency the Minister of War to request my intervention to take measures with a view to diminishing the said evil'.[9]

The state was thus in the vanguard of the Dutch movement to restore regulation. But government circulars could not exert enough pressure to initiate change. It was not until lobbies formed at municipal level and added their voices to the call for regulation that wheels began to turn. The 1851 Municipalities Act provided a fresh impetus to the campaign. This Act stipulated that the power to take measures relating to public order, morality and health, including the supervision of houses of ill repute and prostitutes, henceforth lay with municipal authorities.[10] Some of the latter responded by promulgating local ordinances and police regulations. Prominent advocates of such measures were the local military authorities such as garrison commanders and health officers. Their involvement is clear from the fact that the main municipalities to introduce police and medical supervision (Bergen op Zoom, Brielle, The Hague, Haarlem, Harderwijk, Kampen, Veere and Zutphen) were garrison towns.[11] Gradually, however, the supervisory system left its military origins behind, as it had in France. The later debates that led to the abolition of regulation scarcely betray a sign of the military involvement that had loomed so large at its conception.

In garrison towns, the pressure to break through the existing *laissez-faire* policy and introduce regulation came from various quarters.[12] Army surgeons were one vociferous group. Municipal health committees, which advised local authorities in public health matters, were another. The medical practitioners with the highest profile in these committees were the 'hygienists'. This was a group consisting of the more liberal-minded medical practitioners, together with several representatives of other professions such as teachers and engineers. Hygienists argued that social and sanitary living conditions were clearly related to epidemics and other outbreaks of disease.[13] They therefore drew up ambitious plans for a thoroughgoing programme of sanitary reforms to benefit public health.

The hygienists based their plans on two popular theories of the aetiology of disease: miasma and contagion. According to the theory of miasma, noxious fumes emanating from rank mounds of refuse, polluted water and foul-smelling slums were the chief causes of disease. Theories of contagion focused on infectious substances that the body could produce once it had been poisoned with miasma. Although now discredited, these theories served as a basis for a progressive programme that, while never fully implemented, nevertheless made a more significant contribution at the time to improvements in public health care than did curative medicine.[14]

Views on aetiology were not the same for all diseases. The theory of miasma compounded by contagion was applied pre-eminently to cholera, a disease that was of great significance during the development of ideas on hygiene and the origins of epidemics. In the case of syphilis, for instance, the existence of a syphilitic 'infectant' or 'agent' as the sole aetiological factor was universally accepted. The infectiousness of gonorrhoea was likewise undisputed.[15]

Hygienists concerned themselves with a variety of subjects: the installation of sewers, the drinking water supply, refuse collection, housing for the poor, improvements in nutrition and working conditions – all measures aimed at alleviating largely urban problems. In addition to these activities in the realm of *hygiena publica*, however, they also had plenty to say about *hygiena privata*, which included family life, domestic hygiene and standards of decency and morality. They organized public readings, distributed information on wholesome ways of life, and tried to gain general acceptance for their ideas within the family by addressing themselves to women in particular.

Prostitution, clearly an issue of *hygiena publica*, was a subject on which the hygienists had very definite views. In arguing the case for regulation, they invoked Parent-Duchatelet, their eminent predecessor in such matters, who had maintained that the state must accept prostitution as a regrettable but unavoidable fact of life that was best subjected to strict rules. Municipal supervision could at least help to keep the malady within manageable proportions. The Dutch hygienists' standard work, the *Handboek der Openbare Gezondheidsregeling en der Geneeskundige Politie* (1872) makes several specific suggestions to this end:

> In the first place, all soliciting by prostitutes or their accomplices in the streets, on doorsteps and from brothel windows must be prohibited by law. On the other hand, brothels should be identified as such by a clearly distinguishable sign (such as a coloured lantern or inscription). Brothels must not be allowed to function at the same time as public houses, coffee rooms, inns or suchlike, which are frequented for reasons other than for the women of easy virtue who live there.[16]

In the same way that police ordinances could prevent prostitution from spreading throughout the city in a public and uncontrollable fashion, the hygienists also saw periodic medical examinations of prostitutes as something that could check the spread of venereal disease from the brothels. H.W. Stork was a hygienist whose imagination in this area knew no bounds. In Bavaria, he explained, dogs were subjected to examinations every three months to rule out the possibility of rabies. 'Would one then wish to stand by', Stork demanded rhetorically, 'while the population, in particular that of the large cities, is infected with the poison of syphilis?' Stork advocated brothels, established and maintained at the state's expense, in which prostitutes would have thorough medical examinations every day. This, together with the strict police supervision that he favoured, would make it possible to describe brothels as 'police establishments' that were 'under the unrestricted overall control of medical practitioners'. An organization along these lines was the best way, in the eyes of Stork, to safeguard the health of the urban population.[17]

Hygienists and military doctors together pressured municipal authorities, through the local health committees, to introduce measures in this area. They were not unsuccessful: by the mid-1870s, scores of municipalities had promulgated ordinances and police regulations on the supervision of brothels, although the application of these measures left much to be desired.[18] Both groups accorded more weight to the medical side of supervision than to the element of policing. Military doctors were mainly interested in preventing their troops from becoming infected, and hygienists too favoured regulation chiefly as a way of limiting the negative impact of prostitution on public health. Hence regulation was mainly described in the Netherlands – and increasingly so towards the end of the century – as a way of preventing the spread of venereal disease. In the later debates between regulationists and their opponents, the abolitionists, regulation was almost always used to refer to *medical examinations*. The two terms were used as virtual synonyms.

Given the marked spread of venereal disease in this period, it is scarcely surprising that the issue came to occupy a crucial position within the regulationist creed. The following section will briefly describe the various types of infection that were involved, their incidence and the remedies that were applied.[19]

In the 19th century there were three common venereal diseases: syphilis, chancroid and gonorrhoea. Of these, syphilis and gonorrhoea were by far the most important. Although chancroid was regularly included in the list, it scarcely figured in treatises or statistical tables, and it will accordingly only be touched on here.

The course of syphilis, also known as lues, may be divided into three stages. The disease begins some three weeks after it is contracted with an ulcer at the site of infection, which vanishes spontaneously after some time. This primary stage is followed – after an interval lasting weeks or months – by a secondary stage characterized by a great variety of symptoms. Skin complaints – ulcers, boils, mucous lesions, rashes affecting palms and soles – are the most common, but headache, throat complaints and maladies affecting bones, joints and the sensory organs may also occur. In most cases, these symptoms too disappear spontaneously after a while, after which the disease enters a period of latency that may last several years. Secondary symptoms may manifest themselves again during this period, but they may be altogether absent. In the tertiary stage, which only affects a proportion of sufferers, sometimes after twenty years or more, the most conspicuous symptoms are syphilitic tumours. More serious, however, indeed potentially fatal, is the damage that may be done to organs such as the cardiovascular system, the liver, kidneys, bone marrow and brain. If the latter two organs are affected, paralysis and the well-known phenomenon of syphilitic madness may ensue.

While this three-stage description of syphilis has not been abandoned altogether, it has become more common in present-day symptomatology to speak of only two stages, the dividing-line being the moment at which the disease ceases to be infectious. According to this scheme, primary, secondary and the early latent stages of the disease are called early infectious syphilis. During the second stage, late syphilis, which includes the later period of latency and the tertiary symptoms, the disease can no longer be passed on.[20]

In addition to transmission through sexual intercourse, syphilis can also be communicated during pregnancy, sometimes causing miscarriage or stillbirth. Live-born infants with congenital syphilis generally exhibit secondary symptoms at birth; other abnormalities appear later. The physical and mental damage done in such cases is irreversible. Depending upon the stage of her own disease, it is also possible for an infected mother to give birth to a healthy child.

Gonorrhoea is a disease that can be easily identified in men by a painful inflammation of the urethra that sets in around one week after infection. If left untreated, or treated inadequately, the disease may spread to adjacent organs, including the prostate, ultimately producing sterility. In untreated cases the disease is likely to persist in its infectious form for a long time, although it sometimes clears up spontaneously. In women the infection is more easily overlooked, as it begins painlessly with few if any symptoms. Here too it may spread from the cervix, where the infection tends in most cases to be localized, to the uterus and ovaries, producing chronic abdominal pains and infertility. Childbirth facilitates this internal spread of the disease, so that untreated gonorrhoea infections in women often lead to what is known as one-child sterility. There is no congenital variant of gonorrhoea. The newborn's eyes may, however, become infected during birth, and this may lead to blindness if left untreated.

The third malady mentioned here, chancroid or soft chancre, is less serious than the other two. Chancroid takes the form of an ulcer, which in this case becomes fully developed within a few days after infection. Touching it can easily spread the infection to other parts of the body, in contrast to the syphilitic ulcer, which does not spread in this way. The most common complication in chancroid is the inflammation of neighbouring lymph glands. The spread of this disease is associated, more than the other two, with unhygienic conditions.

Until the mid-19th century, medical practitioners disagreed about the precise connection between these three disorders. Gonorrhoea was not universally recognized as a separate disease, and chancroid even less so, with many classifying both of these maladies as symptoms or stages of syphilis.[21] But even after this myth had been exploded, the criteria used to classify the various diseases remained extremely vague by today's standards. 'Infected' was often the bald verdict of a visiting physician after examining a prostitute. No further details were given. Conversely, a diagnosis of 'syphilis' often meant simply that the patient had a venereal disease of some sort.[22]

It will be clear that such practices make it essential to interpret all statistics on the various venereal diseases with great care. That is to say, when there are any statistics to interpret – we have very few figures at our disposal for this period. Estimates did appear at the end of the century, however, together with research results, concerning the situation in certain specific towns. Great venereologists such as Alfred Fournier in Paris and Alfred Blaschko in Berlin were the most prominent researchers in this field, and they did not flinch from pronouncing over half their fellow-townsmen infected with venereal disease. Towards the end of the 19th century, the incidence of syphilis among the civilian population of the major cities of Western Europe was estimated at 5 to 15%; for gonorrhoea, the estimates varied wildly, from 25% to 75%.[23] These figures generally related to the male urban population, and were intended to convey the seriousness of the problem, so that they will undoubtedly have been inflated.[24] In the Netherlands, little effort was made to collect data: where necessary the findings of foreign studies were quoted, in the pleasant knowledge that these would at least not play the problem down. But we have no figures at all on the incidence of venereal disease among the Dutch civilian population in the latter half of the 19th century.[25]

All we have to go by, as an indication of the extent of the problem in this period, are military statistics. These reveal that in the latter half of the 19th century some 12% of the Dutch army each year contracted one of the three infections named above.[26] The navy was no better off: between 1860 and 1880 the annual proportion of men infected varied from 12% to 28%. The figures for the Dutch East Indies fleet were higher still, with the proportion of sufferers on board seldom falling below 30%.[27]

Although these figures cannot simply be applied to the civilian population, it appears justifiable to conclude that venereal diseases were widespread when regulation was introduced into the Netherlands. We can at least state this for men; where the female part of the population is concerned, we do not have even such unreliable and indirect information at our disposal. It was only later that anyone became interested in such figures. Until approximately 1880 there was only one female character in the debate on venereal disease – the prostitute – and she was brought onto the stage solely in her role as a source of infection. She infected others; but that someone had infected *her* was something that, for the time being, escaped notice.

This imbalance was rooted in certain specific ideas about venereal infection. These ideas can be briefly conveyed in an epidemiological model that describes the mode of transmission that was believed to apply to venereal disease. Such models will be a regular feature of this book. They will assume a variety of forms, as they change to accommodate shifts in the dominant ideas about venereal infection. The regulationists used an epidemiological model that focused on prostitution and that we may visualize as a wheel with spokes. The hub of this wheel was the prostitute, the source from which infection could spread in every direction. On the basis of this model, it was only logical to assume that the further spread of venereal disease should be opposed by removing and treating infected prostitutes. This would not only prevent men from becoming infected, but would be the best way to protect society at large.

The treatment of venereal disease was not a simple matter in the latter half of the 19th century. Some few physicians continued to practise 'syphilisation', which involved inoculating patients – by analogy with the successful immunization against smallpox – with material derived from chancroid, which the physicians in question believed to be a mild variant of the syphilitic toxin. Viewed with hindsight, this deliberate infection of patients with chancroid was a tragically ill-conceived mode of treatment. It was at no time applied on a large scale in the Netherlands, or indeed anywhere else.[28] Most physicians treated syphilis with mercury, administered in a variety of ways. In the course of the 19th century, the common aggressive saliva and smoke cures gave way to ointments, tablets and injections.[29] Later potassium iodide was added, a substance believed to be an effective remedy against tertiary symptoms. At this time a course of syphilis treatment lasted several years, and it was based on the principle of chronic intermittent treatment. This was an approach that had been introduced by Fournier; treatment consisted of periods of mercury or potassium iodide administration alternating with periods of rest. During the first few years, the medication followed a fixed programme, though this programme itself was constantly being changed. It was to be resumed whenever symptoms reappeared.[30] The medical journals all agreed in recommending that this programme be continued for several years; how often patients completed the entire course of treatment in practice is unknown. We do know, however, that prostitutes in whom venereal disease was diagnosed during their medical examination were treated for a far shorter period, lasting at most a few months.[31] Yet this was at a time when it was already common knowledge that syphilis remained infectious for a much longer period of time.[32]

Quite aside from the lax compliance with the regulations that were in force, it is unclear whether the full course of treatment actually had any effect. The medical profession had little doubt as to its efficacy; the vast majority of physicians were convinced of the medical properties of mercury, 'the sole specific against the infection of syphilis' as it was still being called in the 20th century.[33] Even after the introduction of other remedies, many practitioners were averse to relinquishing mercury as part of their treatment of syphilis. Today it is assumed that this poisonous substance may have had a beneficial effect on certain symptoms, but that its administration in large quantities must also have done a great deal of damage. Mercury poisoning can lead, among other things, to excess salivation, loss of teeth, shortness of breath and serious damage to the skin and to internal organs. Whether the remedy had any curative effect in the lower doses that became more fashionable towards the end of the 19th century is still open to question.[34]

The notion that mercury was an effective remedy against syphilis was undoubtedly reinforced by the natural course of the disease.

After all, even without any form of intervention, the symptoms disappeared after a time, as the infection entered the phase of clinical latency. Moreover, more than one-fourth of untreated cases ended in a complete, spontaneous, cure, which meant that tertiary symptoms never appeared at all.[35] That syphilis was a disease that passed through several stages was already known in the mid-19th century. Anyone wanting to learn about its late manifestations could take a look in the anatomical collection at the fair, where amid wax moulds and aborted fetuses in glass jars an abundance of venereal pustules, late-syphilitic deformities and other terrifying items were on view.[36] The French venereologist Philippe Ricord was the first, in his *Traité Pratique des Maladies Vénériennes* (1838) to describe the clinical pattern of syphilis in three stages, each with a distinct array of symptoms. Among the tertiary symptoms to which he referred were damage to the bones and skin, but he did not know about the late manifestations that attracted great attention towards the end of the century: *tabes dorsalis* and *dementia paralytica*. That syphilis could wreck someone's life in later years and even damage the health of his offspring was also known around the mid-19th century. The description of syphilis symptoms in infants and bone deformities in children, one known result of which was the deformed 'saddle nose', dated from this period. In the late 1850s, the British surgeon Hutchinson published his findings concerning the clinical picture of somewhat older children, which has become known as Hutchinson's triad, and consists of certain specific deformities of the teeth, eyes and ears. But it was not until the turn of the century that most of the questions surrounding inherited syphilis, such as the exact mode of transmission and the mother's role in it, had been answered. And it was only then that more effective remedies for syphilis became available.

The main elements in the treatment of gonorrhoea were rinses and irrigation. Particularly popular were the *grands lavages* advocated by the French physician Jules Janet, which consisted of several rinses with potassium permanganate. Later silver nitrate was sometimes used instead, and disinfectants of obscure composition were recommended. At best such remedies achieved some temporary effect, but they seldom vanquished a gonorrhoea infection altogether. The same applied to the thermal therapy that seemed so promising at the beginning of the century. Although gonorrhoea follows a less complex course than syphilis, its treatment was attended by a similar lack of clarity. For instance, when could the treatment, in men, be said to be finished? When the discharge had ceased? When symptoms had been absent for a certain period of time? Or perhaps when the discharge had changed from opaque to clear? In the case of female patients, the complications initially gave little cause for concern, simply because they were unknown; physicians believed that gonorrhoea was not a serious illness for women. Later this proved to be quite untrue, but the consequences of gonorrhoea infections remained largely unresponsive to medical intervention.

In line with this underestimation of the problems posed by gonorrhoea, the measures taken to monitor the health of prostitutes chiefly related to syphilis. The examining physician in Utrecht, Dr L.C. van Goudoever, explained that the chief aim

> [must] be to curb *syphilis*, because this disease is passed on to so many innocent people. ... To fight venereal diseases in general is not the object of the exercise. If this can be done, so much the better, but it is not the responsibility of either the state or the police to prevent persons from contracting gonorrhoea, and the same applies, in fact, to chancroid. As far as these latter two maladies are concerned, one might say that the evil punishes itself.[37]

Articles and treatises published in medical journals on the treatment and cure of venereal diseases contained few references to medical examinations of prostitutes. They generally related to the experiences of general practitioners and dermatologists, whose surgeries were frequented by a different type of patient. These doctors probably treated sufferers – including, of course, the prostitutes' clients – with a good deal more care than did those responsible for routine medical examinations.

That venereal disease was an urgent problem in the latter half of the 19th century is beyond dispute. But that is not in itself enough to explain the determination that arose in the mid-century to tackle it along organized lines, nor the belief that regulation was the most suitable remedy. To gain a better understanding of this new attitude, it will help to look at the main 'narrators' and their 'characters' in the debate on venereal disease, at the time when regulation was introduced.

The various narrators all shared one common desire: to strengthen the nation. Neither the mild forms of coercion used by the government nor the involvement of the military health care authorities can be separated from this desire. Both were motivated by concern about the loss to the armed forces caused by venereal disease. The wars raging through other parts of Europe in the 1860s aroused the concern of the Liberal public authorities and attracted more attention than before to the nation's ability to defend itself. Aside from the concern about the health of the army, this interest also expressed itself in the first debates on compulsory military service and training.[38]

The hygienists certainly saw their efforts as serving the national interest. They viewed the regulation of prostitution as part of a wider programme of public hygiene reforms – reforms to which they accorded a political as well as a medical dimension. Their views of public health could perhaps be defined as the medical expression of the Liberal concept of an enlightened nation. Promoting public health, in their eyes, benefited the progress of the nation; it hastened the correction of social injustice and would greatly enhance the country's economic development. Furthermore, the debate launched by the hygienists at length generated a standard of public health that enabled comparisons to be made between one municipality or region and the next, or even between one 'civilized' country and the next.[39]

All this makes it possible to see the move to contain venereal disease in the latter half of the 19th century as part of a general effort to strengthen the Dutch nation. But this still does not explain why the narrators fixed on regulation as the best way to proceed. We have seen that the regulationists focused entirely on transmission from the prostitute to her male clients; in their scheme of things, the prostitute unquestionably played, so to speak, the leading role. She was the source of infection. Within this general scenario, cleaning up prostitution by temporarily removing infected elements was the best way to halt the further spread of the disease.

This train of thought cemented the long-standing link between prostitution and venereal disease. It was based on specific ideas about the sexuality of men and women, and in particular about the nature of the male sexual urge. For most of the 19th century a man's sexual desire was believed to be a natural urge that he was largely powerless to control. Before standards of decency came 'the demands of nature, which cannot with impunity be resisted. In the whole world of nature there is no urge more powerful than that aimed at the preservation of the species.' These words accompanied an announcement of new regulations on prostitution in The Hague in the 1850s.[40] The suppression of this natural urge was thus not only seen as an impossibility, it was believed to be undesirable. With a view to the health of the man, it was better 'to allow the inclinations that he feels expressed in his sexual organ moderate release in the natural way', as the same preamble to the new regulations explained. Society must make allowance for the fundamental demands of nature as well as the demands of decency. Contemporary observers believed that this dual exigency was indeed met by the institution of marriage, which fulfilled both requirements at once. But it had to be acknowledged that not all men were in a position to marry, and for them an additional facility was needed, which prostitution supplied.[41] These views constituted the foundation on which the edifice of regulation was constructed, and the writings of the advocates of regulation hence called prostitution a *necessary* evil. No one rejoiced in its existence, but given the circumstances in which some men found themselves, that is to say without a wife, it was unavoidable, and moreover prevented a worse evil still. Prostitution could ensure that the sexual urge was satisfied 'naturally', thus preventing its expression by perverse means or through the defilement of decent girls and women.

That the ranks of prostitutes were filled with immoral women who came from the lowest classes of society and were possessed of 'ethical flaws', 'moral insanity' or some such thing that deprived them of all sense of decency was too obvious at this time to need stating, and clinched the argument in favour of regulation.[42] The decent girls and women who were protected by the services of prostitutes were governed by natural laws of a completely different kind: their sexual feelings were believed to be either poorly developed or easily controlled, always assuming a proper upbringing. For such women and girls, there was hence no need to ensure sexual satisfaction, and abstinence before marriage was a strict requirement. While men might be excused their peccadilloes, no such forbearance was in store for the female transgressor – a double standard that was particularly marked, in this period, in the middle classes. The introduction of a supervisory apparatus for prostitution in the latter half of the 19th century was intimately bound up with this double standard.

To sum up, the regulation of prostitution served in various ways as a buffer between prostitution, which society felt bound to tolerate as a necessary though corrupt enclave in its midst, and the 'decent' civilized world round about. This buffer role worked on three levels at once. First, there was the level of the physical environment. Through the registration of brothels and a system of permits, prostitution could theoretically be contained within certain neighbourhoods, although this aspect of regulation was never emphasized in the Netherlands. The second level was medical: the temporary exclusion of infected women from the sexual circuit was designed to protect clients and contain the spread of disease – a form of damage limitation, in the eyes of the regulationists. And thirdly there was the level of the 'sexual order'. Regulation could maintain a healthy, if contemptible, class of women with whom men, chiefly young bachelors, could achieve the necessary release of their sexual energy. This sexual order drew a clear line between 'decent' and 'indecent' women, safeguarding the honour of the former and preventing the need for men to take refuge in masturbation or each other. Regulation thus prevented the defilement of the respectable – i.e. middle-class – sections of society.

The abolitionist offensive

Regulation was introduced in a good number of Dutch municipalities without encountering much resistance. Only an occasional voice was raised in protest. One such voice was that of Dr N.B. Donkersloot, who expounded his objections to the new scheme proposed for The Hague as early as 1856. This is particularly interesting as Donkersloot was a 'hygienist', and thus belonged to a group that was in general eager to see prostitution regulated. Donkersloot contested the principles on which the regulation was based, however, namely that: '1. the recognition of open prostitution is in the interests of public health; 2. the satisfaction of sexual desire is necessary for every person of virile age who wishes to preserve both his bodily and mental health in their normal state, whereas 3. syphilis would spread all the more, were prostitution to be forced into greater secrecy'.[43] For many years, Donkersloot's criticism met with no response at all. But more than twenty years later, a public debate flared up, with many of the same arguments being repeated. By the end of the 1870s, the first signs of a dramatic change in society's acceptance of prostitution began to appear, a shift of climate that would eventually lead to the abolition of regulation in the Netherlands.

Let us first consider the medical profession. The hygienists had had their day, and the regulation of prostitution became an increasingly controversial issue among medical practitioners. Their professional organization, the Dutch Society for the Advancement of Medicine (NMG) made several attempts to define a common approach, but reaching a consensus proved no easy task.[44]

The first report (1879) evaluated the existing legislation on infectious diseases (the 1872 Epidemics Act). Venereal diseases were outside the scope of this Act, and the committee had been given the special task of investigating whether the Act required amendment on this point, i.e. whether supplementary provisions on prostitution should be added. The committee members were apparently much in favour of this approach.[45] Their conclusion was rejected, however, by the General Meeting of the NMG, with the result that another committee was appointed to determine whether it was perhaps desirable instead to enact a *separate* piece of legislation to combat syphilis and establish the supervision of brothels. This committee concluded that venereal infections belonged to the realm of private hygiene, and that there was no need for the state to adopt a supervisory role.[46] This conclusion too aroused fierce protest, and yet a third committee was established. This time even the committee failed to agree, eventually coming up with a majority proposal consisting of draft legislation to establish a strict system of regulation alongside a more moderate minority proposal.[47] When the storm of protest unleashed by the proposed legislation had abated somewhat, a fourth committee set to work. It decided first to hold a questionnaire. This was duly done, eliciting the information that the majority of physicians questioned favoured regulations to curb syphilis. Accordingly, the committee once again advised the NMG to urge the government to take action.[48] At length this recommendation was made,[49] but nothing came of it. Another committee, set up in 1897, did not even issue anything in the nature of a report on its activities. Finally, in 1908 the NMG established one final committee. The report it published, three years later, was welcomed on all sides. By this point, however, regulation had disappeared from the agenda altogether.

This tortuous series of events, with deep divisions forming within the NMG on the idea of institutionalizing medical supervision in an area in which certain physicians had been working for some time, can be understood in the context of De Swaan's theory of medicalization, which he encapsulates as 'the reluctant imperialism of the medical profession'.[50] According to this theory, the expansion of medical authority to embrace an increasing share of life in society is an unintentional consequence of two tendencies. The first is the ambition of physicians, each of whom is endeavouring to increase his or her chances of work, income, prestige and the realization of professional ideals. The second stems from certain other parties locked in conflict, who hope to settle their differences through the intervention of a third party, regarded as possessing special expertise. It is to the advantage of all the parties involved – both the physicians on the look-out for social opportunity and the parties in dispute – to ensure that the controversy is redefined in medical terms, albeit in different ways. If we follow this train of thought, it becomes apparent that the expansion or establishment of a medical 'regime' does not proceed as an automatic consequence of advances in medical science, nor does it stem from the medical profession's unbridled urge to expand its sphere of influence. Instead it is based on a triangular relationship, a 'collusion, a hidden complicity between the parties to the conflict, with one another and with the doctor'.[51] The numerous instances of medical intervention in various areas of social conflict – in 'collusion' with the parties in dispute – constitute the motor of medical expansion, but in the long term this involvement has presented the medical profession with a problem. De Swaan reviews the history of this process:

> In due time, however, the academic and organizational elite in the medical profession were confronted with the accumulated effects of incidental medical intervention. What had gradually become the generally known and accepted practice of individual doctors and separate groupings of doctors in the end required the articulation of a general policy for the profession. But once these socially contested issues became a topic for discussion within the medical profession, almost inevitably problems of legitimation occurred. Whenever the emerging practices could not be fully justified in terms of a consensus of medical knowledge, as many different opinions would appear within the bosom of the profession as existed within the population at large.[52]

This problem of justification underlies the circumspect attitude that is often adopted by medical élites, and it explains why a professional organization such as the NMG, for instance, is hesitant to follow the lead of enterprising members who strive to medicalize more and more areas of life.

This is an apt description of what happened to the regulation of prostitution towards the end of the 19th century. Individual medical practitioners were involved in the supervision of prostitution and had long been employed as medical examiners, but within the profession as a whole it proved impossible to arrive at a consensus concerning the justification for medical authority in this area. Given the subsequent turn of events in the prostitution debate, the regulation introduced in the Netherlands is best understood as an attempt to medicalize prostitution, one that was ultimately unsuccessful. Within the profession as a whole, the differences of opinion proved to be irreconcilable.

It was not solely attributable to dissenting doctors, however, that the medical supervision of prostitution never became fully institutionalized. Any expansion of medical authority is bound to arouse discord, but this does not necessarily block its ultimate success. In this case, however, two other circumstances played an important part. Firstly, one of the points in the 'triangular' situation of collusion described above was missing. The government and the military authorities represented one standpoint, and the medical profession another, but the third 'side' did not stand to benefit from medicalization. That neither prostitutes themselves nor brothel-keepers had anything to gain from an alliance with the physicians undermined the legitimacy of the latter's intervention even more than did the insubstantial nature of the relevant medical expertise. It meant, for instance, that the practice of regulation was extremely susceptible to bribery, and it also meant that prostitutes would do their best to conceal an infection. No one was better aware than they were of the empty promises of medical supervision. Whereas other groups subjected to increased medical attention during this period – e.g. homosexual men, drunks and criminals – benefited to some extent from this development, all that medicalization had to offer prostitutes and brothel-keepers at the close of the 19th century was a possible loss of income.

In the second place, society was immersed in a fierce debate on prostitution at this time, and public opposition to medical supervision was steadily growing. This opposition blocked further medicalization in that it made the profession more reluctant to cooperate, and deepened the divisions among their ranks. At length, the profession's customary restraint stiffened into paralysis. In these circumstances, medical intervention in prostitution, rather than providing a welcome form of conflict control, actually fanned the flames.

A wide range of groups and organizations were caught up in this fierce controversy. The most impassioned arguments came from the Dutch Society Against Prostitution (NVP), which was founded in 1879, marking the beginning of an organized movement to abolish regulation. The NVP was part of an international league that had been established earlier in the 1870s by the English pioneering abolitionist Josephine Butler. It would be hard to overstate the significance to the abolitionist struggle of the NVP's leader, the parson Hendrik Pierson, a man whose keen mind was yoked to an indomitable opposition to regulated prostitution.[53] Pierson and his closest allies belonged to the Réveil tradition, a movement of preachers and laity that evolved within the Dutch Reformed Church between 1810 and 1820 in protest against religious laxity.[54] The writer Willem Bilderdijk, the poet Isaac da Costa and the later founding member of the 'Anti-Revolutionary' party, Guillaume Groen van Prinsterer, are its best-known exponents. These men, largely from patrician backgrounds, opposed what they saw as the arrogance of the *Zeitgeist*, drenched as it was in the rational thinking of the Enlightenment, and encouraged a return to religious values. But the movement was not fired solely by religious zeal. The Réveil had a political dimension, which crystallized into the 'Anti-Revolutionary' ideology. It also engaged in social work, with the Home Mission, a campaign to reach out and help 'sinners' in the Netherlands on the basis of Protestant principles. The Home Mission gave rise to a rich philanthropic practice, founding societies and committees, institutions, asylums and temporary refuges for penitent fallen women, and it was also to a large extent responsible for attacking certain social evils such as drunkenness, immorality and dissolute forms of popular entertainment.

During the initial phase of its existence, the NVP bore the clear imprint of its Protestant roots. In the late 1880s, it moved away from religious orthodoxy and became a broader-based movement; gradually it evolved into an umbrella organization in the struggle against 'legalized vice',[55] as Pierson and his followers called regulation. The dominant influences in the organization were, however, always Protestant ethics and a political affiliation with the 'Anti-Revolutionary Party', with the middle and upper classes clearly in the majority.[56] Catholic involvement in the fight against regulation and against immorality in general was for many years conspicuous by its absence. It was not until the dawn of the new century that the first branches of the NVP were established in the Catholic south of the country, and that the first Catholic took a seat on the board.[57]

Among the staunchest supporters of the NVP's efforts were the Dutch Women's Union for the Promotion of Moral Consciousness (founded in 1884) and the Dutch Midnight Mission Association (founded in 1888), both of which were likewise orthodox Protestant. The former was rooted – more than the NVP itself – in the Réveil; its board members, at any rate, came from the same aristocratic circles. From the 1830s onwards, the Home Mission offered women from these circles an opportunity to take an active part in society. Siep Stuurman has commented that '"feminist energy", attached to a specifically Christian view of social problems in terms of Christian charity and sin, was mobilized here in a religious form'.[58] The same remark holds good for the Women's Union. This association's spokeswomen combined a sense of indignation about regulation with an evangelical devoutness, and had clear ideas about the place of women in the fight to abolish regulation. In the words of the Dowager Klerck-Van Hogendorp, one of the founding members of the Women's Union,

> [A woman] feels intuitively – that cannot be, that must not be! But how things must be changed she cannot know; that, she leaves to men. It is men who have at their disposal the council chamber, the areas of legislation and government, the means to ensure that what is right is done in society.[59]

Within the scope allotted them, the women of the Union played a significant part, however, in the abolitionist struggle. Their society was popular, and they had many times more supporters than the NVP.[60]

The Midnight Mission was to some extent the male counterpart of the Women's Union. Its ranks were just as full of evangelical zeal as were those of the Union, but only men were admitted. Unlike most abolitionists, the Midnight Missionaries addressed their message not to prostitutes, but to their clients, or at any rate to men contemplating a visit to a brothel. They stationed themselves at the entrances to brothels and other suspect establishments, and tried to persuade potential clients to turn back. Passers-by were addressed in fortifying terms, and if the occasion presented itself the Missionaries did not flinch from informing a woman that her husband had been seen near a brothel.[61] Such activities sometimes caused public order disturbances, in which the police – to the Missionaries' disgust – would not infrequently lend the beleaguered brothel-keepers a helping hand. What better proof of the official seal of approval conferred in the Netherlands on immorality? The Midnight Mission distinguished itself from the two societies mentioned earlier not only by its practical bias and readiness to do battle, but also by a tendency to recruit support from the lower classes. This tactic did not boost its membership much, but the organization's militancy nevertheless attracted a good deal of public attention.

These were the three societies most directly involved in the fight against prostitution and regulation. While none was a mass organization, many non-members expressed approval of their activities. The abolitionists were successful because their aims struck a chord in so many larger groups with a wider range of interests.

During the 1880s, this support gained momentum, with action nudging into prominence alongside rhetoric.

One instance of this support was the new line in the abolitionist front formed by feminists who were impatient with the position adopted by the Protestant Women's Union, finding it not radical enough. They echoed the Union's condemnation of the hypocrisy of the regulationists, who saw prostitution as a necessary evil while viewing the prostitute as a contemptible creature. But their polemic went a good deal further. Any man who truly saw it as a necessary evil, they reasoned, would have to take the logical next step and make his own sisters and daughters available for the cause.[62] In contrast to the Women's Union, feminists placed the question of prostitution in a broader framework of social inequality between the sexes, regarding it not in terms of sin, but as an issue directly related to the economic position of women. This is clear, for instance, from a discussion that took place in the National Women's Council of the Netherlands. The impassioned contribution of the feminist Marie Rutgers-Hoitsema would not be contained within lower-case lettering: she insisted that the cause of prostitution was 'ECONOMIC DISPARITY and the ECONOMIC DEPENDENCY OF THE WOMAN to which GIRLS' ENTIRE UPBRINGING is attuned'. Later in the same piece Rutgers-Hoitsema returns to the issue of upbringing. '*Boys* are not taught self-control. The position of dependency occupied by their mother and sisters puffs them up and makes them arrogant.'[63] As we shall see, men's lack of self-control was a recurrent theme in feminist views of prostitution. This was a point of common ground between the Women's Union and the more radical feminists.[64]

Medical practitioners whose one-time fervour for the project of regulation had been dimmed and then obliterated in the harsh light of experience constituted an increasingly vociferous wing of the abolitionist front. In 1880, the medical examiner of prostitutes in Utrecht, Dr L.C. van Goudoever, alerted the authorities to the poor functioning of regulation in major cities, stating that to his knowledge scarcely one-tenth of prostitutes were actually examined. He nevertheless continued to favour medical supervision.[65] But other medics who had previously supported regulation stated publicly that they had changed sides. Dr J. Menno Huizinga, for instance, concluded in 1888 that supervision should be written off as impracticable, and that men and women should be subject to the same moral standards.[66] To seal this U-turn in his convictions he took a seat on the NVP board. A year later Dr J.L. Chanfleury van

IJsselstein also crossed over to the opposing camp. He resigned his supervisory post for the medical examination of prostitutes in The Hague, having concluded that medical supervision was virtually ineffectual as a means of preventing infection.[67] These deserting physicians were a great boost to the abolitionist movement.[68] They combined the argument of the *injustice* of the system of regulation, an argument that was steadily winning ground, with incisive criticism of the medical pretensions to which regulationists laid claim, making it impossible for the latter to carry on dismissing the abolitionists as an unworldly group of laypersons who were unknowledgeable about public health regulations and who were 'hence unable to comprehend the evil, its spread and the facilities provided'.[69]

Public figures spanning the entire political spectrum also increasingly espoused the abolitionist cause.[70] Between the Anti-Revolutionary Party and the abolitionists there was a more or less natural alliance. Two of the NVP's most convinced supporters were the MPs L.W.C. Keuchenius and A.F. de Savornin Lohman; the latter was a personal friend of Pierson's.[71] In 1882 the radical Liberal movement in the person of C.V. Gerritsen entered the controversy,[72] and as the end of the century approached, Catholic leaders joined the growing masses in favour of abolition. Socialists too made their voices heard. Their leader F. Domela Nieuwenhuis was a member of the NVP, and addressed the international conference against prostitution that was held in The Hague in 1883. Moreover, the socialist movement provided many of the speakers for a conference that the NVP organized in collaboration with the Women's Union in 1889.[73]

The socialists' main contribution to the debate was their insistence that prostitution was caused by poverty, and hence directly related to the prevailing capitalist system, a point hammered home in the socialist periodical *Recht voor Allen*: 'Notwithstanding all the spurious arguments to the contrary, the chief cause of prostitution is *poverty and nothing but poverty*. Many are disinclined to hear this, but the truth must be told. Indeed, as long as there is a contrast between rich and poor, between different classes, as long as the exploitation of human beings is an absolute rule, the plague of prostitution will always be with us.'[74] This view of prostitution as an inevitable element of capitalist society that would eventually vanish of its own accord after the victory of the proletariat did not, however, stop socialists participating in the struggle against regulation long before any such victory had appeared on the horizon.

With their uncompromising views about the origins of prostitution, the socialists alienated not only those who favoured regulation, but also many of their fellow-abolitionists. On both sides it was generally acknowledged that prostitution was linked to poverty. But the regulationists saw prostitutes' individual characteristics – which they defined as frivolity, vanity, laziness and a lack of spiritual and moral development – as equally important. Most prostitutes, to their minds, were degenerate creatures without any sense of shame.[75] And among the ranks of the abolitionists, the Protestants in particular distanced themselves from the socialists' stance. Although they did not display the same arrogant insensitivity towards prostitutes as the regulationists, they completely rejected the political analysis on which the socialists placed such emphasis. Not that they could suggest any clear alternative, however. While conceding that prostitution went hand in hand with exploitation, the notion that all prostitutes were mere victims of circumstances was unpalatable to them. Protestants were not averse to using the regulationists' vocabulary – the prostitute's alleged flightiness and craving for finery – but saw such characteristics solely as the signs of a sinful existence, as 'the external symptoms of a deeper disease of waywardness and lack of resolve'.[76] Doing battle against these grave moral defects was something they certainly saw as their responsibility, but unlike the two other main groups in the debate they were somewhat handicapped by the lack of a clear-cut view of the prostitute: they saw her neither as a degenerate nor as a victim of capitalist forces.

Clearly, the movement that aimed to bring regulated prostitution to an end was a broad-based and motley coalition. If we were to include some of the smaller groups involved in the abolitionist effort – the ascetic and single-minded Christian anarchists of the 'Pure Life Movement', for instance – its diversity would be clearer still. In comparison, the regulationists were almost all medical practitioners, and were not united by any formal structure. This small group of hygienists was in effect fighting a rearguard action to rescue medical supervision without the support of any established organizations. Among their main spokesmen were A.P. Fokker and G. Van Overbeek de Meijer, both high-ranking academics in the medical world.[77] In the impassioned correspondence that flared up between the two opposing camps in the debate on regulation, Fokker and Van Overbeek de Meijer defended their position, together with a small group of sympathizers, with considerable verve.[78] But they gradually exuded the courage of despair, as it became increasingly clear in the 1880s that the regulationist project was doomed to failure.

It was around 1885 that the tide visibly turned, as regulationists suffered a series of telling setbacks. Attacks on regulation came thick and fast, and the effectiveness of supervision was widely questioned. Answering the barrage of criticism and endeavouring to quell the doubts became increasingly difficult.[79] The downfall of regulation could no longer be averted, as one municipality after another scrapped its ordinances on prostitution. By 1899, when the Dutch society of dermatologists adopted a motion supporting the abolition of the medical supervision of prostitution throughout the Netherlands, this was an unremarkable stand to take.[80] Supervision had indeed disappeared by then from all but a handful of municipalities. The abolitionists' victory that had been effectively won by the turn of the century was cemented in 1911, with the new morality legislation introduced by the Catholic cabinet minister, E.R.H. Regout. Alongside articles of law – some new, others tightened up – on abortion, pornography, contraception and homosexuality, there were also provisions relating to prostitution. These are commonly clubbed together and called the prohibition of brothels, although they included no such explicit ban. The activities of procurers, pimps and those who traded in women were defined as criminal offences. Prostitutes themselves were not directly affected, although they remained liable to prosecution for public decency offences. The new laws on prostitution were passed by the Lower House of Parliament without the need to count votes.[81]

The NVP was not disbanded when its chief objective had been realized, although Pierson himself saw his mission as accomplished and resigned as leader. When victory had seemed assured several years earlier, the organization had already started to expand its aims, seeking fresh ways of combating immorality and new areas of social work. After 1911 it continued along this path, as did the Women's Union and the Midnight Mission.

There is no need to rehash the entire course of the battle between regulationists and abolitionists in order to understand why regulation ultimately became unacceptable in the eyes of the public.[82] The emphasis here will be on the effective assault staged by the abolitionists on the role of regulation as a 'buffer'. Around the turn of the century, the two most important elements of this role had been disputed more and more hotly. Firstly, the medical protection claimed for regulation was increasingly questioned, with the popular theme of 'innocent victims' as the centrepiece of the arguments. And as for the sexual segregation which regulation had allegedly been helping to maintain, research findings and new theories put paid to all such claims.

Innocent victims

Attacking the claim that regulation could serve as a medical buffer between prostitution and society at large was a pivotal element in the abolitionists' effort. After all, the existing system of supervision had been intended first and foremost as a public health measure, and its advocates had leaned heavily on medical arguments to make their case: regulation would keep the impact of prostitution on public health within manageable limits, they insisted. The issue of venereal disease was obviously central to the efforts to undermine this justification. Abolitionist narrators succeeded in radically changing the usual backdrop of the debate by breaking through the customary obsession with the path of infection from prostitute to her male clientele. They introduced a new character – the 'innocent victim'. This *coup de théâtre*, as it were, transformed the nature of the debate on venereal disease. This was because the innocent victim, the new protagonist, belonged to an entirely different class of characters from the prostitute. The latter was the prototype of an offender, and as such regarded exclusively as a source of infection for others. The innocent victim, on the other hand, belonged to the opposing group of characters, who automatically aroused the sympathy of one and all. By focusing on this victim group, the abolitionists adroitly disengaged themselves from too close an association with the undoubtedly reprehensible character of the prostitute, something that Christian abolitionists were particularly keen to achieve. On the other hand, the emphasis on innocent victims led to the indictment of a new actor in the villain's role, as will presently become clear.

There were basically two types of innocent victim characters in this new dramatization: the wife unknowingly infected by her husband, and the child born infected, who was doomed to live a wretched life without being in any sense to blame. The abolitionists tended to present the events in the form of a pitiful *tableau vivant* of a family whose lot had been little improved by regulation. The father was depicted either away satisfying his own desires, or sitting as a perceptible shadow in the corner, consumed with bitter remorse. The spotlight was on a desperate mother surrounded by her children, whose dull state of mental retardation prevented them from understanding what had been done to them. The general practitioner and fervent neo-Malthusian J. Rutgers still saw this scene before him vividly in the early years of the 20th century:

44

I am filled with sadness, although it all happened many years ago, when I recall the thriving family of a police inspector, a decent man from a respectable background. He had waited for the results of the examination to make sure, but he contracted such a bad case of syphilis that eventually his entire life and career, as well as his family life, were destroyed in the most terrible way, and his wife became a model of silent despair.[83]

These domestic tragedies could hardly be laid at the prostitute's door, maintained the abolitionists. They were caused by a new type of offender to whom the host of innocent victims bore eloquent witness: the male intermediary between prostitution and family, who had previously contrived to avoid censure. That married men visited brothels was not part of regulationists' creed of the necessary evil, and regulationists had indeed always wisely preserved silence on this subject. Their one-sided concern with prostitutes was mere sophistry and proof of prejudice, according to the abolitionists, so it was hardly surprising that they were powerless to prevent the infiltration of venereal diseases into the family home. After all, the character who provided the crucial link in the chain was being let off scot-free. The abolitionist Josephine Butler was one of the first to point this out:

Who is it who brings these loathsome diseases into the family? Is it the prostitute? Where is the home into which she ever finds her way? Is it she, I say, who in her own person brings the poison to the mothers, and through the mothers to the children? Alas! no, it is the man, the husband, the father – and no other – who is directly responsible for the physical and moral sufferings which fall upon the home.[84]

The innocent victims in these homes, of whom the new abolitionist representation of events made the general public painfully aware, exposed the fallacies in the reasoning followed by the champions of regulation, and highlighted the inadequacies of the ways in which regulation was put into practice. The mere existence of these victims demonstrated that the medical buffer much vaunted by the hygienists and their associates was largely a thing of the imagination.

The abolitionists' revised cast of characters – and, as it were, their new script – hence altered the tenor of the debate on venereal disease. And it proved to be a masterful strategy. There were two main reasons for this success. First, in the rough period 1880–1910 medical science gained a far better understanding of venereal

45

diseases, which placed the consequences of these infections in a different light and made the shortcomings of regulation all the more obvious. Researchers learned a good deal about the later manifestations of syphilis. Suspicions that the serious disorders of *tabes dorsalis* and *dementia paralytica* had their origins in a syphilitic infection had steadily deepened in the 1880s and 1890s. In 1894, Alfred Fournier termed these two diseases *parasyphilis*; the former, he claimed, was syphilis of the spinal cord, and the latter syphilis of the brains. Fournier's conclusions were based on clinical observation, as the bacterium *Treponema pallidum*, which causes syphilis, had not yet been isolated.[85] This breakthrough was achieved in 1905 by two German researchers, Erich Hoffmann and Fritz Schaudinn, and one year later the Wassermann test was introduced, a universal blood-serum test for syphilis.[86] Although the direct application of these developments should not be exaggerated, one major advance was that it now became possible to test subjects to check the accuracy of existing fears about the consequences of syphilis. This new possibility demonstrated – overturning previously held beliefs – that the mother of a baby with congenital syphilis was herself always infected prior to the delivery. This discovery meant that the terms *syphilis ex patre*, meaning a direct infection from father to child, and *syphilis par conception*, for a healthy mother contracting the disease from her infected fetus, vanished from use, as they were based on misconceptions. Also significant was the new possibility of demonstrating the existence of asymptomatic periods of latency in the clinical picture of syphilis.

Where gonorrhoea was concerned, the research conducted by New York gynaecologist Emil Noeggerath had far-reaching implications. In the early 1870s he found that gonorrhoea frequently led to infertility in women, which he believed explained the childlessness of many marriages. He wielded some rather dizzying percentages: 80% of married men and 60% of married women had at some time had gonorrhoea. In 1879 the German bacteriologist Albert Neisser isolated the gonococcus, the bacterium that causes gonorrhoea, and demonstrated that *ophthalmia neonatorum*, which produces blindness in newborn infants, originated from a gonorrhoea infection passed on from mother to child during delivery. These new discoveries became generally known among Dutch medical practitioners in the mid-1880s.[87]

In 1881, the German gynaecologist Karl Credé found that a few drops of a silver nitrate solution was enough to prevent gonorrhoeal blindness in neonates.[88] But this was the only advance made in the treatment of venereal infections amid all the new insights into the diseases themselves. This imbalance in progress between theory and treatment caused much shaking of heads, and confirmed many medical practitioners in their suspicions that the medical supervision of prostitution was of no value in protecting innocent members of the family. This is well illustrated by a late 19th-century addition to the nosology of syphilis – *contagion médiate*. This variant exposed the pointlessness of even the most rigorous medical examination; for in *contagion médiate,*

> a prostitute could be visited by a syphilitic man, and the infection could be passed on to her without her falling ill. ... She could thus carry the syphilitic infectant within her body locally, and infect the next man who visits her without suffering any ill effects herself.[89]

Even a healthy prostitute could thus become the 'temporary repository ... of a virus left in her by the previous visitor' and infect others.[90] This left only one solution to the problem of widespread venereal disease: to close down the brothels. The existence of *contagion médiate* has always been controversial, and unsurprisingly we find believers and non-believers in this mode of transmission coinciding with the opponents and supporters of supervision.

The second circumstance that exacerbated public sensitivity to the plight of innocent victims was a growing concern about fertility and the genetic 'quality' of the population. It became commonplace to label venereal diseases, and syphilis in particular, a 'scourge of society'; here was a plague that not only attacked the constitution of the sufferer, but also menaced the body politic.[91] The disruption of the family was the crucial factor in these fears. Venereal diseases took their place alongside alcoholism and tuberculosis as the most feared causes of the degeneration of family life and, as a result, of posterity.[92]

Tragic case histories fuelled these fears. Around the turn of the century Ernst de Vries, a medical practitioner attached to Voorgeest mental asylum, estimated that one-fourth of the patients in this institution were victims of congenital syphilis. His family case history of one ('an idiot since birth') ran as follows:

> 2 of the patient's brothers or sisters are also idiots; 2 idiots are deceased; 2 healthy children died young; 3 children are alive and healthy. The patient's father was formerly a hard-working labourer, then took to drink and died at Endegeest of dementia paralytica ... One of the patient's uncles is an idiot, one aunt insane; another

aunt is normal, but has narrow, uneven pupils that respond poorly; another uncle died at 15 of a disease of the brain. All these are on the father's side. The grandfather was slow-witted, the grandmother vigorous, but miscarried 4 infants besides those listed above.[93]

De Vries did not exclude the possibility of the patient's father having contracted a 'fresh' syphilitic infection, but he thought it more likely, given the general malaise running through the father's generation, that the 'slow-witted' grandfather was the source of all this wretchedness, 'so that our patient belongs to the third generation to be afflicted'.

Around 1900 the disastrous consequences of venereal disease were arousing grave concern in almost every country of Western Europe. This concern has often been described as a fear spreading among the middle classes of 'the degeneration of the race and the depopulation of the nation'.[94] Of the period 1885–1913, Corbin comments in an article about the spectre of congenital syphilis:

> It almost seems as though medical practitioners were induced to supply a scientific version of the delusions that haunted the middle-class of this period; and in so doing, they gave these delusions the seal of approval that allowed fantasy to metamorphose into scientific fact.[95]

Neither the excessive fear of degeneration that Corbin describes nor the fear of depopulation was in fact found everywhere to the same extent. The most fearful were the French. Dutch concern was less high-pitched, but in the Netherlands too, the turn of the century witnessed an upsurge of anxiety about the 'quality' of the population. Much of the French literature about blighted families and their 'inferior' descendants was translated into Dutch, and in the Netherlands too articles were published about wives and children whose health had been irrevocably damaged by a man's thoughtless behaviour. And the medical practitioner and feminist Aletta Jacobs forcefully spelt out the consequences of this damage for society:

> Is it really so very desirable, so much in the interests of our society and of the individual concerned, that he should be able, everywhere and at all times, to hand over a coin to satisfy his sexual urge? Is it not yet sufficiently well-known that prostitution affects not only our domestic circumstances, our personal happiness, that it not only has economic and moral consequences but that it strikes deeper, far deeper into the life of the nation? Is it still not understood that the

physical well-being of each of us, indeed public health as a whole, is under threat from the effects of prostitution? Prostitution is accompanied by terrible infections known as venereal diseases. Because these diseases are so infectious, and because they can be passed on from parents to their children, albeit often in a different form, they exert a profoundly negative effect on our society.[96]

It was the French, however, who most excelled in cataloguing the horrors of congenital syphilis. Fournier, who pioneered many medical theories in the field of syphilis, conducted the most vigorous campaign. With unabating dedication and supplying detailed descriptions of the most varied manifestations of congenital ('inherited') syphilis, he attempted to draw society's attention to the invisible poison that was coursing through its veins. Fournier's reputation extended far beyond the borders of France, and Dutch medical journals frequently included translations or reviews of his publications. Many Dutch commentators endorsed the conclusions set down in his *Syphilis et Mariage* (1880) concerning the rules to be followed by a syphilis patient – or former patient – who wished to marry. Fournier's minimum requirements, to prevent the sufferer's wife and children being infected, were a delay of three to four years subsequent to infection and a complete course of treatment. This was necessary in the interests of 'the prime duty to be fulfilled, which overrides all others ... that of protecting society'.[97]

The results of failing to heed such warnings were represented in the stage play *Les Avariés* (*Damaged Goods*) by Eugène Brieux, who clearly took his inspiration from Fournier. The husband-to-be of this three-act tragedy is unwilling to postpone his marriage for more than six months, and ends up destroying his family. The wider social significance of this sad spectacle is stressed repeatedly in the script: 'You must now rise above your personal distress and attempt to grasp the generalities that are at issue, and think of the thousands who suffer the same fate', the doctor insists to the despairing father-in-law of the reckless young husband.

> 'I tell you, sir, there are thousands, of every rank and station in society. The disease makes its way from the prostitute's couch and the bordello – and often with few intermediate steps – into the marriage bed. To clean up the streets would therefore be to protect ordinary people's homes.'[98]

This play was first published in 1901 in France, where it caused a considerable stir; indeed, it was initially banned from the stage, and it was not put on for Paris audiences until 1905.[99] The feminist Titia van der Tuuk published a Dutch translation (*De Beschadigden*) less than a year after the appearance of the original. The *Geneeskundige Courant* printed it as a serial a few years later, but the play was never performed in the Netherlands.[100]

Better known is Hendrik Ibsen's *Ghosts*. Publishing his play in 1881, Ibsen was one of the first to dramatize the theme of congenital syphilis. This complex domestic tragedy shows the son gradually degenerating into syphilitic madness. Because of his father's actions, his life is 'incurably destroyed'.[101] *Ghosts* was much less explicit about syphilis than *Damaged Goods*, which was after all a deliberate piece of propaganda, but as it jibed mercilessly at certain conventions of middle-class society, the first performances of the play, some ten years after its publication, were greeted with extremely hostile reviews. After the London première of Ibsen's play, an English reviewer compared it to 'an open drain ... a loathsome sore, an abominable piece, a repulsive and degrading work'.[102] *Ghosts* was performed in the Amsterdam Salon des Variétés on 5 September 1890. Here, in contrast to the play's reception in other countries, the performance was open to the general public, and its subject-matter did not provoke an outcry.[103]

It is logical to assume that the flood of publicity linking syphilis to physical decay and the degeneration of society had a deterrent effect. Anyone who reads the terrifying prognoses and sees the repulsive illustrations which some writers of informative material used to reinforce their message ('with 31 colour illustrations of syphilitic genitals and other organs') will immediately conclude that the general reader must have been consumed with dread.[104] While it is difficult to attribute it directly to this scaremongering, there is no doubt that a new form of hypochondria – syphilophobia – emerged at the end of the 19th century.[105] In 1924, the psychoanalyst Alfred Adler devoted an article to this condition, which was common among his patients. He writes: 'I seldom encounter a case of neurosis that does not display clear signs of a fear of syphilis'. His most intractable cases were patients consumed with an unremitting fear of infection, or, having been pronounced cured, of late manifestations of the disease such as *tabes dorsalis* and *dementia paralytica*. Some of his patients, Adler continues, are terrified of the fate awaiting their children yet to be conceived. 'Patients always exhibit a boundless interest in syphilis and everything related to it; the subject is squeezed dry in discussions and in writing.' Adler does not make any connection between his patients' symptoms and the propagandist terror surrounding venereal disease to which they may have been exposed at an impressionable age. He gives no detailed analysis of the phenomenon at all, merely noting (rather strangely) that 'syphilophobia frequently conceals a fear of women, or of men, and in most cases of both'.[106]

Although syphilis was seen as posing the most serious threat to late 19th-century society, some doctors followed Noeggerath and Neisser in denouncing the evils that could be wrought by gonorrhoea. In 1894, a Dr Nijhoff published an article on marriages entered into by male gonorrhoea patients. He emphasized the serious consequences of an infection passed on to the wife, to which 'thousands upon thousands of women' could bear witness: pain, infertility and 'such deformities and displacement of the pelvic organs that even once the inflammations have subsided, functional disorders (incurable infertility), neuralgia, reflex neuroses and psychoses may remain, darkening the rest of the woman's life'.[107] If only the consequences of the seemingly innocuous case of the 'clap' were confined to the men who had contracted it from a prostitute, justice would have been done, according to Nijhoff, but 'since innocent victims are being claimed, the lives of healthy young women are being destroyed and the reproduction of the species is in jeopardy, it is the obligation of us all to try to limit the effects of a disease which is no less of a social evil than syphilis'.[108] The regulation of prostitution, in the eyes of Nijhoff, was completely unequal to this task. Not only was the disease easy to conceal from the examining physician, but gonorrhoea was an ailment that virtually no prostitute could escape, so that a system of medical examinations 'would almost amount to the isolation of all the women who perform this horizontal work'.[109] Nijhoff, like many of his contemporaries, saw sexual abstinence as one of the main weapons against gonorrhoea. In his general advice on health, 'the general practitioner should tactfully emphasise the role played by will power and strength of personality in controlling the sexual urge'.[110]

Advances in medical science coupled with increased concern about women's fertility and the quality of future generations enhanced the poignancy of the innocent victim's fate. Scripts centring on this character were effective means of exploding the inflated claims – medical protection – of regulation as a mere bubble of fantasy cherished by hygienists.

Double standards under attack

Another boon was claimed for the regulation of prostitution, besides the health shield it was supposed to provide for the general population. Regulation was a useful device, its champions assured, for the preservation of what has been termed the 'sexual order': it helped to safeguard the 'respectable' parts of society, the argument went, from sexual defilement. For did not regulated brothels give young men the opportunity to satisfy their sexual needs in a natural way? And did this not protect virtuous women and girls, as well as preventing youths from turning to perversity? The justification for this form of sexual regulation thus lay in well-defined double standards for men and women. Abolitionists attacked these double standards with all the statistics and rhetoric they could muster.

The assault on the double standards that governed sexual morality was the linchpin of the abolitionist offensive; it struck at the very roots of the regulationist project. Whatever the cogency of the points raised about innocent victims and the health of future generations, they could in theory be used to argue for improved, strengthened regulation – perhaps even the state system favoured by many regulationists.[111] Not so the assault on double standards, which accordingly became the rallying cry for all the otherwise disparate parts of the abolitionist lobby. At the anti-prostitution conference held in Amsterdam in 1889, Pierson formulated the common ground shared by abolitionists in a single principle: 'that the same moral standards be applied to men as to women'.[112]

Abolitionists drew on a variety of new information to assail the validity of the double standards underpinning the regulationist cause. Firstly, they publicized new data concerning the brothels' clientele, and secondly, they drew attention to changing views of the male sex urge and sexual abstinence.

In the first respect, a study commissioned by Amsterdam City Council contributed significantly to the debate. 1895 saw the appointment of a committee, its mandate 'to investigate the nature and extent of the prostitution that exists here, and to prepare the measures to be taken by the authorities against public indecency'.[113] This committee published a three-part report in 1897: a general part reporting on the committee's findings and urging the abolition of brothels on various grounds, and two appendices. The first appendix, by C.F.J. Blooker, elaborated on the medical aspects of prostitution. Blooker considered regulation unreliable and impracticable, and saw no health benefits whatever to recommend it. Rebutting regulationists' perennial argument that prohibiting brothels would simply increase clandestine or 'free' prostitution, thus posing a far greater hazard to public health, Blooker concluded that 'the presence or absence of brothels can be termed at the very least a matter of indifference from the point of view of public health'. He too advocated the abolition of brothels. The second appendix was by Dr A. Voûte, and created the greatest stir.[114] Voûte reported the findings of a personal investigation based on visits to 15 brothels, and interviews with several prostitutes working there. This eye-opening experience had revealed certain shocking facts. Voûte discovered not only that the brothels he visited were frequented by a well-to-do clientele, but that this clientele largely consisted of married men of mature years, who moreover had a marked preference for perverse types of sexual satisfaction. Regulationists had always justified the prostitute as a facility for young bachelors who would otherwise be unable to satisfy their sexual urges by any natural means. Voûte dismissed this argument peremptorily:

> It is abundantly plain ... from all these statements that the claim that brothels are a necessary outlet for the tempestuous passions of youth has little substance. Our investigation has revealed once again that brothels are breeding-grounds for the most depraved forms of sexual satisfaction, and exist chiefly by virtue of the sums paid by prosperous citizens of a mature age, often married men, to satisfy their lust.[115]

The municipal authorities responded to this report by amending Amsterdam's General Police Ordinance, outlawing brothels altogether. The law was flouted on such a large scale, however, that in 1902 harsher regulations had to be introduced.[116] Amsterdam had never in fact had formal regulations on prostitution, but a form of supervision existed indirectly before 1897 by way of a system of alcohol licensing and permits for brothel-keepers; prostitutes were registered with the police and required to undergo regular medical check-ups.[117]

The committee's findings became widely known and fuelled the anti-regulationist campaign. Far from preventing undesirable sexual practices, brothels actually appeared to foster them:

> Brothels are clearly the breeding-grounds and schools for the entire catalogue of the most abhorrent forms of sexual perversity, in which present-day brothels are unsurpassed by those of ancient Rome. Such abhorrent and repulsive sexual deviations generally occur in the final phase of a life that has been devoted almost exclusively to lust, and seldom usher it in. This accords with the remarkable fact that brothels almost everywhere are frequented chiefly by married

53

men and the elderly, at any rate by those who are more experienced and seasoned in lust. This finding diminishes still further the arsenal of the regulationists, who so like to regard brothels as necessary institutions to ease the unruly and exuberant passions of young men. Youths are infrequent visitors to brothels, most of whose clients are married or grey-haired men.[118]

This vehement onslaught was part of an exposé of the evils of regulation published in 1906 by the medical practitioner E.A. Keuchenius.

The report's findings supplied the opponents of supervision with a trump card: it enabled them to deride the claim that regulation was a useful safeguard against sexual perversity – one of its stated original aims. Besides spreading sickness and physical decay, brothels were evidently potent sources of moral degeneracy, which threatened to invade even the well-to-do circles that had long seen regulation as shielding them from danger. Abolitionists exploited this point to the fullest. Not only did they fill their 'cast' of innocent victims almost entirely with middle-class characters, but they also tended to portray the prostitutes' clients in a stereotyped fashion, as middle-aged or elderly married, established citizens. The proliferating publicity about the spread of venereal disease all carried the same ominous message: as one writer put it, 'everywhere, the disease of syphilis is more widespread among the well-to-do than among the working classes'.[119] This claim was not substantiated by any clear evidence, but it certainly helped to underscore the importance of the fight against prostitution.[120]

The disclosure of the report's conclusions was a body blow to the supporters of regulation. And compounding this damaging empirical evidence was a change in public attitudes, as the tide was now turning against the double standards that still underpinned the regulationist cause.

This altered climate of opinion stemmed from new ideas concerning male sexuality. The advocates of supervision still held firm to the traditional view that sexual abstinence for men was both unnatural and harmful. As late as 1906, W.H. Mansholt, medical practitioner and staunch champion of regulation, while acknowledging that the only males who suffered serious harm from protracted sexual abstinence were those with an inherited weakness, continued:

> although sexual abstinence does not produce serious disorders in others, it is a fact that men too only reach the peak of their mental powers and their ability to work, the limits of their capacity for

expansion, once they have been able to fulfil their sexual function. As the woman becomes wholly woman only once she is a mother, the man becomes wholly man only with cohabitation. A wholesome society may reasonably be expected to take these demands of nature into account; it will be conceded that our own has many shortcomings in this regard.[121]

This idea of the indomitable male sexual urge, however, was gradually giving way to the belief that custom and disparities in moral upbringing alone accounted for the differences between the sexes. Increasing numbers of medical practitioners were retracting their previously declared views of the harmful effects of chastity. Aletta Jacobs joined in a debate on the double standards of sexual morality being waged in the columns of *Minerva* student periodical:

> Fortunately another fallacy, whereby it was thought harmful for a man to control his sexual urge, is now starting to give way to more clear-headed views. No-one has ever become ill from unsatisfied sexual desire. It is true that patients are seen in hospitals, mental institutions and doctors' surgeries that were once regarded as victims of sexual abstinence, and whom doctors therefore referred – if they were men – to brothels or to prostitutes. But these days such matters are viewed in a different light. Insatiable sexual desire is either the symptom of a disease or the consequence of an ill-conceived way of life, and modern medical practitioners no longer respond to it with the same old prescription. These days, they are more likely to counsel: make sure you take plenty of exercise in the fresh air, keep to plain fare in moderate quantities, refrain from drinking alcohol, rise early and do not retire too late, avoid reading-matter that stimulates the senses and bawdy forms of entertainment. With will power and a wholesome way of life, no young person (whether man or woman) will find sexual abstinence an impossibility.[122]

One significant pointer to this reversal in medical opinion is a motion that was adopted during the second international conference on the prevention of syphilis and other venereal diseases, held in Brussels in 1902. Those present, most of whom belonged to the medical profession, declared that sexual abstinence was not harmful for men's health, and should indeed be heartily recommended from a medical point of view. Pierson spoke with satisfaction of the 'precious truths' that the motion expressed.[123]

This radical swing of the pendulum concerning views of male

chastity was not only based on medical arguments; the clarion call for self-control came from every corner of the abolitionist movement.[124] Groups such as the Clean Living Society (*Rein Leven Beweging*) and feminists never tired of stressing the need for a single standard to be applied to both sexes.[125] Feminists were particularly vehement in denouncing the theory and practice of men's insatiable sex drive. Like women, men should master sexual self-restraint, argued the feminist Annette Versluys-Poelman:

> The sexual urge may perhaps be stronger in men than in women, but this has never been proved. It is certain, however, that men's sexual desire is artificially cultivated, while that of women is artificially repressed. It is certain that no other creatures in the world allow their sexual desire free rein to such an extent, and so uninterruptedly, as do men. There is no reason to assume that this sexual desire would exist to the same unbridled extent in the natural state as in our so-called cultivated Society; but even if this were so, humans need not simply preserve nature in this regard. Self-control is almost the only fixed and unchanging element in upbringing. ... Young men, beware of imagining that no harm is done if you dally with depraved hussies and later marry a pure woman. You can be just as pure and chaste as any woman if you wish, if you do not make yourselves the slaves of your passions.[126]

The numbers of male converts to this new doctrine cannot be ascertained, but it is clear that long-standing views of the male sex drive were increasingly under attack towards the end of the 19th century. Unsurprisingly, the fight against regulated prostitution and the drive to overturn traditional views of male sexuality went hand in hand.

On the one hand, then, abolitionists exposed the medical claims of supervised prostitution as a fiction by highlighting the terrible fate of innocent victims, and on the other hand they swept away the illusion that regulated prostitution was helping to maintain a 'sexual order' in society with their attacks on the double standards of sexual morality on which the whole system was based. Between 1880 and 1900 their efforts were gradually rewarded by a shift in public attitudes: at the end of this period, prostitution was no longer widely viewed as an acceptable element of society. In 1902, the National Women's Council was unable to find a speaker to defend the merits of regulation. 'And this is not the first time we have discovered that no-one is willing to defend the preservation of this system in public', Klerck-Van Hogendorp observed in her introductory address, adding that this signalled a change in public opinion 'that we have observed with great satisfaction'.[127]

The anguish of an age

One question about the demise of regulated prostitution remains to be answered: why did it occur at this particular time, in the last decades of the 19th century? Bearing in mind that regulationists and abolitionists were partly driven by the same concerns and motives, we need to explain why the remedy proposed by the former became increasingly unacceptable. After all, the limited effectiveness of the regulatory system was well-known from the outset: even the founder and most vociferous champion of supervision, Parent-Duchâtelet, had to concede that fewer infections were transmitted by way of clandestine prostitution than through its regulated equivalent.[128] And to the consternation of the regulationists, this awkward statistic – to the extent that relevant comparative research data were available – refused to change. Nor can we deny that medical science was far enough advanced in the mid-19th century to question the usefulness of supervision. So it is curious that it was several decades before the fight against regulation began in earnest, with a widespread public debate on prostitution and venereal disease.

To explain why the change occurred when it did, we should first examine changes in prostitution that were giving rise to increased public concern – changes in the Netherlands and other countries, which had nothing to do with either government measures or the actions of the abolitionists. Most importantly, the traditional brothel was being increasingly marginalized.[129] Corbin described this *fin-de-siècle* trend as a European and possibly even global phenomenon. It did not produce any overall decline in prostitution, as it was accompanied by a proportionate rise in non-regulated, 'free' prostitution.

Corbin has very definite views about the reason for this change, which he ascribes to a change in the clientele. The nature of prostitution, according to Corbin, is determined first and foremost by sexual frustrations. The demand produced by these feelings completely determines the supply. In the mid-19th century, he argues, such frustrations were concentrated largely in the lower regions of society; most of the prostitute's clients belonged to the urban proletariat, being migrants and seasonal workers who were largely dependent on prostitutes for the satisfaction of their sexual needs. As these classes gradually became more fully integrated into society, however, and the uneven balance between the sexes in these groups was somewhat restored, the need for prostitutes diminished. On the other hand, Corbin continues, the middle classes were increasingly plagued by sexual frustrations in the latter half of the 19th century. The late 19th-century romantic idealization of the respectable woman and wife as someone who was pure, chaste and sexually restrained, made prostitution an attractive recourse – Corbin goes so far as to call it necessary – to middle-class men.[130] He also dwells on the increasing incidence of forced celibacy in this group, as a result of marriages being postponed and many people failing to marry at all.[131] Combined with their increased financial resources and a somewhat more pleasure-oriented lifestyle, the frustrations generated by such factors, Corbin concludes, fanned the need for erotic recreation outside the home.

The increase in demand by middle-class men – Corbin describes it in terms of a need for seduction, with all the accompanying overtones of adventure and conquest – altered the structure of prostitution. The joyless satisfaction of the sexual needs of the proletariat made way for a new style of prostitution, in which the client's illusion of genuine conquest was preserved to the fullest extent.[132] The regulated brothels, with their predictable rituals and their supply of passive prostitutes, were absolutely not equipped to meet this new demand. Those that stayed in business developed exotic specialities to satisfy the wishes of their new clientele. But clandestine, 'free' prostitution profited far more from the changing trends. New institutions such as department stores and modern bars, new careers such as that of shop-girl and waitress, facilitated the spread of new forms of prostitution, tailored to the middle-class market. In short, the demise of the brothel was accompanied by a greater, and above all more diffuse, dissemination of debauchery.

Some of the changes that Corbin describes would also appear to be valid for the Netherlands. Here too, the number of regulated brothels dwindled, with the most expensive and lavishly decorated establishments having the best chance of survival.[133] Foreign girls were hired here in increasing numbers.[134] At the same time, clandestine prostitution was on the increase. The burgeoning of rendez-vous establishments, café-chantants, variety theatres, bars with waitress service and other meeting-places of this kind all contributed to this trend.[135] Corbin's theory that these changes stemmed from a shift in clientele is not implausible, but leaves many questions unanswered. Even if we adopt it wholesale, the reasons for the change in clientele and for the development of the demand for sexual gratification remain fairly obscure.

One of the reasons for the sexual frustration among middle-class men cited by Corbin is that the well-to-do had taken to marrying relatively late. In the Netherlands, too, this tendency was said to be increasing the demand for prostitution.[136] The general trend in the last two decades of the 19th century, however, is contrary to that described by Corbin for France: after 1870, the number of new marriages increased slightly, and the age of marriage actually fell, even among men of the higher social classes.[137] Although a discrepancy remained in the age at which men of different classes married, there was no question in the Netherlands of an increase in the tendency among the well-to-do to postpone or renounce marriage. Moreover, positing a link between the age of marriage and a tendency to visit prostitutes is in itself a questionable assumption, particularly when we bear in mind the discovery that the majority of clients were in fact married men.

Nor is it possible to make any unequivocal statements concerning the desires of the prostitutes' new clients. We can find oblique suggestions, however, that the demand for paid sexual attentions indeed changed much as Corbin describes. For instance, the following account appears in one of the reports on prostitution commissioned by the NMG:

> The 'brothel problem' has become less significant, because the brothels, at least in their old form, are becoming far less numerous, quite independently from the attitude adopted by the government. While it is true that many of the common places where prostitutes congregate bear a resemblance to actual brothels, it cannot be denied that such establishments lack the essential character of brothels (the passive acquiescence of the prostitute in relation to her client, the large number of visitors that the prostitute is compelled to receive) and hence cannot be placed in the same category.[138]

It is reasonable to view the presence of increasing numbers of foreign prostitutes in late 19th-century Dutch brothels, with Corbin, as a response to changes in demand. This element may have given a visit to the brothel the tinge of adventure that the client was looking for. Far more research would be needed, however, to establish a clear link between a change in clients' social origins and the changes in the demand for prostitutes' services.

Notwithstanding all these reservations, Corbin's theory of a shift in social class among prostitutes' clients in the latter decades of the 19th century may well be relevant for the Netherlands. It seems clear, at any rate, that prostitution was witnessing the same differentiation that took place in other areas of social and economic life in this period. Viewed in that light, the prostitution debate could be seen as the reaction of middle-class groups that felt threatened by the diminishing gap between prostitution and their own world. This is not a particularly compelling argument, however. The struggle against *regulated* brothels, as conducted in the Netherlands, can scarcely be described as an adequate response to the changes that have been outlined here. Moreover, similar – but far more pronounced – developments in France produced quite different consequences. There, in combination with other, largely demographic circumstances, they led to a dread of degeneration and depopulation, an obsessive preoccupation with the dangers of venereal infection and an extreme form of sanitary supervision, which took the place of traditional regulation.[139]

I therefore conclude that while the unforced decrease in numbers of traditional brothels and the growing differentiation within prostitution probably hastened the end of regulation in the Netherlands, these factors do not satisfactorily explain the late 19th-century tumult surrounding the twin issues of prostitution and venereal disease. The storm about supervised prostitution was completely out of tune with the times: regulated brothels were long past their prime, and were indeed on the way out.

If the public alarm about prostitution and venereal disease cannot be adequately explained by developments in prostitution itself, another logical explanation springs to mind – that the incidence of venereal disease suddenly soared at the end of the 19th century. We have few statistics at our disposal in this regard. Those we do have – again, army statistics provide most information – display a decline from the mid-19th century onwards. Around 1850, the annual number of cases of venereal disease accounted for about 12% of the troops, while by the 1880s this figure had dropped to 9%. Around the turn of the century it had fallen to a mere 3%, and on the eve of the First World War it was less than 2%.[140] That these statistics only relate to the army is of course a considerable limitation. Given the more diffuse spread and diversification of prostitution, it is entirely conceivable that venereal disease affected larger numbers of civilians in the late 19th century. On the other hand, however, this period also witnessed important advances in hygiene, which make it more plausible that the incidence of venereal disease among the civilian population gradually fell from the mid-century onwards. Any such conclusion must remain, however, in the realm of conjecture.

Judging by the available information, neither prostitution itself nor the incidence of venereal disease adequately accounts for the sudden eruption of the debate on prostitution in the latter half of the 19th century. It is clear, however, that both these evils were *popularly perceived* as far more significant, and in this sense they were in fact responsible for the explosion of public concern. To understand the roots of the debate, we therefore have to investigate why the public became increasingly *indignant*, at this time, about the twin evils of prostitution and venereal disease. I shall draw on various readings of late 19th-century social and political trends in the Netherlands to illuminate the background to this changed climate of opinion.

One salient change was in the political balance of power. Visible cracks appeared in the bastion of Liberal domination in the last quarter of the 19th century. A religious camp emerged in political life, with the formation of Christian parties and the mustering of churchgoing grassroots opinion into a considerable force in society. Protestants organized themselves first, establishing the ARP ('Anti-Revolutionary Party') as a modern political party, and Catholics followed suit at a later stage. The new Protestant activists focused on several key issues. Their chief concern was to establish schools based on Protestant principles, but they also made their influence felt in issues impinging on morality, marriage, family life and sexuality. They wanted a new politics of personal values, in which government would have far more broad-ranging responsibilities than under the Liberals.[141]

The Liberals' fierce opposition to extensive government powers to intrude into people's private lives did not mean that they abandoned the field of morality to the religious parties. New political alliances were formed, with Catholics and Protestants naturally gravitating towards each other when moral issues were at stake, but Protestants and Liberals finding each other more congenial in other areas. As the Liberals' dominant influence crumbled, they were obliged to shift their ground somewhat in the direction of their religious rivals. As a result, in the 1880s the Liberals and Anti-Revolutionary Party often joined forces in a drive to strengthen the moral fibre of the nation. Despite the Liberals' temporary revival of popularity in the 1890s, their ties with the ARP were further consolidated after 1900. In their reaction to the social revolutions that marked the turn of the century, both the conservative and progressive wings of the now fragmented Liberal movement – departing from traditional Liberal standpoints – emphasized the importance of a deep sense of morality. Issues of moral standards and decency were now the subject of political debate within the new Liberal parties. The fight against immorality and lack of discipline thus commanded attention, at the beginning of the century, across the political spectrum. Although the majority of Liberals voted against the morality legislation, as being flagrantly at odds with Liberal principles, they acknowledged the political importance of the issues dealt with in its regulations.[142]

The fragmentation of traditional Liberalism and the rise of the Christian parties not only reflected the changing attitudes to morality around the turn of the century, but also tended to reinforce them, as witnessed by a variety of social initiatives. Protestant activists formed the vanguard of the new movement: in countless societies, foremost among which were the NVP and the Women's Union, they decried places associated with debauchery, such as brothels and fairs, and other objectionable excesses, from contraception to pornography. Viewed in this light, the prostitution debate was part of a broad-ranging review of society's moral standards which was launched around 1900, and which culminated in the morality legislation of 1911.[143]

Alongside alterations in the political landscape, there were other more general changes in Dutch society during this period. These can best be characterized as a closing of the gap between different social groups in terms of the power they wielded – sometimes labelled 'functional democratization'.[144] The gap was narrowing between social classes, and also between men and women.

Prior to 1850, the world of paupers and workers had few points of contact with that of the well-to-do.[145] In the latter half of the century, urbanization and industrialization increased the amount of contact between the two worlds, and helped to inculcate a sense of mutual dependency. This new situation, in which the urban proletariat and middle classes were to a certain extent thrown together, triggered reactions on both sides.

This increasing mutual dependence galvanized the middle classes into action in the long term, and they stepped up their efforts to improve the lot of the common people. The hygienists were among the first to draw attention to the appalling living conditions of urban workers, but their pleas initially fell on deaf ears. It was not until the 1870s that the prosperous middle classes became convinced of the need for special provisions in the province of public sanitation and of measures geared towards improving the living conditions of the working classes.[146] With the onward march of industrialization, the well-to-do acquired a keener sense of the need for the civilization of the workers. Their efforts were to a great degree responsible for the changes in lifestyle among the working class. Ali de Regt (1984) describes what happened as a civilizing process, a process that expressed itself in a more disciplined way of life, a stronger work ethic and a greater emphasis on family life and domesticity. But other influences were making themselves felt, besides the civilizing drive instigated by the middle classes. Many workers were eager to transcend the traditional boundaries of their class; this too led to increased differentiation, with organized groups and skilled workers tending to emulate middle-class patterns of behaviour. Their efforts to cast their lives in a mould of respectability, marked by regular habits, were supported by the labour movement.[147]

Both middle-class civilizers and working-class climbers emphasized the virtues of cleanliness and domesticity. The struggle to live a decent life was largely a struggle to obtain adequate, clean living accommodation and a fight against the prevailing ills, of which alcoholism and prostitution were considered the most pernicious. In this light, the fact that prostitution was attracting the attention both of persons in the foremost ranks of society and of workers' leaders, who were often socialists, can be seen mainly as part of a civilization process involving the working classes.

Simultaneously with this abridgement of the power gap between social classes, a similar process took place between men and women, with the appearance of the first organized feminists. The shift in relations between the sexes has been explained in a variety of ways. In his book on the emancipation of women in a number of countries, Evans (1977) refers to changes in the class structure triggered by the rise and expansion of the middle classes as the most important causative factor. As social relations changed, so too did the position of women, both within the family and on the labour market, affecting the balance of power between the sexes.[148] As far as the Netherlands is concerned, the demographic factor is also often cited – in particular the 'surplus' of unmarried women in the latter half of the 19th century – as having helped to increase women's power base. The middle classes in particular saw the 'surplus' of women as a matter for concern. In all probability, the presence of this group, for whom fathers or brothers were traditionally expected to assume total responsibility, provided an added incentive to many champions of economic autonomy for middle-class unmarried women.[149]

Whatever the underlying causes may have been, women undoubtedly acquired more power in the latter half of the 19th century, and their combined efforts took the visible form of the first feminist movement. Although the movement's primary concerns were to gain access to public life, the emphasis being on education, decent paid employment and suffrage for women, its assault on the prevailing sexual mores was of dual importance: as the English feminists quipped, their main aims were 'votes for women, chastity for men'. Feminists disputed the uncontrollability of the male sexual urge, and firmly advocated self-restraint. This element of the feminist programme can be regarded as a specific variation of the *fin-de-siècle* drive towards civilization, one that, rather than being targeted at the working classes, pursued the sexual education and moral elevation of *men* of all classes. We have no evidence of any increase in male chastity as a result of this campaign, but by adopting this vantage-point women certainly succeeded in giving a new slant to the debate on prostitution and venereal disease, one that had a broad appeal and that helps to explain the sudden increase in the public interest in these matters. The controversy surrounding prostitution was hence in part a logical consequence of women's increased power and of the rise of feminism as a significant factor in social change.

As the process of functional democratization continued, both between social classes and between men and women, people became sensitized to signs of inequality that had previously been taken for granted. In the last decades of the 19th century, social issues became a popular preoccupation. Enlightened middle-class people became shocked about the wretched conditions in which other people lived their lives, and no longer accepted them. As Jan Romein puts it, 'the middle-classes acquired a bad conscience' and started to question their own 'right to exploit others'.[150] At the same time, ideas concerning women's subordinate role in society gradually started to shift ground. These two trends came together in the debate on prostitution. As the great gap in power between social classes and between men and women narrowed, the system of regulation – which was essentially the formalized exploitation of women from the lower classes – came increasingly to be seen, from the 1870s onwards, as unacceptable social injustice, an anomalous relic of the past. The denigrating tone in which the first generation of hygienists – whose concern about social issues far outstripped that of the public at large – spoke of prostitutes in the 1850s did not reappear in the rhetoric of their successors. Pierson expressed the

64

new attitudes when he observed, in response to the regulationists'
view that outside marriage, prostitution was the least harmful means
of satisfying the male sex drive:

> Even were we to accept the truth of the view that prostitution is the
> least dangerous form of gratification, who gives you the right to
> sacrifice some one else to your insatiable desire? Who gives you the
> right to use for this purpose the daughters of the poor, who, for lack
> of education, have none of the vital supports to steady their morality
> and chastity that surround girls of the higher social classes?[151]

One reason for the rapid spread of abolitionist views was their
close alignment to these new sensitivities. Abolitionists were a
good deal more 'modern' than their opponents in this regard, and
they seized every opportunity to highlight the anachronistic nature
of regulation.[152]

The 1880s and 1890s were an era of great change, both in
politics and in society at large. In addition to these, there was a third
area of change, that indirectly affected attitudes to prostitution and
venereal disease. This was the realm of international relations, which
enhanced competition between nations. States indulged to a greater
extent in mutual comparisons, around the turn of the century, in
terms of military capability, economic productivity, colonial
expansion and population growth, and this led in several European
countries to a striking preoccupation with the health of their
population. Many were gripped in particular by fears that
widespread tuberculosis, alcoholism and venereal disease would
result in an overall degeneration of the population. Although, as we
have seen, the Netherlands was not one of the most fearful nations
in this regard, around 1900 it was a Dutch commonplace, inspired
by a general concern about a decline in moral standards and the
nation's inadequate military capability, to say that the country
needed healthy citizens. The resulting concern for new generations
strengthened efforts to oppose infection and what had been dubbed
'germ damage'. Although these efforts in reproductive hygiene were
as yet ill-defined, they did sometimes help determine points of
emphasis in the prostitution debate. This did not necessarily swing
in the abolitionist direction. The views of reproductive hygiene are
somewhat chameleon-like in nature; in France they were indeed
seized upon to strengthen the regulationists' hand. In the turn-of-
the-century climate of opinion in the Netherlands, however,
concern about health and procreation tended to embrace
abolitionism. The threat posed by venereal disease to families and to

posterity added weight to the demand for a ban on brothels. The prostitution debate was thus in part rooted in the concern for the health of future generations. In the early years of the 20th century, this concern intensified, with a campaign starting up to introduce medical examinations for those planning to marry. The history of venereal disease thus crossed the path of semi-eugenic endeavours once again. In this period too, military health care was a particular area of concern, as will become clear in chapter 2.

The developments sketched in this chapter could be schematically summarized in a staged structure. The main axes of change were in political life (rise of the religious parties), functional democratization (emancipation of the working classes and of women) and heightened international rivalry. Against this background, certain campaigns were waged: a largely Christian-based morality campaign, an intensification in the middle-class drive towards 'civilization', the labour movement, the first generation of feminist activism and a broad-based coalition striving to protect the quality and size of the population. Within these movements, certain groups emerged that have been defined here as narrators in the prostitution debate: orthodox Protestants, hygienists, middle-class 'civilizers', labour leaders, feminists, military surgeons and population hygienists. These narrators were found on both sides of the regulationist/abolitionist divide. Though diametrically opposed in their aims, regulationism and abolitionism had grown from a partial overlap of concerns, and hence shared certain basic assumptions: in particular, both believed that prostitution and the related problem of venereal disease were no longer private matters, but issues that were deeply embedded in the sphere of social life and that were highly relevant to political decision-making. Whatever their diverse reasons, for each of the various narrators, prostitution and venereal disease were clearly politically charged issues.[153]

Those who struggled to abolish regulated prostitution, in particular – and the majority, as has become clear, came down on the abolitionist side – saw themselves as waging a political battle. This highlights the different origins of the two sides: many of those who had promoted regulation in its early stages, such as hygienists and military surgeons, wanted prostitution to be controlled, but they were too bound up with the dominant Liberal ethos and the social balance of power of an earlier age to see anything objectionable about *regulated* prostitution. Later generations tended to see regulation itself as the very embodiment of everything they opposed: the sanctioning of indecency and immorality by the

Liberal public authorities, the unmitigated exploitation of the lower classes, and the supremacy of the male sex drive. Regulated prostitution – even more than prostitution in general – was the perfect metaphor for all these evils. This, above, all, explains why such an impassioned campaign was fought in the waning years of the 19th century, by so many people of different persuasions, to consign regulated prostitution to the rubbish-heap of bygone legislation.

Notes

1. A variety of theories have been proposed to explain the sudden appearance of syphilis in Europe in or around 1495. See Rosebury 1971:Chapters III-VIII; Quétel 1986:Chapter II.
2. The first signs of this rupture in the discourse on venereal diseases, and syphilis in particular, have been described for Belgium in Rebmann 1991.
3. The following section draws on several previous studies: Lewandowski & Van Dranen 1933:Chapter VI; Van Slobbe 1937; Stemvers 1981; Huitzing 1983; Kam 1983; Stemvers 1983; Stemvers 1985 and Hekma 1987.
4. Especially in France, the establishments set up for the treatment of infected prostitutes resembled penitentiaries more than hospitals; cf. Corbin 1978. For the care of syphilitic patients during the regulatory period in the Netherlands, see Van Lieburg 1982:166-75.
5. The same development has been noted in other countries. The Netherlands is of course dealt with here. Judith Walkowitz has described the process in England, where the specific military context of the Contagious Diseases Acts lost its significance between the first Act passed in 1864 and the last in 1869; see Walkowitz 1980:71-9.
6. See Stemvers 1981:24.
7. Van Slobbe 1937:43-50; Kam 1983:23-4.
8. Berigten Binnenland, *NTvG* 4 (1860):303-4.
9. Berigten Binnenland, *NTvG* 4 (1860):303. The average figure cited in the memorandum of 2,665 soldiers annually afflicted with venereal disease is equivalent to 12% of garrisoned troops. Cf. G.D.L. Huet, 'Voorloopig verslag door den gecommitteerde tot onderzoek naar de werking der reglementering op de prostitutie hier te lande', *NTvG* 9 (1865):337-56.
10. Article 188 of the Municipalities Act provided that 'the policing of the theatres, inns, public houses and all premises and gatherings that are open to the public, all public amusements and houses of ill repute shall be the responsibility of the Burgomaster. He shall guard against

any activities that conflict with the public order or morality'; see Van Slobbe 1937:64; Kam 1983:146, n. 7.

11. For a more detailed survey of municipalities that regulated prostitution, see Van de Bergh 1879.

12. Cf. Stemvers 1981:5-6.

13. For a brief outline of the Dutch hygienist movement, see Van Daalen 1990 and Houwaart 1991. The following section also draws on Verdoorn 1965, Hekma 1987 and Mol & Van Lieshout 1989.

14. The role of curative medicine and that of the new body of knowledge generated by bacteriology are in general deemed to have played a very limited role in the improvements in public health in the 19th century as discussed in the Introduction; see Verdoorn 1965; McKeown 1976a and 1976b.

15. See Houwaart 1991:362, n. 11.

16. Ali Cohen et al. 1872, II:551-57; this reference is on 553.

17. H.W. Stork, 'Iets over prostitutie', *Geneeskundige Courant* 28 (1874), no. 25.

18. The various authors do not entirely concur as to the number of municipalities that introduced regulation; the average hovers around 35.

19. This topic is discussed in greater detail in Prakken 1948; Stolz & Suurmond (eds.) 1982; and Cassel 1987:Chapter I.

20. See Stolz & Suurmond (eds.) 1982:Chapter X.

21. For a more detailed survey of the history of venereal disease, see A.A. Fokker, 'Geschiedenis der syphilis in de Nederlanden', *NTvG* 4 (1860):419-46. See also 'De syphilis in de Nederlanden', *NTvG* 4 (1860):451-72; Van der Valk 1910; Flegel 1974; Helwegen 1987.

22. Cf. Kam 1983:73.

23. See Cassel 1987:17-18.

24. As early as 1873, Herbert Spencer pointed out the unreliability of observations where the observer's interests are at stake: 'Where personal interests come into play, there must be, even in men intending to be truthful, a great readiness to see the facts which it is convenient to see, and such reluctance to see opposite facts as will prevent much activity in seeking for them. Hence, a large discount has mostly to be made from the evidence furnished by institutions and societies in justification of the policies they pursue or advocate. And since much of the evidence respecting both past and present social phenomena comes to us through agencies calculated thus to pervert it, there is here a further impediment to clear vision of facts.' Spencer goes on to cite the example of people involved in the fight against venereal disease who, carried along by the force of their own convictions, believed the

incidence of venereal disease to be far higher than it actually was: 'while venereal disease has been diminishing in frequency and severity, certain instrumentalists and agencies have created a belief that rigorous measures are required to check its progress'; Spencer 1873:83-84.

25. Some studies were conducted at a later stage, however; e.g. A.P. Fokker, 'Rapport der commissie van onderzoek naar de frequentie van syphilitische en venerische ziekten in de gemeente Groningen', *NTvG* 29 (1893) I:285-95; C.P. Schokking, 'De geslachtziekten te Leiden, in 1912-1930', *NTvG* 74 (1930) IV:6153; J.J. Zoon, 'Het voorkomen van syphilis en gonorrhoe in Utrecht en omgeving sinds 1910', *NTvG* 75 (1931) II:2162.

26. See Stemvers 1981:5, based on Mounier 1889; Stemvers 1985:41. Haustein's army statistics (1927) do not begin for the Dutch army until 1880.

27. Haustein 1927:798, 800. See also Van Deinse 1918; Bottema 1931.

28. See J.R. Prakken, 'Syphilisatie', *NTvG* 114 (1970) I:1019-23.

29. See Voorhoeve 1951.

30. See M. Gutteling, 'Het tegenwoordig standpunt der syphilisbehandeling', *Geneeskundige Bladen* 3 (1896):109-48; 'R.', 'Geregelde behandeling van de syphilis', *Geneeskundige Courant* 59 (1905), no. 10:76-7; R.G.C. Schröder, 'De kwikverbindingen der Ed. IV', *Geneeskundige Courant* 60 (1906), no. 50:405-7 and 61 (1907), no. 1:3-5.

31. Selhorst (1899, p. 80) observed that prostitutes were admitted to hospital only for short periods, until the external symptoms had gone. Cf. also Keuchenius (in Mansholt & Keuchenius 1906:37): in contrast to the prescribed five years of medical supervision, the 'syphilitic prostitute was discharged ... after four months'. Furthermore, Kam's study revealed that many prostitutes with a diagnosed venereal infection simply packed their bags and moved to another town, without undergoing any treatment at all; Kam 1983: Chapter 17.

32. Cf. the regulations, discussed below, that applied to those contemplating marriage.

33. See R.G.C. Schröder, 'De kwikverbindingen der Ed. IV', *Geneeskundige Courant* 60 (1906), no. 50:405.

34. See J.R. Prakken, 'Mercurialisten en antimercurialisten', *NTvG* 116 (1972) I:30-5.

35. Data on the course of untreated syphilis are available, because the Norwegian dermatologist Caesar Boeck refused to give the syphilis patients admitted to his clinic any form of medical treatment. He considered the existing mercury treatment to be worthless, so that

between 1891 and 1910 a group of almost 2,000 untreated patients passed through his clinic. The material relating to this group has since been analysed on several occasions. See Clark & Danbolt 1964, Rosebury 1972. A second study of the consequences of untreated syphilis is known as the Tuskegee Study, and culminated in a national scandal. Between 1932 and 1972, a group of 400 black men with tertiary syphilis in Alabama, U.S.A., were – completely without their knowledge, and in some cases without their even knowing that they had syphilis – left untreated. Yet during this very same period, various remedies, including penicillin, became available. The group regularly underwent medical examinations and received placebos. This experiment caused an uproar when it was made public in 1972, and it was immediately stopped. See also Jones 1981.

36. See Keyser 1976:196.
37. L.C. van Goudoever, 'Een veel besproken onderwerp', *NTvG* 16 (1880):181-92; here:187.
38. See Te Velde 1992:41-9.
39. For these aspects of the hygiene movement, see Houwaart 1991:307-18.
40. Quoted in N.B. Donkersloot, 'Moet de staat het bestaan van openlijke prostitutie erkennen?', *Geneeskundige Courant* 10 (1856), no. 44.
41. A particularly radical variant of this view is elaborated by the German physician Hulsmeyer, whose book was translated into Dutch; see Hulsmeyer 1893. He saw it as the State's responsibility to formally regulate sexual relations outside marriage. 'All human life', he stated boldly, 'relates essentially to these two things – earning money and the enjoyment of sexual intercourse' (109). While the first of these activities was suitably channelled by countless ordinances, rules and acts of parliament, the only action undertaken by the State in the realm of sexual intercourse was the enactment of legislation on marriage that was woefully inadequate. To fill this gap, Hulsmeyer devised a plan for the establishment of communal brothels with detailed regulations for prostitutes and staff as well as for visitors.
42. See e.g. the comments about prostitutes made by the police surgeon D.J. Admiraal, in 'De prostitutie en de burgerlijke overheid; een rapport en nog wat', in *Medisch Weekblad* 3 (1896/97), no. 29:369-76.
43. See N.B. Donkersloot, 'Moet de staat het bestaan van openlijke prostitutie erkennen?', in *Geneeskundige Courant* 10 (1856), no. 44.
44. See Festen 1974:152-9.
45. Carsten, Van der Horst, Huizinga, *NTvG* 15 (1879):321-36, esp. 331-6.

46. Donkersloot, Egeling, Huet, *NTvG* 17 (1881):34-8.
47. Van Overbeek de Meijer, Fokker, Huizinga, *NTvG* 18 (1882):161-8.
48. Kuhn, Godefroi, Guye, *NTvG* 20 (1884):377-82.
49. Stokvis, Guye, *NTvG* 20 (1884):963-4.
50. De Swaan 1988:238-44; 1990:57-71.
51. De Swaan 1990:69.
52. De Swaan 1988:242.
53. Part 3 of the biography of Pierson (Schram 1968) deals with his struggle against regulated prostitution.
54. See Sijmons 1976; Stuurman 1983. Kluit 1970 discusses the Réveil at length.
55. See the pamphlet with that title [i.e. 'Gewettigde Ontucht'] published by Pierson in 1878.
56. See Sijmons 1976:43-7; Noordam 1991:173 notes that the professional groups best represented in the NVP's membership were preachers, theologists, jurists and school-teachers. Those who played an active role within the NVP came from a variety of professions: J.C. van Schermbeek was chief of police, G.J.D. Mounier was a mathematician, O.Q. van Swinderen and A. de Graaf belonged to the legal profession, S.R. Hermanides and P.J. Idenburg were physicians, and J.W. Gunning was a university professor.
57. The relative lack of Catholic involvement at this stage of the struggle against immorality is discussed in Sijmons 1976:35-6, 43-4; Stuurman 1983:218-24.
58. Stuurman 1983:212. De Bie & Fritschy (1985) likewise acknowledge the Protestant Réveil, albeit somewhat hesitantly, as one of the roots of present-day feminism. This conclusion has little to do with the charitable activities that women could perform within this movement, but relates to the critical attitude that prevailed, which helped to sharpen the emerging feminist mind.
59. Klerck-Van Hogendorp 1883-84 II:6. The actual role of the Women's Union in the fight against prostitution was probably a good deal more substantial than the modest references recorded by its spokeswomen suggest. Klerck-Van Hogendorp (1883-84 III:12) wrote, for instance, that the Women's Union would leave the public fight against prostitution, and the taking of whatever measures proved necessary, to the NVP. She continued: 'We wish only to support it [the NVP], and to gain public support for it by presenting women's arguments in a woman's way.' In fact, the Women's Union did get involved in public actions to abolish regulation, and in the early years of the century a conflict arose with the NVP because the women of the Union expressed a desire

to have women appointed to the board of the NVP. Pierson
opposed this idea; he saw the struggle against regulation as one of
men pitted against men. See Schram 1968:202-3. On the activities
of the Women's Union, see also Beelaerts van Blokland-
Kneppelhout & Van Hogendorp 1909.

60. See Sijmons 1976:84.

61. See Dekker 1989:112. On the Midnight Missionaries, see also Schram
1968:223-30; Sijmons 1976:69-72. A first-hand account of their
activities can be found in Van Munster n.d. and Van Munster 1901.

62. Josephine Butler, quoted by Klerck-Van Hogendorp 1883-84 I:10;
see also Jacobs 1924:181-2.

63. Rutgers-Hoitsema; see National Women's Council of the Netherlands
1902:15, 19. For the feminist view of the issue of prostitution, see
also the contribution by Jacobs, *idem*:33-42; Van der Tuuk 1898;
Versluys-Poelman 1902; Jacobs 1902.

64. The special position that women occupied in the abolitionist camp is
discussed in Schwegman 1989b. In her view it was a paradoxical
position characterized by a distance in one sense, and a lack of
distance in another, between the champions of abolition and the
objects of their concern, namely fallen women. In social terms, the
two groups were undoubtedly worlds apart, but at the same time the
reputations of women abolitionists – unlike those of their male
companions in the struggle – could be tarnished and dishonoured,
like those of all women, if they abandoned themselves to passion. In
this respect, the views of sexuality that were raised in the prostitution
debate concerned all women.

65. L.C. van Goudoever, 'Een veel besproken onderwerp', *NTvG* 16
(1880):181-92. More devastating criticism still was provided by two
other supporters of regulation concerning the situation in Rotterdam.
They qualified the system in use there as completely inadequate. See
T. Broes van Dort & F.A. Rietema, 'Het sanitair toezicht op de
prostitutie te Rotterdam', *NTvG* 33 (1897) I:836-8.

66. J. Menno Huizinga, 'Theoretisch of practisch?', *NTvG* 24 (1888)
II:537-9.

67. Chanfleury van Ijsselstein 1889.

68. Cf. the observation made by Dr Aletta Jacobs, the first woman to
gain a degree in medicine (indeed, the first female student) in the
Netherlands: 'The opponents of sanitary supervision consisted at first
only of men – and some few women – who were *not* physicians;
representatives of the medical profession were purely exceptional.
And their objections to this action on the part of the Government
were largely based on legal, religious and ethical grounds. It is easy to

understand, however, that medical practitioners, who at that time believed medical supervision to be in men's interests, were not persuaded by arguments of this kind. Regulation had to be fought on health-related grounds.' See National Women's Council 1902:38. See also Rutgers 1906:348.

69. This particular quotation is from Van Overbeek de Meijer 1883:24.

70.. For a survey of MPs and Ministers who expressed views on the issue of prostitution, see Sijmons 1976: Appendix I.

71. Not to be confused with the lawyer W.H. de Savornin Lohman and medical practitioner E.A. Keuchenius, who also belonged to the abolitionist camp; cf. De Savornin Lohman 1881; Keuchenius, in Mansholt & Keuchenius 1906.

72. Gerritsen 1882.

73. See *Handelingen van het nationaal congres tegen de prostitutie* 1889:129-34; 164-5.

74. *Recht voor Allen* 5 (1883), no. 30. See also: 'Moeten de dochters der arbeiders ten prooi worden aan de wellusten der rijken?', *idem* 7 (1885), no. 43 and 'En de oorzaak van dat alles?', *idem*, no. 49.

75. See G.D.L. Huet, 'Vervolg van het voorloopig verslag', *NTvG* 10 (1866); Mansholt in Mansholt & Keuchenius 1906.

76. De Graaf 1923:281-2.

77. Fokker was professor of hygiene at Groningen University, and Van Overbeek de Meijer's chair was in health sciences, at Utrecht University. Other advocates of regulation were J. van Dooremaal: *NTvG* 15 (1879) I:497-9; *NTvG* 16 (1880) I:49-51; *Nederlandsch Militair Geneeskundig Archief* 7 (1883) 666-85; M.J. Godefroi, 'Getuigen en redden. Open brief aan de Weleerwaarden heer H. Pierson', 1880. In *De Prostitutie-kwestie* I, n.d.; L.C. van Goudoever, 'Een veel besproken onderwerp', *NTvG* 16 (1880) 181-92.

78. Much of this correspondence can be followed in the pages of the monthly journal of the NVP, *Het Maandblad. Getuigen en Redden* (1878-1911). The debate between advocates and opponents of regulation was also conducted in the columns of the *NTvG* and in numerous pamphlets, some of which have been collected in *De Prostitutie-kwestie*, 2 vols., n.d.

79. The Achilles' heel of medical supervision had always been the complete lack of convincing proof of any salutary effects attributable to its introduction. In 1889, the mathematician G.J.D. Mounier, who was on the board of the NVP, put an end to many years of impenetrable juggling and counter-juggling with statistics by using the figures that had been recorded for garrison towns with and without regulation. His statistical analysis of these figures established

that the presence of supervision did not diminish the likelihood of
contracting a venereal infection: see Mounier 1889.

80. S. Mendes da Costa, 'Verslag van het wetenschappelijk gedeelte der
    werkzaamheden over het vereenigingsjaar 1897-1898', *NTvG* 35
    (1899) I:192-6.

81. See Schram 1968:245-52; Sijmons 1976:90.

82. For an overview of the arguments, see Lewandowski & Van Dranen
    1933:Chapter VI; Van Slobbe 1937; De Vreese [1942]; Prakken 1973;
    Schram 1976:171-252; Sijmons 1976:50-5; Hekma 1987:154-6.

83. Rutgers 1914:9.

84. Butler 1913 [1875]:25. We find a similar argument in e.g. Savornin
    Lohman 1881:10-11; The report to the NMG drawn up by Van
    Overbeek de Meijer, A.P. Fokker and Menno Huizinga was evaluated
    in W. van den Bergh, J.W. Gunning, S.R. Hermanides, H. Pierson
    and O.Q. van Swinderen 1882. In *De Prostitutie-kwestie*, 2 vols.,
    n.d.:36-8 (Gunning), 68-70 (Pierson); Jacobs 1902:72-3.

85. Fournier's theories were eventually confirmed in 1913 by the
    Japanese microbiologist Noguchi.

86. There is an interesting discussion of the development of the
    Wassermann test, from the vantage-point of the sociology of science,
    in Fleck 1981 [1935].

87. See G.T. Haneveld, 'Bij het eeuwfeest van de gonokok: het belang
    van zijn ontdekking en de ontvangst daarvan in Nederland', *NTvG*
    123 (1979) II:1875-8.

88. Wain reports that this discovery gained acceptance only very
    gradually (1970:349). Shame and ignorance combined to retard the
    universal application of Credé's discovery.

89. Keuchenius in Mansholt & Keuchenius 1906:28. For a discussion of
    contagion médiate, also called *médiate contagion*, see Hermanides
    1883:38-41; Rutgers 1906:348.

90. *Rapport van de commissie tot onderzoek naar den omvang en den aard
    der hier bestaande prostitutie* 1897, Memorandum by Blooker:102.

91. Many writers have remarked on this: in addition to Temkin [1977]
    the subject is also discussed in Corbin 1981 and Nye 1984:158 ff.

92. See Rénon [1904]. See also Van den Belt 1988.

93. Ernst de Vries, 'Syphilis in het zwakzinnigengesticht "Voorgeest"',
    Geneeskundige Bladen 20 (1918):73-102 (this ref.:76).

94. Velle 1987:340. See also Corbin [1978]; Nye 1984; Quétel 1986.

95. Corbin 1981:146.

96. Jacobs: see *Nationale Vrouwenraad* 1902:35.

97. Fournier [1880]:231. This quotation has been translated from the
    Dutch translation of Fournier's book *Syphilis et Mariage* (*Syphilis en*

Huwelijk), published in 1905.

98. Brieux [1901]:159.
99. Westland 1915:21. The play was performed in Brussels and Liège, however, soon after publication.
100. See Westland 1915:71.
101. Ibsen [1881].
102. Quoted in Clurman [1977]:1; see also 118-26.
103. See Vergeer 1990:87-8.
104. The 31 illustrations, advertised in fine lettering on the cover, were included in Galtier-Boissière [1906]. Among present-day writers, Van Ussel [1968] devotes most attention to the fanatical hyperbole that characterized the fight against venereal disease in the Western Europe of the late 19th century. He places it on a par with the excesses of anti-masturbationists in the 18th and 19th centuries. 'In both cases we find the same pathological features, such as the exaggeration of the seriousness of the situation, moralistic and sadistic elements of treatment motivated by an aversion to sexual pleasure etc.' (308).
105. Kern 1975:42; Corbin 1981. Van Ussel [1968:308] uses the term 'syphilophobia' in a different sense. It is his term for the pathological features of the late 19th-century war on syphilis.
106. Adler 1924:108, 114. For present-day manifestations of phobic complaints of this kind, see Jeannette Kok & Ad Beckeringh, 'Venereofobie: overmatige angst voor geslachtsziekten', *SOA* 5 (1984), no. 1:4-5; G.F. Koerselman, 'Geslachtsziekten-hypochondrie', *SOA* 5 (1984), no.3:2-5.
107. G.C. Nijhoff, 'Het huwelijk van den gonorrhoïcus', *Geneeskundige Bladen* 1 (1894):227-46 (this ref.:242).
108. *idem*:243.
109. *idem*:244.
110. *idem*:244.
111. See e.g. the pro-regulationist arguments of Schultetus Aeneae (1889), who exploited the theme of the innocent victim effectively; [A.] P. Fokker, 'Rapport der commissie van onderzoek naar de frequentie van syphilitische en venerische ziekten in de gemeente Groningen', *NTvG* 29 (1893) I:285-95, in which he stresses the dangers threatening the middle classes; and Mansholt (in Mansholt & Keuchenius 1906) on the health of future generations.
112. Pierson, Opening address; see *Handelingen van het nationaal congres tegen de prostitutie* 1889:16-20.
113. See *Rapport van de commissie tot onderzoek*, 1897.
114. Voûte's report was originally confidential, but his findings leaked out all the same. They are referred to in the *NTvG*: 'Prostitutie-rapport

aan den Gemeenteraad te Amsterdam', *NTvG* 33 (1897) I:276.

115. *Rapport van de commissie tot onderzoek* 1897, report by Voûte:21.

116. See Van Slobbe 1937:90-8.

117. See Van Slobbe 1937:56.

118. Keuchenius, in Mansholt & Keuchenius 1906:34-5. For the link between prostitution and perversions, see the paper that Voûte presented to the anti-prostitution conference: 'De prostitutie en de tegennatuurlijke geslachtsbevrediging', in *Handelingen van het nationaal congres tegen de prostitutie* 1889:44-7.

119. G.J.E. Ruijsch, 'Prophylaxie tegen syphilis', *Tijdschrift voor Sociale Hygiene* 10 (1908):118-24, this ref. 118. See also P.A. de Wilde, 'Eenige beschouwingen over Syphilis, in verband met levensverzekering', *Geneeskundige Courant* 61 (1907) 1:1-3.

120. The only research that could perhaps be cited in support was Fokker's study in the city of Groningen. Cf. [A.] P. Fokker, 'Rapport der commissie van onderzoek naar de frequentie van syphilitische en venerische ziekten in de gemeente Groningen', *NTvG* 29 (1893) I:289-95. Almost all the cases collected by the committee involved middle-class subjects.

121. Mansholt, in Mansholt & Keuchenius 1906:2. See also Van Overbeek de Meijer, who endorsed the statement of the German medical practitioner W.O. Focke that 'no means of satisfying the (ungovernable!) sexual urge outside marriage [is] less harmful than prostitution'. In the view of Van Overbeek de Meijer, repressing prostitution would serve merely to 'expand the filthy cesspool in which – in addition to those with venereal disease – mutual masturbators, pederasts, sapphists etc. seek each other out'. See 'Geneeskundig toezicht op de prostitutie', *NTvG* 25 (1889) I:60-3.

122. Jacobs 1902:71-2.

123. Cf. the second Brussels conference, 1-6 September 1902: *Het Maandblad. Getuigen en Redden* 24 (1902) no. 10; Schram 1968:222. The motion read: 'That the most important and most effective means of preventing the spread of venereal diseases consists of publicizing to the fullest extent the dangers and effects of these diseases. Male youths in particular must be taught that chastity and abstinence are not only unharmful but that from a medical point of view these virtues are highly to be recommended.'

124. See Corbin [1978]:333; Velle 1987:339.

125. See Pierson, 'Tweeërlei zedewet?', 1889, in *De Prostitutie-kwestie* 2, n.d.

126. Versluys-Poelman 1902:42-3.

127. Klerck-Van Hogendorp, Introduction; see *Nationale Vrouwenraad van Nederland*:2. See also Mansholt (in Mansholt & Keuchenius

1906:13) who defends his pro-supervision stand in the pamphlet published in 1906, in the series *Pro en Contra*, and complains that 'the opponents of regulation are triumphing on virtually every front; it is becoming almost indecent – at least, it is not modern – to still find that it has a useful role to play'.

128. See *Rapport van de commissie tot onderzoek* 1897:99. That the introduction of regulated prostitution influenced the number of syphilis infections negatively rather than positively could also be inferred, for instance, from Huet's reports: G.D.L. Huet, 'Voorloopig verslag door den gecommitteerde tot onderzoek naar de werking der reglementen op de prostitutie hier te lande', *NTvG* 9 (1865) 337-56; Huet, 'Vervolg van het voorloopig verslag', *NTvG* 10 (1866) 315-32. Huet had great difficulty accounting for these findings.

129. Corbin [1978]:172-3. For a discussion of this phenomenon in the Netherlands, see e.g. L.C. van Goudoever, 'Een veel besproken onderwerp', *NTvG* 16 (1880) 188; *Rapport van de commissie tot onderzoek* 1897, Blooker Memorandum:100; Rutgers 1906:344; *Rapport der commissie tot onderzoek* 1911:1736. See also Stemvers, 1985:67-72.

130. Corbin [1978]:287-91.

131. Corbin [1978]:291-6.

132. See Corbin [1978]:249: 'All these new behavioural patterns in prostitution mean that *the prostitute gives her client the impression that she is allowing herself to be seduced* rather than being a mere creature without the freedom to refuse'.

133. See Stemvers 1985:69-72.

134. The 1897 Amsterdam prostitution committee report recorded that the 19 brothels that were registered with the police employed 11 Dutch women and 99 foreign women.

135. Huitzing 1983:25-6; for developments in Dutch night-life, see also Vergeer 1990.

136. See Huitzing 1981:239.

137. See Van Poppel 1993.

138. *Rapport der commissie tot onderzoek* 1911:1736.

139. See Corbin [1978]:386-405.

140. For the 1850 figures on infections, see Stemvers 1981:5; for the later period see Haustein 1927:702-3. The decline in incidence discussed here is somewhat exaggerated by the fact that after 1850 recurrences of the disease in an individual were no longer included in the statistics.

141. See Stuurman 1983:Chapter V.

142. This issue is dealt with at greater length in Te Velde 1992. In the realm of social policies, too, Liberals and religious parties sometimes

found themselves unexpectedly in agreement. De Rooy illustrates this in relation to the legislation on children that was enacted in 1901. See De Rooy 1992:53-6.

143. For this interpretation, see Stemvers 1985:78 ff.; Hekma 1987; Stuurman 1983. For similar trends outside the Netherlands, see Pivar 1973; Weeks 1981.

144. See Elias [1970]:75-6.

145. Brugmans [1925]:Chapters IV-V; Festen 1974:36-37.

146. See Houwaart 1991:324-5.

147. For these changes in workers' lives, which were in part imposed by middle-class measures and in part the consequence of a mode of rivalry between different groups of workers, see De Regt [1984].

148. Evans 1977:28-32. Evans also sees feminism as having had certain religious roots, in Protestantism, and as having derived political and ideological roots from 19th-century Liberalism.

149. See Blok et al. 1978:20; Stuurman 1983:211; De Bie & Fritschy 1985:38.

150. Romein 1967:281.

151. Pierson, 'Tweeërlei zedewet?' 1889:10, in *De Prostitutie-kwestie* 2, n.d.

152. They preferred, for instance, to speak of 'medical examinations' instead of 'sanitary supervision', because 'we prefer to call something by its proper name, instead of concealing its defilement and disgrace beneath a label with extremely doctrinaire, linguistic, and even aesthetic overtones'. See 'Aphorismen tot aanbeveling van de Nederlandsche Vereeniging tegen de Prostitutie', 1883:17, in *De Prostitutie-kwestie* 2, n.d.

153. Other issues became similarly politicized around the turn of the century, e.g. reproduction (cf. the resistance to the doctrine of neo-Malthusianism and the rise of eugenics), alcoholism and paternity research. On this latter subject, see Sevenhuijsen 1987.

2

Two Separate Debates (1900–1930)

When the regulationist project withered around the turn of the century, there was no obvious alternative to take its place. In 1908 the Dutch medical association, the NMG, appointed the last in a string of committees mandated to propose new ways of tackling venereal disease. Every previous committee had failed to unite the ranks of the profession; each report in turn had merely fanned the flames of discord. But times had changed, and the bulky report that appeared in 1911 was warmly welcomed on all sides.[1] Its success cannot be attributed, however, either to any incisiveness of argumentation or to a sudden spirit of concord in the medical establishment. Part of the explanation lay in the fact that the prostitution issue had already been resolved; the report was able to refer dismissively to the 'old system of regulation' without arousing protest. For the rest, the report probed such a broad range of possibilities – sex education campaigns, personal precautions, measures to curb prostitution, medical treatment and statutory regulations, encompassing minority and majority views alike – that everyone found in it what he or she was looking for.

The committee set out systematically – though not to any great extent programmatically – ways of filling the gap left by the failure of regulation. This gap was most noticeable in the realm of medical treatment. Moreover, the long prostitution debate had increased awareness so that more people than ever were classed as needing treatment: with the recognition of innocent victims came an obligation to help them.

Every bit as urgent as the question of how sufferers should be treated was deciding who should bear responsibility for implementing the new measures. This question too was in effect raised by the demise of regulation. After all, if the fight against venereal disease was no longer synonymous with medical supervision, the long unchallenged reign of the medical profession over this territory was renegotiable.

Medical treatment

The medical treatment of VD sufferers attracted an increasing amount of attention at the beginning of the new century. With regulation moribund, the need to expand available modes of treatment was one of the few things about which regulationists and abolitionists could agree.[2] Many physicians were already focusing on ways of improving medical provisions before the old system was finally abolished. Besides the need for expansion, facilities had to be made easily accessible to everyone who needed them. Such accessibility was far from guaranteed under the existing provisions. On top of the financial problems – the bodies administering public health funds often refused to cover the costs of treatment and sickness allowance in the case of venereal disease – there were the additional barriers erected by shame and ignorance. Some medical practitioners campaigned against the contempt and moral condemnation that was generally meted out to sufferers of venereal disease. While conceding that syphilis and gonorrhoea could not be called entirely 'normal' diseases, the NMG committee's report pointed out that these infections were often contracted through no fault of the patient, so that continuing to associate them with vice and prostitution was unjust:

> The view that debauchery and excess are to blame must go; instead, the public must be made to understand that syphilis is caused by an infectant that can be contracted at any time, and in any place. Once this becomes known, the person infected with syphilis will be judged less harshly by the people, who will have no grounds for regarding him as morally inferior.[3]

The report urged that every person afflicted with venereal disease, rich or poor, male or female, should seek medical attention as soon as possible, and that it must be made easier to do so. Ultimately this would benefit society as a whole as well as the individuals concerned. In Rotterdam, the 1903 prohibition of brothels was followed almost immediately by the establishment of the Netherlands' first municipal VD clinic, providing treatment free of charge.[4] Before this, the only comparable facilities had been parts of the dermatology wards of certain teaching hospitals. Other towns soon followed suit, and by 1917 there were forty-five functioning clinics, over half of which were in the three major cities of Amsterdam, Rotterdam and The Hague. By 1925, their numbers had increased to sixty-eight.[5]

The debate that accompanied this change of direction in the fight against venereal disease highlighted a hitherto neglected aspect of venereal disease – the shame felt by the characters. In the past, the narrators' preoccupations had scarcely left room for such feelings to be taken into consideration. Regulationists had in fact seen the lack of any sense of shame as one of the chief character traits of the protagonist – the prostitute – while the characters in the abolitionists' tragedies ultimately remained fairly bloodless, allegorical constructions, whose emotional lives were presented in highly artificial and theoretical terms. Besides, this genre was dominated by emotions of a very different kind – the disgust and indignation of the narrators themselves.

In the early 20th century, patients' feelings of shame also made their first appearance as a practical problem, as an obstacle to seeking proper medical attention. Anti-venereal disease activists had to address this problem. As well as the continued efforts to destigmatize these infections, there was a fresh interest in making the new clinics less clearly identifiable as such and in exercising greater discretion when naming them. In a questionnaire that the NMG conducted among its members in 1911, inspired by the report, all the branches approached favoured comprehensive medical treatment of venereal disease. One branch, however, was against the establishment of special clinics, because 'it fears that the clinic's patients may be seen going in: "Fama ruit [rumours spread fast]."' Another branch expressed the same fears, and recommended that 'such clinics not be too clearly labeled as such'.[6]

Fear of a loss of social status loomed large among patients' concerns. Although the clinics were in principle open to all, in practice only a small group – the poorest – used them. Dr Muller, who worked at one such establishment, suggested that the overwhelming preponderance of poor people at the clinics was simply due to the disproportionate number of sufferers in this section of the population, but he did not supply any evidence to back this up.[7] A more plausible explanation is that those who could afford it preferred to consult their general practitioner or a private dermatologist, rather than mixing with the 'common' people of the clinics. The clinics' *modus operandi* and cramped conditions probably acted as a deterrent to anyone who could afford to go elsewhere: time and discretion were in short supply. 'At every clinic, the rule is to admit patients in groups; one patient is examined while another is still getting dressed and two more are undressing for their turn', wrote Dr Van der Hoog. Practices of this kind, he continued, would particularly deter those who did not belong to the poorest sections of society, but for whom free treatment at the clinic would have been a great boon:

> And here again, it is the large group of the less well-off middle classes that are worst affected by this. The workers do not feel these indignities to the same extent, they can more easily shrug them off, but the lower middle classes, the teacher, the minor official, the small merchant, are too sensitive for that. Therefore we see everywhere that clinics for venereal disease are visited only by the poorest members of society.[8]

For the 'lower middle classes', the financial benefit of free treatment was evidently outweighed by the disgrace of having to jostle with the impoverished people in the waiting-room or surgery of the clinic. They shunned the clinics not so much because of a difference in income – which may not in fact have been so great – but because of a subtle though essential distinction in social status. People who had fought their way up from the lowest rungs of the social ladder did their utmost, precisely by observing middle-class values such as cleanliness, frugality, domesticity and self-control, to distinguish themselves from those less attached to these values. For them, a venereal infection held out the dire prospect of social degradation. This particular type of disease was all the more shameful because it was not easily reconcilable with the virtues they had embraced. By steering clear of the free facilities the damage could be somewhat limited and a desirable social distance preserved from the clinic's motley crowd.

Some anti-venereal disease campaigners understood the great significance of a financial contribution, and advocated the establishment of other clinics, alongside the free facilities, that would charge a fee. Private treatment was extremely expensive, but 'does that mean that treatment ought to be available to everyone free of charge?' demanded Dr Veldhuijzen of Amsterdam rhetorically.

> Not a bit of it. A few free clinics will doubtless be needed in the large cities, but apart from this, experience has amply demonstrated that anyone suffering from venereal disease who has been informed about the seriousness of this condition will be inclined to seek

treatment and will be willing to pay a reasonable price for it. Indeed, many would be loath to mingle with the riff-raff that turns up at the free clinics. This applies doubly where women are concerned. Furthermore, we know from experience that many people are less appreciative of treatment that is given free of charge than of that for which they have paid.[9]

Between the old days of the prostitution debate and these discussions on financial contributions, the treatment of syphilis – gonorrhoea was still generally treated with disinfecting irrigations – had been transformed. The period 1910–1930 saw several major advances, the most spectacular of which being the discovery made by the German chemotherapist Paul Ehrlich. After an almost endless series of experiments, Ehrlich and his colleague Sahachiro Hata finally found a drug with a specific action against syphilis. This compound, first found to be effective in human subjects in 1909, was the 606th preparation that the indefatigable team had tried out, and for some time it was known as 'Ehrlich–Hata 606', or simply '606'. When released for general use in late 1910 it was named arsphenamine, and marketed under the trade name of Salvarsan. This remarkable new arsenic compound acted rapidly and dramatically upon syphilitic skin conditions and swiftly reduced the number of spirochetes in the patient's blood. These astonishing results fuelled hopes that Salvarsan would be the 'magic bullet' that would kill *Treponema pallidum*, the spirochete that causes syphilis, without damaging the body's cells. The popular press hailed the new compound as a revolutionary discovery in the treatment of syphilis.[10] In contrast to this enthusiasm, the Dutch medical establishment was initially sceptical of the new drug. The medical journals gave it a cool reception, with practitioners proving reluctant to abandon their traditional mercury and potassium iodide treatment.[11] Against some syphilitic disorders – in particular the neurological variants – Salvarsan appeared relatively ineffectual, and some neurologists even maintained that it exacerbated the symptoms of these maladies.[12]

Salvarsan indeed proved to be far from harmless. Its basic constituent, after all, was the deadly poison arsenic, and any error in application or allergic reaction could easily have dramatic results. When it was first introduced, several serious accidents occurred, and adverse side-effects ranging from nausea and shortness of breath to muscular cramp and severe damage to liver and kidneys were not uncommon. For some few patients, a course of Salvarsan actually proved fatal. In 1912, Ehrlich produced an updated version, 914 or 'neo-Salvarsan', that was slightly less effective but far less toxic. Salvarsan (the 'neo' was soon dropped again) gradually conquered the reservations of the medical establishment to become the main anti-syphilitic drug, although some doctors continued to combine it with a traditional mercury treatment. From our present-day vantage-point, Salvarsan was the first anti-syphilitic of proven effectiveness. It acts against the disease extremely fast, reducing it to a level at which it is no longer infectious. Whether Salvarsan can effect a complete cure, however, is still a matter of controversy.[13]

That it took so long for medical practitioners to accept Salvarsan was undoubtedly related to the compound's initial anti-climactic results after Ehrlich had vaunted its qualities as a wonder drug; neo-Salvarsan had even been called 'Hy' for a while, which was short for 'hyper-ideal'. Inevitably, this raised hopes that were quickly dashed in medical practice: one dose, it appeared, was never enough, on some variants of the disease the preparation had almost no effect, and errors in application could have damaging consequences. In this light, the somewhat disappointed tone of the international medical community's initial experience with the new drug, reported at length in the Dutch press, is understandable. Moreover, to those who stood by the beneficial effects of mercury, Salvarsan was regarded more in the light of a welcome addition than a radical departure in syphilis treatment. Added to this was probably a degree of plain conservatism. Whatever its merits as an improved mode of treatment, the new drug also made new demands on medical practitioners. The constituent arsenic was toxic, so that dosages had to be calculated and measured out with unusual precision, and careful records had to be kept of the doses already administered in each course of treatment. Furthermore, Salvarsan was one of the first drugs that had to be injected intravenously, a procedure with which most doctors had virtually no experience. Patients on the receiving end of a bungled intravenous injection of Salvarsan would have a painful swelling that could persist for several days.[14]

One final reason sometimes given for the medical profession's grudging acceptance of the new drug was that certain doctors feared the threat to their livelihood. As one observer commented in 1910, after German doctors had objected to the introduction of Salvarsan:

> It will be a blow to doctors and their assistants, institutions, indeed
> entire health resorts that have up to now lived on and profited from
> the chronic condition of the unfortunate syphilitics. In their circles,

the seeds of suspicion are being sown concerning the new drug, and a mood of hostility prevails. ... Reliable sources have it that 'in some cities there are even entire groups of doctors whose suspicion of the new treatment, ostensibly on principle, cannot be explained in any other way'.[15]

Objections of this kind may perhaps have played a minor role, but this should not be exaggerated. It is illogical to suppose that 'entire groups of doctors' would have upheld for any length of time a position that would have sent patients scurrying to their rivals.

In contrast to the hype that had surrounded the advent of Salvarsan, suggesting that a single dose would work a cure, a course of treatment generally lasted frustratingly long, but even so, results came far more rapidly than with the traditional mercury method. One or more Salvarsan injections could often produce a considerable improvement. But this was far from the end of the story: to banish the disease altogether, another course of treatment would sometimes be needed, and in any case a long period of medical supervision was essential. It would be two or three years before a patient could be pronounced definitely cured, so that even in the best cases, Salvarsan could only reduce the period during which marriage was forbidden from five years to three.[16] The new drug therefore brought only a limited improvement, and introduced several new problems. As the injections generally eliminated the unpleasant symptoms of the disease quite quickly, it was not always easy to persuade patients to complete a course of treatment that was both painful and expensive.

The 1920s witnessed several new advances in treatment. Firstly, in 1921 the element bismuth, which shares certain properties with arsenic, was found to have a curative effect, especially on the later stages of syphilis. With the advent of bismuth, the old mercury and potassium iodide method finally became obsolete. Around the same time, the 'malaria treatment' was introduced. The Viennese psychiatrist Julius Wagner von Jauregg had discovered as far back as 1890 that a patient suffering from *dementia paralytica* had rallied strikingly, though temporarily, after a bout of typhoid fever. After a long series of experiments in which patients were deliberately infected with tuberculin and later with malaria, this therapy was introduced into medical practice in the early 1920s. It was used chiefly to combat neurosyphilitic disorders such as *dementia paralytica*, which were still common in the first few decades of this century.[17] A syphilis patient would be injected with a small amount of blood taken from a malaria sufferer, and after eight to ten attacks of fever, quinine would be given to suppress the malaria. To increase the likelihood of a complete cure, Salvarsan was also administered after every attack of fever.[18] The results of this treatment ultimately justified the considerable ordeal it involved for the patient: 'Persistent vomiting, not infrequently continuing during the periods without fever, unbearable headache, sometimes symptoms of collapse and substantial weight loss indicate the seriousness of the disease introduced. The heart should be monitored closely and supported in its struggle with tonics',[19] wrote a physician concerning this treatment, which he had administered to a patient. In 1927, Wagner von Jauregg received the Nobel prize for his contribution to the treatment of syphilis.

It is time to consider the impact of these innovations – Salvarsan in particular – on the incidence of syphilis in the Netherlands. What figures we have suggest a slight drop in incidence after 1912, but this trend was completely reversed by the First World War. After 1920 there was another conspicuous decline, which persisted for some considerable time. The drop in patient numbers that various dermatology clinics recorded after 1912 had been generally attributed to the impact of Salvarsan treatment, but the increase around the First World War tempered this optimistic view.[20] So when it came to making a retrospective interpretation of the second decline, in the 1920s, there was far less agreement. The sanguine hopes that had accompanied the first results of the new drug, at any rate, were no longer thought justified:

> people were quick to attribute a drop in the incidence of syphilis to
> the general availability of arsphenamines, but a variety of other
> possibilities present themselves, and the fact that the gonorrhoea
> and syphilis curves follow a roughly parallel course strongly
> militates against treatment having been the dominant influence.[21]

The availability of better treatment probably did affect the incidence of syphilis, but Ehrlich's discovery was far from the watershed hailed by lyrically-minded journalists when it was first made public. Moreover, Salvarsan had no effect whatsoever on syphilis mortality rates.[22] The following comment – by no means exceptional – was made by a doctor in 1917, five years after the introduction of Salvarsan: 'The suffering that results from syphilis is all too often appalling. It destroys many a person's happiness and health, ruins lives and obliterates futures.'[23]

Warriors in the fight against venereal disease

Another issue that raised its head around 1900 was that of who was best qualified to tackle the problem of venereal disease. As already noted, the collapse of regulation meant that supreme medical authority in this area could no longer be taken for granted. Although medical practitioners were at no point in danger of being pushed aside, their dominant role had nevertheless been somewhat diluted. The last NMG committee, for instance – the one appointed in 1908 – was also the first to include members from outside the profession.[24] Deciding where responsibility would lie for the revised approach to venereal disease was a vexed question, as is clear from the committee's mixed response to the idea of a separate anti-venereal disease society being set up. Societies of this kind already existed in Germany, France and the United States, and the committee cautiously favoured the founding of one in the Netherlands. But it had definite reservations:

> The most obvious danger is that, if local branches were founded consisting largely of laypersons, they would feel the need to be 'active' and do all kinds of things that would have only a remote bearing on disease control and would be far more likely to foster an unhealthy interest in sexual matters. Lectures on prostitution in the middle ages or exhibitions of venereal diseases are all things that the committee cannot condemn harshly enough, believing that if they have any effect at all, it is more likely to be adverse than favourable. Nevertheless, the committee does not view these objections as so compelling that it feels obliged to advise against the establishment of such a society. It is of the opinion that, provided it were set up soundly from the outset and were to consist of more medical practitioners and persons directly involved in disease control than interested laypersons, the aforementioned dangers may be averted.[25]

This muted recommendation was issued by the NMG committee in 1911, and it was three years before the Dutch Anti-Venereal Disease Society was finally founded. Perusing its membership will identify the groups that – alongside the medics – became influential in the fight against venereal disease. First, however, a brief explanation is needed of this three-year delay.

The delay was caused mainly by a new dispute that had arisen, with the dust stirred up by the debate on regulated prostitution scarcely settled on the ground, concerning one of the potential weapons to be deployed. This new controversy centred on the advertisement and use of a variety of prophylactics – to be discussed at length below – that were designed to prevent venereal disease from being passed on. The NMG committee too had been divided on this issue, with a small majority favouring the admissibility of these remedies while several members remained firmly opposed on grounds of principle. During the formatory period of the Anti-Venereal Disease Society, prophylactics proved to be a divisive issue once again. It was generally agreed that the board of the Society should contain a variety of views, not only ranging from medics to experts from other walks of life, but also including people for and against prophylactics. Indeed, 'the society [was] established with the express aim of organizing the campaign against venereal disease by ensuring cooperation between people with greatly differing views concerning the nature of the measures that should be taken'.[26] Under these conditions, it proved anything but simple to find someone who would be willing to lead the new society.

The man who eventually agreed to take on this daunting task was the lawyer Andrew de Graaf, who was already well known as the Chairman of the National Committee against Trade in Women and as someone committed to the fight against prostitution and against immorality in many areas of life. De Graaf's agreement was conditional, however: he insisted that the new committee should contain eminent specialists in dermatology and venereal disease and that its statutes should eschew all references to propaganda on behalf of either regulated prostitution or prophylactics. Any recommendation directed towards either type of propaganda would cause De Graaf and his associates to resign on the spot.[27] After some time it proved possible to compose a board that met both conditions. The advocates of prophylactics agreed to the adoption of statutes in which the Society's objective was defined only in general terms as the combating of venereal disease, and which included only formal provisions on matters such as the holding of meetings, the issuing of recommendations and the distribution of publications. De Graaf was never compelled to put his threat of resignation into practice; under his leadership, the Society at no time erred by either encouraging immorality (by encouraging open propaganda for prophylactics) or advocating its legal sanctioning (by a return to regulated prostitution).

These careful preparations produced a new, workable and enduring coalition between medical practitioners and one specific section of the abolitionist victors: the Protestant activists. Of the various groups that had joined to form the abolitionist front, this was the sector that had best succeeded in finding some common ground with the medics. The two groups were in fact so well attuned to each other that not a single note of discord was sounded in the Society's early life. The executive board was dominated by Protestants, and half of its members came from the medical profession: Professor T.M. van Leeuwen, Dr D. Snoeck Henkemans and W.F. Veldhuyzen. The remaining members were H.A.M. van Asch van Wijck, A. de Graaf and G. Velthuysen Jr. It was Van Leeuwen who best embodied the marriage of medicine with religion. He was both professor of dermatology at the University of Utrecht and a devout Christian, and was able to combine these two dimensions of his life impeccably as the Society's secretary. To him, venereal disease was an issue that had to be tackled at the level of morality at least as much as at the level of health, if not more so. He and De Graaf – a lawyer, abolitionist and rescuer of lost souls who openly avowed his religious aversion to the 'one-sided tyranny of medicine' – determined the face of the Society well into the 1940s.[28]

During the establishment of the Society, discussions revolved largely about the issues with which it would *not* concern itself. This raises the question of what it did do. During the first few years of its existence, the Society was particularly active in organizing lectures, distributing informative leaflets, improving medical training and, most importantly of all, building up a system of advice centres.[29] During the 1920s a system of this kind grew up alongside the existing outpatient clinics. The Hague opened the first centre in 1919, and several other cities – starting with Amsterdam, Utrecht and Haarlem – followed suit. The prime responsibility of these centres was to provide advice; although they performed medical examinations, patients were referred to their GPs, dermatologists or clinics for treatment. The centres were well placed to play a mediating role: where difficulties arose between doctor and patient they would intervene, and where necessary they would urge patients to complete the course of treatment. They also lent such tangible support as was needed in these cases, sometimes paying travel expenses or medical bills.[30] Conversely, GPs and dermatologists were supposed to send patients to the centres for the non-medical aspects of treatment. Only in a handful of university towns was the advice centre attached to a dermatology clinic, with the various tasks being performed in the same organization.

The muddled organizational structure found in most of the country, with a division of responsibilities between advice, mediation and social work on the one hand and medical treatment on the other, irritated all those concerned. Advice-centres, at which a dermatologist made diagnoses and gave advice with the support of a nurse-cum-social worker, often resented their forced dependence on the cooperation of the physicians treating the patients. Conversely, the physicians were irritated by what they viewed as unfair competition, as their own patients were receiving advice at the centres without their knowledge. Indeed, physicians feared that their patients were on occasion even receiving treatment there. In some cases these fears were quite justified: certain advice-centre doctors were also practising physicians, and hence could refer patients to their own surgeries. Understandably, relations between advice centres and practising physicians were decidedly frosty. Staff at advice centres often complained about the lack of cooperation they received from practising physicians, which hampered their work. Advocates of advice centres – and their staff – therefore tried to emphasize the unacceptability of unprofessional tactics such as exploiting the centres to bolster individual practices.

The fight against venereal disease thus gradually took on a different form after the final abandonment of the regulation project. The year 1911 witnessed the statutory abolition of regulated prostitution and the almost simultaneous appearance of outpatient clinics, new and fairly successful modes of treatment and the establishment of an anti-venereal disease society. In the meantime, the high-pitched public consternation of the 1890s had largely subsided. Nevertheless, this period too had its debates, centring on two more or less distinct 'circuits' of venereal infection – domestic life on the one hand and the world of soldiers and sailors on the other. These two circuits involved different characters; understandably enough they were discussed by different narrators who had different remedies to propose.

In general, the concerns voiced were not dissimilar to those of the 19th century, and the prostitute, while receding somewhat into the background, was still seen as the ultimate source of infection. The victims of prostitution were the central figures in both scenarios. So while the 'wheel' model of epidemiology was still adhered to at the beginning of the 20th century, the narrators' attention was starting to move along the various spokes of the wheel, rather than remaining fixated on the hub.

The family

When venereal disease came up for discussion in well-informed circles, attention soon centred on the family, which was deemed to be under threat from marital and congenital infection alike. As far as the incidence of venereal disease passed on between married partners is concerned, we can be brief: nothing at all is known about it. Afflicted children, however, are somewhat easier to trace in the statistics. Between 1901 and 1920, almost 2% of all still-births were the result of syphilis. In major cities this figure was a good deal higher; between 1910 and 1914 it was as high as 6%. In absolute figures, out of every 10 000 newborns in the major cities in the period 1901–1920, 19 died of syphilis.[31] The available information does not allow us to translate into figures the wretchedness of the children that survived – with ailments ranging from gonorrhoeal blindness to syphilitic slow-wittedness – but it suggests that this was still a common problem at the beginning of the 20th century.[32] Over the next few decades, however, as treatment improved and the incidence of venereal disease started to fall, it is probable that the number of congenital afflictions gradually decreased.[33]

Despite this downward trend, the suffering inflicted on families as a result of venereal disease still commanded a good deal of attention in the first few decades of the century. We can find this concern reflected in literary references. In *Vergelding* (*Retribution*, 1906) for instance, a story written by Pieter van der Meer, the protagonist makes a dreadful discovery: 'the day after he had written Jeanne the love-letter, asking her in tender words if she would consent to be his wife, [he noticed] the first signs of infection on his body of the dreadful disease that ravages mankind, the scourge inflicted by a wrathful God'.[34] Having long led a dark existence in which much was sordid, he has now mended his ways, partly through the attentions of his bride. Intoxicated by alcohol and evil influences, however, he has had one final relapse into thoughtlessness, which will haunt him for the rest of his days. Himself a doctor, he is only too aware of the obdurate nature of the disease and the poor prospects of full recovery. Nevertheless he decides – without informing his bride of his condition – to go through with the marriage, but never to touch his wife until confident that he is completely cured. From the first day of their marriage, this stifling knowledge transforms their former carefree intimacy into a 'strange and terrible life together' and eventually into a veritable hell. Consumed by 'fiendish desires', the protagonist is appalled, feeling 'his determination slipping away, his power to resist diminishing, and more and more often tempestuous desires overpowering him and depriving him of his will-power'.[35] He sees only one way out of this hopeless situation: with a bullet through his temple he puts an end to his suffering.

The writer Cora Westland deals with a similar story in her novel *Levenswond* (*Fatal Injury*, 1913), which she dedicated to the playwright Brieux. Again, the protagonist is a man whose intended marriage is impeded by an old syphilis infection that has stubbornly defied treatment. This time, after a painful inner struggle, the candidate conjures up the courage to inform his future wife of their predicament. Together, they decide to marry anyway in the conviction that they are strong enough to maintain chaste relations. This proves unduly optimistic, however: the marriage soon succumbs to the increasing pressures on it, and at length a syphilitic child is born ('a small, skinny little girl with the face of an old woman') who dies shortly after birth.

These literary descriptions of the havoc that venereal disease could wreak upon a newly established family reveal a fairly complex grasp of the material. While it is true that the male protagonists act ill-advisedly, and could be accused of a certain degree of selfishness, it is all within the bounds of plain human fallibility. This is especially true as the reader is allowed a glimpse of their crisis of conscience, their feelings being stretched to the utmost limits, and their sincere remorse. In contrast, many propagandist treatises that appeared on this subject presented matters in a greatly simplified form. The main characters in such treatises, rather than being endowed with recognizable human frailty, are mere stereotypes. In the first place there are the *ignorant*, encompassing not only women and children but sometimes also naïve young men who have been seduced. But the vast majority of the males presented in these tracts are the *thoughtless*, those who through indifference or on occasion through an evil constitution untroubled by any qualms of conscience have a fateful influence upon the health and happiness of others.

The early 20th-century efforts to inform women and youths properly and to attack male indifference and selfishness were a natural sequel to the beliefs and activities of those who had opposed regulated prostitution, a few decades earlier, on the basis of feminist principles or out of concern about the quality of the population. Their Protestant comrades in this struggle had entrenched themselves in the Dutch anti-venereal disease society, and adopted a different approach. It was not until the 1920s that Protestants returned to the forefront of the ranks of narrators. One thing was clear: the way feminists, eugenists and other radicals were portraying the drama of ignorant women whose lives were being ruined by unscrupulous men was completely beyond the pale for the Protestants. The most extreme pronouncements of all came from the physician J. Rutgers, who had the effrontery to contend that neo-Malthusianism held out the best answer for both the individual home and society as a whole. This solution, of which widespread contraception was the key component, would produce a sincere and healthy climate for sexual intercourse that would render prostitution obsolete.[36] To a devout Christian, this cure was scarcely any better than the disease. But many other activists grappling with the problem of how to prevent venereal disease being passed on in the home, it should be said, were also sceptical of Rutgers' solution.

The main instrument that narrators advocated to curb infection in the family was ensuring that the public was properly informed. Much suffering could be prevented in this way. One well-known spokesman in this camp was Brieux, who had given the doctor in *De Beschadigden* (*Damaged Goods*) these words to say:

> The true medicine, you see, consists in a change of morality. Syphilis should no longer be treated as a mysterious disease that should not even be named out loud ... . The public are allowed to remain ignorant of the true nature and consequences of this disease, and this exacerbates it and helps it spread. People generally contract the disease because "one did not know", and then they infect others because "one did not know". People must know – and the young must learn – their responsibilities, and they must become aware that in their youthful years they may pave the way for future disaster.[37]

The most deprived group in this respect were the women who, kept naïve and ignorant by all those around them, often walked blindly into their own downfall. They simply had no idea what might befall them. Hence information addressed specifically at women was of crucial importance.

> Women must know the hazards that beset their sons once they fly from the nest. ... They must know what it is that is ruining their happiness, has destroyed their health, is bringing their children into the world in a sickly state. Many a sweet illusion will be rudely shattered by this knowledge, but this must not deter us from informing women, as the only way to banish this cancer from our society is through the power and the will of women.[38]

Aletta Jacobs wrote these impassioned words in 1902. Other feminists too judged the time ripe for a new clarity on matters sexual, which would decrease women's helplessness in relation to men, since, to quote Titia van der Tuuk (the feminist of the Pure Life Movement who translated Brieux' work into Dutch): 'the childlike dependency and extreme ignorance of women in the realm of sexuality constantly helps and encourages men to put their selfish intentions into practice'.[39] Women would continue to bear the burden of these intentions, she maintained – whether in the form of shattered ideals, a sickly existence or permanent infertility – until a radical sexual reform had been achieved. Not that infertility was in itself such an unfortunate outcome, Van der Tuuk went on, 'since infected cells are bound to produce infested offspring', but even this case reveals the same underlying pattern: 'here, too, the woman is the innocent victim of the rash or unscrupulous man'.[40]

Other women who identified themselves less explicitly with feminism than Jacobs and Van der Tuuk also protested against the inequality that existed between the sexes. In 1913, for instance, M. Schoemaker-Frentzen's pamphlet *Mogen wij zwijgen?* (*May we Remain Silent?*), which was entirely devoted to the 'conspiracy of silence' and its consequences, had a warm reception. Schoemaker-Frentzen set out to shatter this conspiracy, just as Cora Westland had expressed in her novel *Levenswond* an explicit desire to rid the world of the 'convention that forbids a woman to know about life, or, if she does know, obliges her to conceal this knowledge behind a mask of innocence or ignorance'. Schoemaker-Frentzen believed that wives and mothers should take their lives into their own hands, starting by defying the conspiracy of silence in the upbringing of their children.

Alongside the pleas advocating information addressed specifically to women, education reformers from feminist or socialist circles were also proposing sex education for young people, so that those contemplating marriage would be better prepared for adult married life rather than having their eyes crudely opened, like previous generations, when it was too late. Sex education for young people was not in itself a new idea.[41] What was new, however, was the idea of using it as an instrument in the fight against venereal disease, which added a pragmatic inducement to the more idealistic arguments advanced in the past.[42] This issue still had to be approached with extreme delicacy, however. To avoid the risk of arousing an unwholesome interest in sexual matters, which some feared would result from injudicious or premature education, it was deemed of immense importance to select as educators only 'the most serious of persons'.[43] The last thing people wanted was for sex education to take place in an atmosphere of levity or prurience. The earnestness of the matter had to be impressed above all on parents, who bore prime responsibility for educating their children, although schools and GPs also had important parts to play. While mothers, in particular, were expected to ensure that their young sons were well versed in the facts of life, GPs could provide additional information and help prevent the young men from going astray later on.[44] Self-control and abstinence were to be the twin beacons of this education; on that score, physicians were to leave no room for doubt. '*Abstinence* must be the cornerstone of any programme of sex education',[45] decreed the physician Schoonheid in a series of articles on sex education as a weapon against venereal disease. At the same time, it was the GP's task to rouse married men and those with marriage plans from their nonchalance, whether this sprang from selfishness or from plain naïvety, and to alert them to the possible repercussions of their indifference on wife and offspring.

One measure of reproductive hygiene introduced in this context was the pre-marital medical examination, one of the first specific applications of the eugenic ideal. Its objective was to inform prospective spouses about each other's state of health, and if necessary to give couples the medical advice to postpone or even abandon their wedding plans. This would go some way towards preventing infection within marriage and restricting the conception of sickly and deficient offspring. In the course of time, the arguments used to promote this scheme – and the arguments within the eugenic movement as a whole – tended to place greater emphasis on genetic deviations and inherited disease, but initially the main aim was to prevent mutual infection and damage to cells. The scheme was indeed primarily intended to contain the damaging effects of tuberculosis, alcoholism and above all venereal disease,[46] although there was also a desire to impose certain restrictions on marriages involving other persons ranging from the insane to epileptics and deaf mutes. In the propaganda for the medical examination the consequences of free and rash marriages were laid on very thickly; the never-ending sadness of infertility as a result of gonorrhoea was stressed almost as much as the terrible symptoms of syphilis and the risk to future offspring.[47] What could be more sensible, under these circumstances, than for those contemplating marriage to exchange recent bills of health before finally committing themselves, thereby excluding a future of endless disorders and unwanted childlessness?

The medical examination was a measure that would protect women from the 'selfish intentions' of their future husbands, would make the men themselves aware at an earlier stage of their responsibility to their future family, and would moreover help prevent them, too, from later disappointment. In short, it could forestall a good deal of domestic tragedy. Viewed within a broader context, the postponement or cancellation of impetuous marriages could curb the physical and mental deterioration of the population in an effective and rational manner. And to be assured that the degenerative influence of venereal diseases was still a matter of concern, one need only look upon the child-sufferers of syphilis. Johan van Breukelen conducted his readers on an imaginary tour past all the imperfections arising from ill-advised marriages: sickly and bed-ridden little victims of parental alcoholism, tuberculosis or venereal disease. Here is his description of one case belonging to the latter category.

> This child's arms and legs were white, waxlike sticks; only its belly was round. It had what looked like the white plaster-cast of a monkey's face; the nose, a broad, blunt feature implanted some distance below the forehead, resembled an animal's snout. The drooping eyelids, the wrinkles surrounding the mouth – the overall impression was of a regression into the animal kingdom.[48]

Van Breukelen was a fervent believer in the need for pre-marital medical examinations.

Disagreements among the supporters of such a system produced a variety of proposals. The idea that the outcome of a medical examination could lead to a ban on the marriage was unpopular.[49] The Committee for the Promotion of Medical Examinations before Marriage, founded in 1912, did not favour a ban on marriage, but strongly advocated a compulsory medical examination. People should be free to ignore the medical advice proffered, the Committee argued, but at least they would know what they were doing. But many balked at the notion of a formal obligation to undergo the examination, even presented in this form, preferring voluntary compliance based on a purely moral obligation.[50] In the event, medical examinations prior to marriage were never made compulsory in the Netherlands; as a voluntary institution they aroused little opposition, though some questioned their usefulness.[51]

Protestant groups within the anti-venereal disease movement were as scathing of medical examinations as they were of sex education. 'Ineffectual, exaggerated, in many respects disadvantageous – in short, unworthy of further consideration', was Van Leeuwen's verdict on pre-marital medical examinations. His objections, though in part based on practical considerations, were rooted more firmly in an antipathy to the combination of rational expediency and medical presumption exuded by the eugenic project. Furthermore, measures of this kind distracted people's attention from what the Protestants saw as the true problem, which was the nation's moral health:

> To seek to reduce the number of mental defectives, of idiots, of the incurably insane and the unbalanced in our society, which alcohol, syphilis, avarice and pleasure-seeking are rotting away, by advising certain individuals against marriage, may be likened to the issuing of a prohibition on smoking in a burning house.[52]

A more effective way of attacking common diseases, in Van Leeuwen's view, would be to foster chastity, sincerity, proper hygiene, self-control and sobriety.

At the beginning of the 20th century, the contraction of venereal disease within the family was thus a subject that commanded the attention of a small but varied section of society, including medical practitioners, population hygienists, feminists and the early eugenists. Although these different groups of narrators were united in their desire to preserve the health of the family, their mutual relations were far from uncomplicated. Feminists and physicians looked on each other, for instance – unavoidably given the terms of the debate – with mutual suspicion. Feminists saw medical practitioners as complicitous in the prototypical tragedy of the time, as the latter so often failed to intervene because of a tacit gentlemen's agreement between their profession and male patients with venereal disease who wished to marry, or who declined to inform their wives. By preserving silence in such cases and by hiding behind the vow of professional confidentiality, physicians themselves helped to sustain these criminal practices of men and to keep women trapped in their ignorance.

In a broader context, too, relations between the different groups were often more hostile than cordial. Eugenists saw feminism, for instance, as a dysgenic factor in society, and they seized every opportunity to deride feminists' efforts to achieve higher education, employment and economic independence.[53] That these groups have been considered here together under a single heading should therefore not be taken to imply a common fund of principles and ideals, but at most a partial overlap of concerns amounting to a similar view of the problem of venereal disease at this stage in time. They agreed in their identification of the main characters, and all wished to combat the pernicious problem of venereal infection within the family using various forms of public information.

The specific way in which the narrators of the domestic 'circuit' presented the problem, and their clear-cut casting of the main roles in the tragedy, tell us more than simply the route of infection that they saw as posing the greatest hazard. They allow us to reconstruct a wider theme, a particular view of society. In the first place, such descriptions related – just as in the earlier debate on prostitution – to men and women, and to views of the differences between the sexes. Women accounted for the majority in this debate on the contraction of venereal disease in the home. They contrasted women's ignorance and innocence with the carefree egoism of men, and thus continued an important line of argument from the prostitution debate – the attack on men, albeit less directly an attack on the free rein allowed to his sex drive and more on his unthinking attitude and self-centredness, against which the family had to be protected. The obvious distinction between the sexes undoubtedly helped to underscore the clarity of the message: offenders and victims could be distinguished without the slightest difficulty. And where innocence and naïvety were threatened by uncaring self-centredness, it was not hard to take sides, nor to decide on the most necessary remedies: women needed to be properly informed, and men should refrain from extra-marital sexual intercourse. Thus we can see the characters that featured in this debate largely as allegorical figures whose actions in the domestic tragedy are of chiefly symbolic significance. The criticism of men that is explicit or implicit in this representation of events was a continuation of the feminist civilization campaign that had been launched towards the end of the 19th century.

The concern about the size and quality of the population that had focused many views in the prostitution debate likewise resurfaced in the debate on venereal infection in the home. More than before, however, the early 20th-century interest in infertility and the damage to posterity was based on, and structured by, a eugenic ideal that was initially geared towards finding fresh, more rational ways of tackling familiar social problems. Not only the prospect of an 'inferior' generation but also the waste associated with the insidious spread of venereal disease was a thorn in the eye of the new eugenicists. In view of the 'appallingly large numbers' of hospital patients suffering from congenital syphilis, the medical practitioner Ernst de Vries, who was involved in the earliest attempts to launch a Dutch Society of Eugenics, dwelt in passing on this point:

> a third of these patients are profound idiots, in whom all vestige of mental life has been extinguished, and who therefore prolong a useless existence at the cost of society. While it is true that they do not live to a great age, the decent care that the institution provides lengthens their lives to no insignificant degree.[54]

The eugenist movement did not win over large numbers of supporters in the Netherlands, but during the initial phase of its existence, in which the hygiene of reproduction played a dominant role, it clearly coloured public attitudes to the problem of venereal disease. The specific measures advocated by the eugenists, however, were never adopted.

Relations between the social classes attracted relatively little attention among the narrators in the domestic 'circuit', who were themselves largely drawn from the middle classes. Although pre-marital medical examinations, for example, were in theory designed to prevent domestic misery at every level of society, the narrators here were in fact largely concerned with the bourgeoisie: the ignorant woman of their scenarios was a middle-class character, as was the carefree man who held her future in his hands. But this was not the whole story. Some of the sex education proposals, for instance, could be regarded as part of the wider-ranging civilization process in which middle-class groups endeavoured to model the family lives of working people along the lines they preferred. Sexual self-restraint went along with respectability and an orderly family life, and where this did not come naturally, it had to be taught. This could be done by introducing pupils at state primary schools to middle-class values and instructing them in the value of a happy family life, by organizing public lectures, by providing lessons in good hygiene, and by alerting people to the serious consequences of uncontrolled excess. The emphasis in these modes of instruction was not so much on 'sex education' in its modern sense as on the inculcation of a certain attitude to sexuality, of which self-control, respect and a sense of responsibility were the key ingredients.

Predictably enough, the clash of cultures between different social classes often generated friction. The gynaecologist Jeanne Knoop found it impossible to engage the schoolgirls' attention during her scheduled hours of instruction at the state school of domestic science. Where they had not already been prematurely informed about the coarsest aspects of sexuality – at home, in the street, or in their surroundings – and had learnt to find vulgarity in everything, there was another reason for their lack of interest. 'They were serious, they were not vulgar and yet it did not work', mused Knoop after one such lesson. 'It is my belief that the reason is a lack of development. ... My method is based on imparting knowledge infused with certain ethical concepts. These children are simply not interested in acquiring such knowledge. In retrospect, it was foolish to imagine that they might be.' Knoop continued her classes at the school attended by middle-class children, but stopped teaching at the state school.[55] Even so, she remained convinced that working-class girls too needed to be properly informed, albeit at a somewhat later stage:

> The lower-class child may be addressed later, once it has grown to adulthood and has learnt the seriousness of life, in public lectures describing the dangers that exist in the sexual domain, including for instance the hazards posed by venereal disease. One need scarcely, if at all, refer to individuals' sex lives in such a context.[56]

Whether Knoop and her associates succeeded better when they introduced their ethical concepts at this later stage we cannot say, as they did not report on it.

Stained uniforms

Another route of infection that attracted a good deal of attention in the first few decades of this century was linked to the armed forces and the merchant navy. Prostitution obviously springs to mind most readily, but attention now focused far more than in the past on prostitutes' male clientele, a group easiest to tackle in its densest pockets of concentration.

This focus on the armed forces was in itself no newer than the concern about the family. In the 19th century, anxiety about the physical and moral state of the troops had provided the main backdrop for the drive to regulate prostitution. The renewed focus on the armed forces a few decades later cannot be explained simply by statistics. While the incidence of venereal disease in army and navy was undeniably higher than in other professions, this had been true for as long as anyone could remember.

What was new was the approach to the problem: society displayed an increasing tendency to seek rational solutions, the emphasis being on expediency and efficiency. In social issues this preference was exemplified by the eugenics movement, which favoured a scientific approach to the population problem and which endeavoured, on the basis of rational calculations, to solve the problems that 'defective' individuals posed to society.[57] Aside from this advocacy of social efficiency, the new drive to remedy society's problems rationally also took the form of a movement for 'national efficiency', similar if less powerful than its British counterpart.[58] Domestic concerns combined here with a desire to bolster the Netherlands' international position. The Dutch effort at the beginning of this century to create a strong and efficiently organized nation should be viewed in the context of the battle against indiscipline and lack of backbone fought largely by the Liberals,[59] who greatly disapproved of the idleness and dissipation they saw as triumphing in certain parts of society.

The armed forces were one such area of concern. A healthy nation had the right to expect at the very least a solid army, but the Netherlands had little to boast of in this regard. This was the gist of a report by the Defence Council, established in 1908, whose criticism on the wartime fighting potential of the Dutch army was devastating. The Council went as far as to conclude that the army's usefulness was virtually non-existent. Discipline was ragged, duties were performed in a slipshod manner, the men's attitudes were poor, their officers exercised too little authority, and in combat the troops were clumsy and indecisive. In short, the forces were completely unfit for any serious task whatsoever.[60] There is no reason to assume that this deplorable state of affairs was a recent development, but while the situation had been overlooked or shrugged off in the past, it was now a source of irritation.

The traditionally high incidence of venereal disease in the army and navy was a clear sign of abuses that no self-respecting nation could allow to continue. In relation to the army, the concerns on this score were voiced at the outbreak of the First World War. While the Dutch army was not directly involved in the war, fit and healthy troops were of crucial importance when it might prove necessary to defend the country. In fact the soldiers' state of health left much to be desired. Mobilization lasted many years, and an increase in the number of venereal infections was one of the consequences. Between 1913 and 1918 the number of cases per thousand men rocketed from eleven to over thirty. Then the number rapidly fell again; by 1925 it had dropped to five. It should be noted that in comparison to the other armies of Western Europe, the increase in VD in the Dutch army between 1914 and 1918 was of decidedly modest proportions.[61] In the French army, the number of infections per thousand men exceeded eighty, and in the US forces, incidence was over 10%. This caused large numbers of men to be withdrawn from active service for longer or shorter intervals, with the resulting loss of millions of working days, certainly where the US army was concerned.[62]

In the Dutch navy, mobilization had a less dramatic impact. While it is true that the number of new infections per thousand men was higher than in the army – in the period 1914–1918 it averaged forty each year – the steady decrease that had set in around the turn of the century was scarcely deflected by mobilization. A far more serious situation – and one that was particularly unfavourable from an international perspective – existed in the seaborne forces bound for the Dutch East Indies. Here, the war years – with over 300 new infections for every thousand men who had set sail – were not exceptional. These appalling statistics had been standard for several decades. The number of new cases seldom fell below 30%, and in some years more than half of the men were registered as suffering from venereal disease. This was exceptional, however, even for the navy in the Dutch East Indies.[63]

With the exception of the mobilized army in the Netherlands, venereal disease was not in general becoming a more serious problem. But the climate of opinion had changed: just as the Defence Council now castigated the army for its lack of military discipline, a level of infection once tolerated with resignation now became a source of irritation. In the first decades of the century, army surgeons stressed 'the need to combat [venereal disease] vigorously in the interests of military efficiency'.[64] Expenditure was a particular area of concern: detailed calculations were regularly made of the proportion of the total number of working days lost through illness that was due to venereal disease, the number of days' nursing this group of sufferers required, and how much all this was costing.[65] Such calculations, which formulated the waste of manpower and money in numerical terms, had never been made before. Now, however, these bald figures highlighted the need to take decisive action to reduce venereal disease within the armed forces.

The army's old preference for regulated prostitution occasionally resurfaced, but without gaining any support. With thousands of Dutch soldiers gathering in the country's border regions, many of these areas witnessed an increase in prostitution. Frequently, military authorities urged town councils to pass special ordinances in this area, but the vast majority of such requests went unheeded.[66] The navy occasionally called for regulated prostitution in ports, but their pleas too fell upon deaf ears. More importantly, however, the military authorities themselves were gradually changing their attitude towards the problem of venereal disease. Even they were abandoning their traditional emphasis on regulation as a panacea or even the best option. Army surgeons were increasingly coming to appreciate the value of prophylaxis.

Prophylaxis came in various forms. One effective item, simple to use and a prophylactic in the truest sense of the word, was the condom. Even so, it was not the most widely promoted. This may have been because the condom was also a contraceptive device, and as such it fell under the ban on advertising introduced by the 1911 morality laws. No clear distinction was drawn between the condom's two virtues, which made overtly singing its praises in the armed forces a tricky business. But condoms had other drawbacks too, as discussed by Van Deinse, a naval surgeon:

> Condoms are unpopular with many men, partly because of the dampening effect they have on the libido, and partly because of the fairly high costs incurred by regular users. For these reasons, the need is felt for something that would be capable of neutralizing the consequences of *coitus impurus* without the use of a condom.[67]

The neutralizing substances referred to here were so-called 'chemical prophylactics'. These had modest enough beginnings, as Van Deinse assured his readers that 'urination immediately *post coitum* followed by thorough cleansing with soap and water has a splendid prophylactic effect'.[68] But these initial ablutions should be followed by more stringent cleansing, for instance with bichloride of mercury, a powerful antiseptic. To prevent gonorrhoea, there was protargol, a compound of silver. This was available in the form of ointment, but a protargol solution either injected into the urethra or introduced into it in the form of drops was far more common. A specific prophylactic against syphilis was calomel ointment, a compound of mercury which was to be rubbed all over the sex organ preferably prior to each suspect sexual act, and in any case afterwards – as soon as possible after the event, if the preventive effect were to be maximized. The longer one waited, the less chance of success; to go through the procedure twelve hours later was considered virtually pointless.[69] Pocket-sized prophylactic kits were accordingly available for the man who wished to be prepared.

The navy introduced a system of voluntary prophylaxis as early as 1904: when going on land, anyone who wanted could take a kit with him; alternatively, he could go through the necessary procedure in a designated cabin afterwards. Some army barracks introduced similar disinfecting rooms. This practice was abolished in 1908 after representatives of the Christian political parties had objected to prophylactic substances being supplied officially.[70] Some years later, under the influence of war and mobilization, the pendulum swung back to the arguments of military efficiency, and in 1914 prophylaxis was reintroduced on a semi-voluntary basis.

These measures were largely targeted at the fleet in the Dutch East Indies, with its appallingly high levels of infection. Given the rise of Japan as a strong power in the region around the turn of the century, the Netherlands was taking a close look at all the chinks in its own armour. The fleet's readiness for battle was of crucial importance. Since Japan's defeat of Russia in 1905, the Dutch government had become greatly concerned about the continuing Japanese expansion, which posed a threat to the Dutch in the East Indies territories that seemed likely only to increase over the next few years.[71] The Netherlands government endeavoured to temper this threat through diplomacy, while at the same time seeking to consolidate its military strength. From 1909 onwards, the navy's heavy *materiél* was destined for the East Indies, and in 1912 the first plans were made to expand the fleet for the defence of the colonies.[72] The anxieties concerning the defence of the empire gave the anti-venereal disease campaign in the Dutch East Indies a somewhat grim character: nowhere was the need for healthy, vigorous troops felt more keenly, and nowhere did all the measures adopted seem so ineffective. The high level of venereal disease was a direct and continuous reminder of the weakness and powerlessness of the Dutch armed forces at a time when a vigorous image was needed more than ever before.

The results of the voluntary use of the preventive procedures described above did little to justify military surgeons' initially high hopes of prophylactics. Effectiveness varied enormously: medical practitioners saw condoms as the best preventive measure, offering almost complete protection from gonorrhoea and the maximum possible protection from syphilis, although in the latter case there was always a possibility that a 'condom chancre' might develop. In the case of chemical preparations, the gonorrhoea prophylactic protargol scored highest. This compound could not be kept for long, however, due to a rapid loss of effectiveness. Less perishable products had certain unattractive features, however, as naval surgeon De Mooij observed:

The perishability of protargol solutions might prompt recourse to a different product; a silver nitrate solution may be given, although it should be noted that this creates permanent stains in underwear; in the tropics this is a more serious problem, as the white trousers too may become stained.[73]

A more pressing problem than the imperfections of the prophylactics themselves was that of their application. To achieve an optimum effect, these substances had to be used correctly, and as soon as possible after intercourse. Both conditions were often disregarded. The men did not always have the kit with them at the essential moment, and they sometimes lacked the necessary instruction to use it properly. More important still, as the naval surgeons observed in disappointment, was the general lack of motivation. In the period 1903–1908 and after 1914, prophylactics were available to crew members free of charge, but the demand for them was so low that nothing definite was achieved.[74] The statistics for the navy in the Dutch East Indies, where the need for prophylactics was felt most keenly and where they were introduced most energetically, do not indicate any clear drop in incidence for these periods. In 1917, because of these disappointing results, the use of prophylactics was made compulsory: instead of kits being distributed to crew going on land, the men were treated by the surgeons after re-embarkation. Treatment was 'compulsory' in that men who refused it and later developed symptoms of venereal disease could be disciplined. Whether this new scheme was any more effective than the voluntary one is unclear. The decrease in numbers of sufferers after 1920 is so universal that there is little basis for ascribing it wholly, in the Dutch navy, to the compulsory use of prophylactics.

Whatever the truth may have been about the efficacy of prophylactics, the navy's faith in them survived for decades. Right up to the 1980s, medical staff stood poised with their protargol and calomel ointment in the prophylaxis cabins to disinfect men coming back on board or to ensure that they did so properly themselves. All the disadvantages of these procedures persisted too: a high percentage-rate of failures, extra work for medical staff, and the impossibility of treating men on leave. And right up to the end it was 'well-known that a large proportion of the crew were little motivated to apply the disinfection procedures adequately'.[75] Yet the crew were apparently even less motivated to use condoms, as it was not until the advent of AIDS that the navy finally abandoned the use of chemical prophylactics. These substances give no protection against the virus that causes AIDS. Even so, prophylactic treatment remained available sporadically until 1988, when the Inspector of the Maritime Health Service instructed all ships and establishments with medical services to close down their prophylactic anti-venereal disease facilities for good.[76]

Given the quiet disappearance of prophylactics from the scene a few years ago, it is interesting to look back on the furious controversy generated by their use and promotion in the early part of the century.[77] In general, the argument was one between military spokesmen on the one hand and civilians on the other. The debate revolved around two fundamental differences of opinion.

In the first place, the army and navy surgeons that formed the majority among the supporters of prophylaxis had a pragmatic approach that jarred on the sensibilities of civilian society.[78] As the majority of soldiers and sailors would not be deterred from having sexual intercourse, military surgeons were solely concerned to arrange effective damage limitation. While conceding that the men should be admonished about the moral repugnance of premarital and extra-marital sexual relations and warned about the dangers associated with such conduct, they observed that one could not expect this to have much effect. Military spokesmen paid lip service to principles of moral education and standards of decency in certain set phrases, but a certain note of weary mollification often crept into their discourse. Some ventured to express a more open hostility to moralizing. Bromberg, a dermatologist and specialist in venereal diseases who had been called up into the armed forces, expostulated:

> When one realizes that a soldier who has contracted gonorrhoea has to be withdrawn from active service for 4 to 6 weeks, it is time to leave off admonitions and sermonizing that experience has shown to be useless and to take *medical* measures instead. Personal prophylaxis should be the first of these measures.[79]

In the issue of morality, these champions of prophylaxis found themselves facing a formidable – largely Christian – opposition. The bottles of drops to prevent gonorrhoea had long been available even outside the armed forces, but their use, or, to put it more accurately, the promotion of their use, encountered great resistance. It has already been noted that the first chairman of the Dutch Anti-Venereal Disease Society came out clearly against the use of prophylactics during the early stages of the society's existence, and maintained this position for years. Prominent spokesmen of the

Society, such as De Graaf and Van Leeuwen, backed by a substantial proportion of the medical profession, seized every opportunity to express the revulsion with which they regarded prophylactics. It was not so much the adverse side-effects of the chemical products that disturbed them, but the consequences of promoting them. Propaganda on behalf of prophylactics – indeed, the very knowledge of their existence – would inevitably encourage extra-marital sexual relations and more visits to prostitutes, and would thus actually aggravate the problem of immorality. Anyone who went out with a prophylactic in his pocket would feel a constant urge to use it. The opponents of prophylactics saw any benefit to be gained from such products as being completely outweighed by the seductive influence of the pocket-sized kits and of what they imagined would be the next stage – the dreaded condom dispensers that would soon be dotted around the public highways. These opponents included the Dutch government, which first became involved in the venereal disease debate after the First World War. In 1918 the Dutch Anti-Venereal Disease Society requested a state subsidy. The government granted it, but attached one condition, namely that the organization should refrain from promoting the use of prophylactics.[80] The Society obviously had no difficulty agreeing to this, as it had adopted this position from the outset.

The few physicians who openly favoured the use of prophylactics by civilians wielded little influence.[81] That individual medical practitioners – possibly in large numbers – did in fact give preventive treatment subsequent to a possible exposure to infection was something no one could prevent, and was accepted as a kind of compromise, a far lesser evil than open propaganda. Many physicians too saw preventive treatment given by themselves as preferable by far (not to mention more lucrative) than the unrestricted sale to laymen of chemical substances for self-administration. Nor was this treatment open to the main charge levelled against prophylactics, namely that if they were purchased 'with malice aforethought' and carried about in one's pocket, they would actually invite fornication. Even the military spokesmen found this idea a little unpalatable.

'There is and remains something distasteful about carrying about your person some preparation, before feeling any need for sexual intercourse, just in case the urge should arise',[82] wrote the naval health officer Von Römer in 1913. This is why it was easier to defend compulsory than voluntary prophylaxis in the navy: the former did not involve anything being handed out; action was taken upon the men's return, after they had unfortunately succumbed to a moment of weakness. Many found this a more acceptable practice than the distribution of prophylactic kits, even though in practice the difference was minimal. The distinction will undoubtedly have been exaggerated in an effort to placate the opponents of prophylactics. For instance, the new term 'early treatment' (*vroegbehandeling*) was coined, to indicate that there was no question of encouraging lechery by handing out preventive supplies beforehand.[83] One could scarcely take issue with treatment, even 'early' treatment.

To a confirmed opponent such as the dermatologist Van Leeuwen, secretary of the Society from 1914 until the early 1930s, even the preventive 'early treatment' by medical practitioners was going too far. As he dourly observed, 'I for one shall never regard it as my duty to be available at all hours of the day and night to disinfect whomsoever presents himself for this purpose, and I shall take such action only in the most exceptional of circumstances and for highly exceptional reasons'.[84] He deemed it preferable to postpone treatment until the first symptoms of venereal disease had appeared.

The fundamental and tenacious opposition to prophylactics of which Van Leeuwen was the leading spokesman can best be understood as a remnant of the view that one cannot with impunity indulge in extra-marital sexual intercourse or other forms of immoral conduct. The notion that venereal diseases were punishments for sins may have lost ground since the turn of the century, but it had certainly not disappeared altogether. Particularly in Christian circles, people still discussed the issue in judgemental terms such as sinfulness and guilt, and prophylactics were anathema to them. To Van Leeuwen and those like him, the nonchalant ease with which men could indulge in fornication if they went out armed with a prophylactic kit was simply unacceptable. These men were not innocent victims that one wished to help with all available means, but a group that wilfully sought out vice and for whom the old adage in fact applied with undiminished force: no cure without repentance. Military surgeons, on the other hand, had never had much truck with religious rhetoric. To them, the troops' effectiveness in times of need was always more important than their virtuousness, which made guilt an irrelevancy.

There was another issue that divided the advocates and opponents of prophylactics. This was their view of the regulation of male sexuality. Military circles persisted far longer than the outside world in their belief that sexual abstinence could be damaging to a man's health and that it ran counter to man's essential being. Military surgeons, as they often reminded whoever was listening, did not need to be told about masculine nature. They understood it as no one else did, and the response of the military authorities to the problem was more or less attuned to this view. Certain exalted individuals, they conceded, might be able to control their sexual urge, but in the everyday life of the army and navy the thing was impossible.

More strongly opposed than anyone else to this justification of prophylactics were feminists. Their central proposition concerning male sexuality led naturally to the rejection of any prophylactic ointment or bottles of drops, whose only purpose was to make possible the unbridled satisfaction of the male sex drive. Physicians who prescribed such products, contended the feminist and gynaecologist Catharine van Tussenbroek, were on the wrong track. In her review of a book by the German medical practitioner Bumm, in which he had welcomed the use of prophylactics, she wrote:

> There is one hope for the future: a better upbringing for young men. An upbringing that focuses on chastity, a sense of responsibility and self-respect will do more to prevent gonorrhoea infections than the prophylactic bottle of drops that Bumm would like to give our youth as he sets out for the brothel. That a prophylactic of this kind should have been recommended by an excellent physician such as Bumm, and that this recommendation should have aroused no powerful protest from within the medical profession, proves that the educator who is endeavouring to strike at the roots of the evil must regard the physician of this day and age as an enemy rather than an ally.[85]

Titia van der Tuuk made a similar comment some ten years later concerning products used to prevent infection.

> [The man] also takes refuge in bottles of drops, which the authorities of army and navy, with a woeful failure to appreciate the need for the stronger sex to exert self-control and with profound contempt for the female sex, the members of which, in their eyes, are always to a greater or lesser extent objects and necessary sources of pleasure for the man, have made available in dispensers for a nominal sum of money. In this way the authorities foster the view that sexual intercourse is something to which men are entitled at all times.[86]

In the view of feminists, prophylactics provided no solution; if anything, they served to exacerbate the acceptance of unbridled male sexuality that they were trying to change.

Other opponents of prophylactics such as the Society, inspired more by religious than feminist values, likewise advocated the inculcation of higher moral standards and sexual self-control, but they tended to acknowledge the difficulty for men, somewhat more in line with their military adversaries, of attaining these ideals. It was wrong to tempt men by encouraging them to carry prophylactics around with them. Once a certain idea came into their heads, it was bound to end in one way, so the important thing was not to give them that idea in the first place. An extra sanction in the form of a fear of venereal disease was indeed virtually indispensable in the control of male sexuality. Men's conduct in difficult situations was more likely to be affected, it was believed, by external sanctions than by inner convictions.

The idea of the irrepressibility of the male sex urge, once aroused, may be regarded as the counterpart of the views concerning female virtuousness and chastity that were central to the other controversy that has already been discussed above, with its different frame of reference, characters and narrators, focusing on the family. In fact, when we compare the domestic and military debates, we are struck by the fact that the self-control so firmly advocated for men as well as women within the domestic circuit vanished from sight in the all-male setting of the armed forces. This difference between a 'mixed' and a single-sex debate can be explained using the theories of Norbert Elias, in which the development of self-control is influenced by the intensification and expansion of human chains of interdependency.

The social pressure to which this expansion gives rise leads to a controlled and orderly regulation of impulses and desires, to increased self-restraint and to the need to take others into account and to reject immediate satisfaction in favour of goals that are further off.[87] In this context, the changes in relations between the sexes, which both helped to produce and were themselves the product of the first generation of feminism, made it possible for women to articulate their complaints and grievances – and their demands and desires – and made it necessary for men to take more account of women's wishes than before. In the realm of sexuality, this meant that men too could be expected to exercise self-control. But a few male preserves remained that – either because of their special composition or their marginal position – could ward off the demands of the new sexual order. One such preserve was the military 'circuit', in which both the narrators and the characters were male. This was the determining factor in the debate about

110

venereal disease in the armed forces: the discussions took place within the enclosed world of a male preserve – a sanctuary for unimpeached male supremacy.

Somewhat similar to this, albeit less overburdened with sexual ideology, was the situation in the Dutch merchant navy. Here too, the high incidence of venereal disease after the First World War was a cause for concern. On the whole these were balmy days for the merchant navy. The total amount of transport by water rose sharply between 1920 and 1930, and the merchant fleet was modernized, acquiring faster ships with a larger cargo capacity.[88] Under these favourable circumstances, and against the backdrop of the desire for an efficient management, the losses sustained – here too – as a result of infectious diseases were more and more of a thorn in the eye of modern shipping companies.

The expansion in this sector increased the economic value of a healthy and well-functioning shipping industry. But that the physical condition of the men was far from perfect had been known for a long time. A questionnaire that the Central Health Council conducted in 1914 among medical practitioners confirmed yet again the high incidence of venereal disease in ports – roughly three times the national average. In May 1914, the number of registered cases in men per 100,000 of the male population for the country as a whole was 6.3; the figures for municipalities were 1.2, 8 and 18, in ascending order of population size. In the ports, which included smaller ones such as Delfzijl, Velsen and Maassluis, this figure averaged 18.7.[89] Other sources too revealed the uniquely unfavourable state of health of seafarers. In the years 1920–1925, several outpatient clinics reported a drop in the number of civilian patients suffering from venereal disease, but among sailors – in Rotterdam at any rate – this number remained stubbornly high. The men flocked to the free outpatient clinic there; one out of every three male patients was a sailor.[90]

The merchant navy was no more interested than the armed forces in pondering the reasons for this high level of infection – whether it had to do with poor discipline on board, a less than pleasant atmosphere, boredom in the foreign ports, the flood of provocative temptations for those on shore leave, the exceptional way of life or the poor example set by older shipmates. All it wanted – and wanted urgently – was to put an end to the drain on money and working days caused by the lax policy on venereal disease in this sector. This pragmatic objective took little account of concepts such as guilt or immorality. Of prime importance was that the men should have easy access to medical treatment. On disembarkation in Amsterdam, for instance, all crew members were issued with a map of the city indicating the locations of clinics and how to get there by tram.[91] In the mid-1920s, with the financial support of shipping companies, the port of Rotterdam acquired its own clinic and hospital, where sailors could go for treatment not only for venereal disease but also for tropical and internal disorders.[92] But a policy confined to the territory of the Netherlands was inadequate to deal with the problems associated with transcontinental voyages. From time immemorial, ships had been carriers of disease, and this was still the case at the beginning of the 20th century: cholera, plague, yellow fever, scabies and other diseases spread from one port to the next, and from one country to the next. Venereal diseases were simply one among many categories of infectious disease that the sailors imported when they came ashore. This was common knowledge, and for centuries local or national governments had imposed quarantine regulations when an epidemic was feared, to protect the population from infectious diseases that could be imported from ships.[93] It was no coincidence that trading centres and ports had a far higher incidence of venereal disease than would normally correspond to their population size, nor was it surprising that the relatively uncommon soft chancre and the non-indigenous lymphogranuloma inguinale turned up most frequently in major ports. Nicknames such as *Spaanse pokken* (Spanish pox) in the Netherlands, 'French disease' in Britain and *mal de Naples* in France (all meaning syphilis) show that every country preferred to locate the origin of its scourges elsewhere. But all this understanding about the connection between international contacts and the spread of infection had never produced anything beyond local measures to curb venereal disease.

In the 1920s, for the first time, this changed. The expansion of trade made most states increasingly dependent – whether directly or indirectly – on international shipping, and therefore gave them a greater interest in effective health regulations. After all, the transmission of germs within this international network not only affected the sailors themselves but also menaced the inhabitants of the ports, and after them the rest of the country. These secondary consequences, sometimes referred to as 'external effects', had always existed. Quarantine measures and *cordons sanitaires* from bygone eras had served to contain the external effects of trade and international contacts, but with the new intensification of such ties and modern means of transport, these effects increased in terms of

112

both quantity and range. Haphazard local measures introduced in ports were no longer sufficient. They would only work if similar efforts were made in ports in other parts of the world.[94]

Gradually, these developments – the increased mutual dependency of states as intercontinental ties intensified, and the resulting extension of 'external effects' – seeped into the collective consciousness. As a result, the treatment of infected sailors became the subject of the first international agreement to contain venereal disease. In 1924, the Agreement of Brussels was signed; the signatory states undertook to provide medical examinations and treatment for sailors suffering from venereal disease free of charge, regardless of nationality.[95] Treatment could be continued from one port to the next with the aid of a special medical booklet. Rotterdam had set up its special port clinic for VD sufferers as early as 1925, but the Netherlands did not accede to the Agreement until 1930. From that moment on, the care of seamen was the responsibility of the Dutch state.

In conclusion, we may note that the fight against venereal disease among certain specific professions was tackled pragmatically and resolutely. Those most directly concerned with this 'circuit' were military surgeons and physicians attached to port clinics. The solutions they favoured were prophylactics for military men and additional, free facilities for the treatment of sailors. Under the motto of 'national health is national wealth' and against the background of society's far broader need to put its house in order and to regulate matters rationally and efficiently, the high incidence of venereal disease within these sectors attracted grave concern. Just as the influence of feminists and population hygienists who had first expressed their ideas in the prostitution debate now helped to define the problem of venereal disease in terms of 'ignorant women' and 'thoughtless men', the quest for efficiency in its turn defined the armed forces as 'high risk' professions that required attention.

'"Promiscuity", as it is called'

Alongside the two circuits of attention – domestic and military – that have been discussed in this chapter, quite a new note sounded in the fight against venereal disease in the 1920s. At first sight, this note was apparently linked not so much to a particular sector of society, but to a specific sexual practice – relations with a number of sexual partners. At the advice centres of the Dutch Anti-Venereal Disease Society, promiscuity and unpaid sexual activity were given increasing emphasis as vehicles of venereal infection. Outside the

Society too, the increase in promiscuity was regularly bemoaned, but those who adopted the role of narrators in this new area, and who wrote at length in the columns of the Society's periodical *Sexuele Hygiëne* about promiscuous living and its consequences, were largely members of the Society's own staff.

According to the commentators, the new trend of non-exclusivity in sexual relationships was not a uniform or worldwide phenomenon. The main (and usually sole) focus of interest was an increase in *female* promiscuity, which was gradually taking the place – and serving the previous purpose – of prostitution. Whereas around 1910, prostitution was still without a doubt 'the major source ... of venereal infection',[96] in 1920 Van Leeuwen repeated this observation, but this time with the following reservation:

> that prostitution is gradually changing in appearance, in the sense that engaging in a variety of sexual relationships is becoming increasingly common, and far more women and girls engage in extra-marital relations not as a livelihood, but do so in addition to some other employment. So while the professional prostitute may be the most highly infectious source of venereal disease, she is no longer the main source; alongside real prostitution there is now "promiscuity", as it is called.[97]

The first complaints about an increase in promiscuity among women were heard in the First World War, when despite the increased efforts to monitor the state of health in the Dutch mobilized army, large numbers of soldiers still went on contracting venereal disease. Some of these infections originated from 'real' prostitutes, but more and more were coming, the military authorities suggested, from women and girls who were content with some minor favours and a little amusement, and who belonged either to the local population of garrison towns or to the host of Belgian refugees who had come to the Netherlands. The warnings issued to soldiers not to associate with women of dubious character, even combined with the disinfecting facilities in certain barracks, made so little impact that the army authorities, entirely in line with their traditions in this area, asked the government to take action against the Belgian refugees to prevent a further deterioration of moral standards and public decency. On this occasion they were successful: pursuant to a ministerial decree promulgated in 1915, it was allowed by law, if necessary, to intern Belgian women against their will.[98]

After the war, complaints about changing patterns of behaviour among girls continued to be voiced. Sometimes this change was interpreted as an expression of a complete degeneration of moral values, sometimes it was viewed as a sign of an underlying shift in the relationship between the sexes or of premature sexual maturity.[99] Whatever the explanation, a change had undeniably taken place. As the dermatologist Van der Hoog observed,

> As specialists, we have noticed that these days, the female persons who, although they do not always seek it, unquestionably need our help, do not belong to the same categories as before. In the past, there were mainly two large groups – firstly the prostitutes, women who engage in sexual activity for a living, and secondly married women who had been infected by their husbands, very often unaware of the nature of their disease – that together formed the largest contingent of regular visitors to the gynaecologist's surgery. These days we see an immense number of young girls, mostly girls belonging to the middle classes.[100]

It was these girls who now attracted most attention within the Dutch Anti-Venereal Disease Society, and who were increasingly identified as the source and vehicle of venereal infections. In the 1930s, they would seldom be absent from the scenario, as will be discussed in greater detail in the following chapter.

Notes

1. *Rapport der commissie tot onderzoek* 1911:1709-808.
2. See e.g. *Rapport van de commissie tot onderzoek* 1897, Blooker appendix:103.
3. *Rapport der commissie tot onderzoek* 1911:1771. A few pages later, incidentally, it appears that the tolerance urged here was not intended to apply in equal measure to all VD sufferers. Because of the undesirable influence emanating from the unseemly and loud conduct of prostitutes, the ostracism disdained for other patients was still deemed necessary for this particular group: 'We thus believe that ostracism of this nature, not of the patients of venereal disease as such, but of some of them, owing to their characters, will be unavoidable.' (1774)
4. See Rutgers 1906; C.H. van Herwerden, 'De geschiedenis der stichting van de gemeentelijke kostelooze polikliniek voor huid- en geslachtsziekten te Rotterdam', *Tijdschrift voor Sociale Geneeskunde* 2 (1924), no. 10:215-6. See also J.J. Bloemen, 'De kostelooze gemeentelijke polikliniek voor huid- en geslachtsziekten te Rotterdam', *SH* vol. V, no. IV (1927):186-90.

5. See the chief medical inspector's report for the year 1925, in *Verslagen en mededelingen betreffende de volksgezondheid* 1926:1278. For a survey of municipal committees and negotiations that preceded the expansion of the numbers of clinics in Amsterdam, see De Haan 1991.

6. For this questionnaire, see *NTvG* 56 (1912) IA:577-82, and for its results, see *NTvG* 56 (1912) IB:2040-65; these quotations are from 2061.

7. 'It is also undoubtedly the case that the persons belonging to this group [i.e. the poorest] by far outnumber the more prosperous persons who seek help either as private patients or that are entitled to avail themselves of hospital facilities': Muller 1939:63.

8. Van der Hoog 1922:75.

9. W.F. Veldhuyzen, 'Het ontwerp van wet op de ziekenverzorging en de bestrijding der geslachtsziekten', *SH* vol. 1, no. 1 (1921):60.

10. See Voorhoeve 1951:121-2; Greiling 1955:169-70.

11. E. van der Hoop, 'De nieuwste syphilistherapie met het middel van Ehrlich-Hata', *Geneeskundige Courant* 64 (1910), no. 41:321-2; S. Mendes da Costa, 'Mijn ervaringen over de behandeling van syphilis met salvarsan', *NTvG* 55 (1911):5-12; A.H.M.E. Lommen, 'Mijn ervaringen met de salvarsanbehandeling', *Medisch Weekblad voor Noord en Zuid-Nederland* 18 (1911/12):27-31. See also Greiling 1955:170-5. Elsewhere there are references to a marked enthusiasm among medical practitioners that gave way to a period of cooling-off and disappointment; see Dowling 1973:243-6. I have been unable to trace any such enthusiasm in the Netherlands; even relatively positive articles (e.g. Van Leeuwen 1911) are fairly lukewarm in their appreciation.

12. Wolffensperger, 'Beteekenis van Salvarsan voor de aandoeningen van het centrale zenuwstelsel', *Medisch Weekblad voor Noord en Zuid-Nederland* 18 (1911/12):461-3.

13. See Brandt 1987:130. In the Netherlands, Salvarsan emerged from clinical trials conducted in the 1930s as vastly superior to other forms of treatment; see Bottema 1931:55.

14. Cf. Dowling 1977:94; Brandt 1987:41; Cassel 1987:67.

15. *Geneeskundige Courant*, vol. 64 (1910), no. 36:287.

16. 'Syphilis en huwelijk', *Medisch Weekblad voor Noord en Zuid-Nederland* 29 (1922/23):539.

17. *Rapport der commissie tot onderzoek* 1911:1709-808.

18. See A. Gans, 'De behandeling der dementia paralytica met malariaënting volgens Wagner-Jauregg', *NTvG* 66 (1922) IB:1693-7; Voorhoeve 1951:135-53.

19. K. Edel, 'Behandeling van syphilis door middel van malaria', *NTvG* 72 (1928) IV:5911.

20. See C.P. Schokking, K. Beintema & J.J. Zoon, 'Voorkomen en
    uitbreiding van geslachtsziekten in het gebied, bestreken door de
    dermatologische klinieken in Leiden, Groningen en Utrecht', *SH*,
    fifth series, no. 1 (1938):16-31.
21. Prakken 1948:260. See also Schokking, Beintema & Zoon,
    'Voorkomen en uitbreiding', *SH*, fifth series, no. 1 (1938):24 and 28.
    Idsoe & Guthe (1967:233) likewise reached the conclusion, on the
    basis of international comparisons, that the introduction of Salvarsan
    had no immediate impact on the epidemiological development of
    syphilis. The effective use of Salvarsan was not widespread until the
    1920s, when it consolidated a tendency that had already set in.
22. Cf. Bijkerk 1969, II:36-7. During the entire period 1900-1950,
    annual syphilis mortalities oscillated between 400 and 500; this rate
    did not decline until after the Second World War. However,
    McKeown (1976a:103; 153) reports that Salvarsan did reduce
    syphilis mortality rates.
23. Schoonheid 1917:3.
24. The committee was made up of the following persons: D. Hudig
    (Director of the Central Bureau for Social Advice), T.M. Roest van
    Limburg (Chief of Police in Rotterdam), G. Velthuysen (member of
    the board of the Dutch Midnight Mission society) and the medical
    practitioners P.H. Schoonheid (specialist in dermatology and venereal
    disease), D. Snoeck Henkemans (M.D. and board member of the
    NVP), R.A. Tange (health inspector in the Royal Dutch Navy) and
    C.L. Wijn (dermatologist).
25. *Rapport der commissie tot onderzoek* 1911:1786.
26. T. M. Van Leeuwen, 'Twintig jaar bestrijding der geslachtsziekten in
    Nederland', *NTvG* 78 (1934), IV:5162. See also Veldhuyzen,
    'Inleiding', *SH* vol. 1, no. 1 (1921):3-10.
27. De Graaf 1929:90-1.
28. See the first issue of *SH* vol. 1, no. 1 (1921): Van Leeuwen:2-3; De
    Graaf:38-54; this quotation from 54.
29. See W.F. Veldhuyzen, 'De consultatiebureaux van de Ned.
    Vereeniging tot bestrijding der geslachtsziekten', *SH* vol. III, no. II
    (1923):53-63.
30. See Veldhuyzen, 'De consultatiebureaux van de Nederlandsche
    Vereeniging tot bestrijding der geslachtsziekten', *NTvG* 63 (1919),
    IIB:1640-2; Van Steenbergen 1950:79-83.
31. Haustein 1927:267-8. Haustein points out that part of the
    explanation for the difference between large cities and small towns
    relates to superior diagnoses in the former. For some comparative
    figures on the cause of death in still-births for the period 1920-1925,

see D.G. Wesselink, 'Bijdrage tot de oorzaak van den dood van het levenloos geboren kind', *NTvG* 70 (1926), 3:2714-6. Of the thirteen causes of death cited by Wesselink, a syphilis infection in the mother occupies the tenth place.

32. For material on the consequences of congenital syphilis, see 'Verbreiding van de geslachtsziekten', 1921:14-8; 35-41; W.F. Veldhuijzen, 'De sociale balans der geslachtsziekten', *SH* vol. I, no. 1 (1921):11-21.

33. See the figures on the proportion of venereal disease responsible for eye diseases and blindness, in *Verbreiding van de geslachtsziekten* 1921:21; cf. also Haustein's figures on the number of syphilitic still-births during the period 1901-1920: Haustein 1927:267-8.

34. Van der Meer 1906:43.

35. Van der Meer 1906:132.

36. Cf. Rutgers 1914.

37. Brieux 1902:169.

38. Jacobs 1902:73.

39. Van der Tuuk 1915:117.

40. Van der Tuuk 1915:151.

41. See Röling 1990 on earlier proposals.

42. See e.g. Wibaut-Berdenis van Berlekom, in Wibaut-Berdenis van Berlekom & Nathans 1909:13.

43. *Rapport der commissie tot onderzoek* 1911:1716; see also Wijnaendts Francken 1920:18: 'But such education should at any rate be provided in an absolutely dignified manner as befits the seriousness of the subject. Any frivolousness or suggestion of sensuality or humourousness must be avoided altogether.' For the lofty tone of many sex educators, see also Röling 1990.

44. See G.C. Nijhoff, 'Het huwelijk van den gonorrhoïcus', in *Geneeskundige Bladen* 1 (1894):244; Schoemaker-Frentzen 1913:26-7.

45. P.H. Schoonheid, 'Sexueele paedagogiek als middel van bestrijding der geslachtsziekten', *Medisch Weekblad* 19 (1913), no. 46:543-6; no. 47:555-9; no. 48:570-3, this quotation 555; see also 573. See also *Rapport der commissie tot onderzoek* 1911:1780.

46. Van Praag 1976:103; Noordman 1989:56.

47. See Greidanus 1904; Nijhoff 1908; Berdenis van Berlekom, in Berdenis van Berlekom & Bles 1914.

48. Van Breukelen 1911:12.

49. This idea was proposed in Wijnaendts Francken 1901.

50. A detailed account of this controversy is given in Noordman 1989:37-56.

51. Doubts were raised, for instance, in the NMG committee's 1911

report; see *Rapport der commissie tot onderzoek* 1911:1734-5.

52. Van Leeuwen 1924:803; for a similar line of argument, see Bakker 1925.
53. See Noordman 1989:79-80; Everard 1992.
54. De Vries, in *Verbreiding van de geslachtsziekten* 1921:15.
55. See Jeanne Knoop, 'Sexueele opvoeding', *SH* vol. III, no. 1 (1923):1-20; this quotation from 18.
56. Jeanne Knoop, 'Sexueele opvoeding', *SH* vol. III, no. 1 (1923):20.
57. See Noordman 1989:255-9.
58. See Searle 1971. For the influence of the ideology of national efficiency on the fight against tuberculosis in Great Britain, see Bryder 1988, chapter I.
59. On this subject see Te Velde 1992:220-1, 273.
60. See Smit 1971 I:149-50.
61. See Haustein 1927:665; see also Hirschfeld & Gaspar (eds.), n.d., esp. chapter VII.
62. Verdoorn 1972, II:601. This high level of infection was in itself difficult enough to deal with, but the armed forces also found themselves confronting an offshoot of this problem: the feigning of venereal disease. A venereal disease was scarcely regarded as shameful in a military context, and the prospect of a spell of rest and some respite from the mortal danger of battle made some soldiers decide to induce symptoms of venereal disease. The German writer Pick estimated the number of men feigning venereal disease during the First World War to be over 5% of the total. Men wanting to create the desired symptoms did not shun the crudest of methods. The most common trick was the simulation of a gonorrhoea infection, achieved by introducing a soap solution or another substance such as turpentine into the urethra. Deliberate authentic gonorrhoea infections were also not unknown, for which purpose the soldier would transfer to his own body the pus of a sufferer. The imitation of syphilis was often achieved using chemical substances that caused ulceration on the skin or mucous membranes. But other methods were sometimes used, such as cigarette burns in the mouth or the rubbing of genitalia with garlic, which produced an injury resembling certain specific symptoms of syphilis. Although the military authorities of the warring armies were well aware of the phenomenon of simulated venereal disease, they did not succeed in 'eliminating this evil, roots and all'. See G.A. Prins, 'Simulatie van geslachtsziekten', *Militair Geneeskundig Tijdschrift* 21 (1917):411-2; T.E. Kempers, 'Simulatie van huid- en geslachtsziekten', *Militair Geneeskundig Tijdschrift* 24 (1935):174-9.

63. See Haustein 1927:797-801.
64. H. Peeters, 'Militair hygiënische vraagstukken. Het vraagstuk der geslachtsziekten te velde', *NTvG* 78 (1934) I:125-33, this quotation from 127.
65. See e.g. Van Deinse 1918:108-9; P. de Mooij, 'Beschouwingen over de prophylaxis tegen venerische ziekten in en buiten de Marine', *Geneeskundige Bladen* 23 (1923):148-9. Van der Hoog (1922:221) estimated the annual cost of the nursing and treatment of infected soldiers in the Dutch East Indies Army in 1919 at between 3 and 4 million guilders.
66. See Kleijngeld 1983:160-3.
67. Van Deinse 1918:56-7.
68. Van Deinse 1918:57.
69. See E.H. Hermans, 'De praeventie van venerische ziekten', *NTvG* 84 (1940) IV:4397-402.
70. Objections were raised as soon as the navy's budget came up for discussion in parliament: the free supply of bottles of preventive drops was alleged to encourage fornication. Wentholt, Minister for the Navy, answered that he had called a halt to the practice as soon as it had come to his attention. See *Bijlagen van het Verslag der Handelingen van de Tweede Kamer der Staten-Generaal* 1908–1909, Annex A, vol. I, Chapter VI, no. 29:9-10 (draft report) and Annex A, vol. II, Chapter VI, no. 30:25-7 (Memorandum in Reply). According to Van Deinse (1918:84) the whole navy was dismayed by this abolition, which was motivated by 'solely theoretical moral considerations'.
71. See Smit 1971 I:201-6.
72. See Smit 1971 I:190 and 206-8. Because of the outbreak of the First World War, the expansion of the fleet did not in fact take place.
73. P. de Mooij, 'Beschouwingen over de prophylaxis tegen venerische ziekten in en buiten de marine', *Geneeskundige Bladen* 23 (1923):147-72; this quotation from 164.
74. See Van Deinse 1918:79; P. de Mooij, 'Beschouwingen over de prophylaxis tegen venerische ziekten in en buiten de Marine', *Geneeskundige Bladen* 23 (1923):150.
75. H.J. Dirksen et al., 'Over een proefneming met een nieuwe vorm van prophylaxe tegen geslachtsziekten bij de koninklijke marine', *Nederlands Militair Geneeskundig Tijdschrift* 24 (1971), July-Aug.:186-92; N.J. Kruijer, 'Het condoom ter vervanging van de protargol', *Nederlands Militair Geneeskundig Tijdschrift* 44 (1991), April:45-9; this quotation from 45.
76. N.J. Kruijer, 'Het condoom ter vervanging van de protargol',

Nederlands Militair Geneeskundig Tijdschrift 44 (1991), April:45-9.

77. The heat of this debate is indicated by the fact that not one of the committees that issued recommendations at this time was able to formulate a common position on the admissibility of prophylactics. See *Rapport der commissie tot onderzoek* 1911:1726; *Centrale Gezondheidsraad* 1919:55-6.

78. That there was a need for the general introduction of prophylactic measures in the armed forces was clear; there was less consent, however, about the way it should be done. See e.g. the debate between various health officers in 'Venerische ziekten bij de zeemacht', *Marineblad* 27 (1912/13):1089-101, 1102-8; 28 (1913/14):236-46, 247-53.

79. R. Bromberg, 'Over huid- en geslachtsaandoeningen bij strijdende of gemobiliseerde legers', *Militair Geneeskundig Tijdschrift* 20 (1916):243-4. See also J.M.C. Mouton, 'Oorlog en geslachtsziekten', *Militair Geneeskundig Tijdschrift* 19 (1915):222: 'The bald fact is that while it is possible to make extra-marital sexual intercourse a little more difficult, there can be no question of any significant reduction, certainly not in the communications zone, and in view of this, we are left with only one method of preventing the associated negative consequences, namely venereal disease, and that method is personal prophylaxis.'

80. See T.M. van Leeuwen, 'De bestrijding der geslachtsziekten', *NTvG* 64 (1920) IA:203.

81. That is not to say that civilians did not use them. The pocket-sized gonorrhoea prophylactic must have been quite popular, judging by the large variety of types and brands that were available (Samariter, Phallokos, Viro, Protector, Sanitas etc.; see P.H. Schoonheid, 'Sexueele paedagogiek als middel van bestrijding der geslachtsziekten', *Medisch Weekblad* 19 (1913), no. 47:556-7 n. 1). That the use of condoms to ward off venereal disease was also no longer uncommon may be inferred from the novel *Een Liefde* (*A Love*) by Lodewijk van Deyssel (1887, vol. II:23), in which the main character reflects that 'he desperately needed a shag. He could go to a whorehouse but he had no liking for rubbers, and without one he found it too risky.' See also Van der Mey in his reaction to Aletta Jacobs in the debate on double standards described in the previous chapter: 'A man will almost certainly protect himself from infection by using a condom and bichloride of mercury' (99). See R. van der Mey, 'Wat Mevrouw Jacobs in 't midden te brengen had', *Minerva. Algemeen Nederlandsch Studenten Weekblad* 27 (1902), no. 8:97-9.

82. L.S.A.M von Römer, 'Venerische ziekten bij de zeemacht', *Marineblad* 28 (1913/14):245.
83. See e.g. Bottema 1931:3.
84. T.M. van Leeuwen, 'De bestrijding der geslachtsziekten', *NTvG* 64 (1920) IA:205.
85. Catharine van Tussenbroek, *NTvG* 39 II (1903):1152-4 (this quotation from 1154).
86. Van der Tuuk 1915:157.
87. Elias [1939], esp. II:239-60.
88. *Geschiedenis van het moderne Nederland* 1988:371-3.
89. See J.J. Bloemen, 'De gevaren, die de openbare gezondheid van de zijde der koopvaardij bedreigen', *SH* vol. V, no. IV (1927):173-85; cf. also Haustein 1927:654.
90. J.J. Bloemen, 'De gevaren, die de openbare gezondheid van de zijde der koopvaardij bedreigen', *SH* vol. V, no. IV (1927):180.
91. See Van Slobbe (1937:118) for a map of this kind.
92. Hermans 1976:56-9; Van Lieburg 1992, Chapter 3.
93. See Houwaart 1991:38-9.
94. These observations are based on De Swaan's theory of the development of collective action, in which interdependency and the extension of external effects are of crucial importance. See De Swaan 1988. For an interesting account of the impact of changing patterns of contact between societies on the spread of infectious disease, see McNeill 1976.
95. See Agreement of Brussels 1958:47-51.
96. *Rapport der commissie tot onderzoek* 1911:1783.
97. T.M. van Leeuwen, 'De bestrijding der geslachtsziekten', *NTvG* 64 (1920) IA:202.
98. See *Vluchten voor de groote oorlog* 1988:45-6.
99. On the notion of a degeneration of moral standards, see L.M. de Buy Wenniger, 'Is de onzedelijkheid gedurende de mobilisatie toegenomen?', *SH* vol. II, no. I (1922):36-8. Lammerts van Bueren (1931:129) also expressed his disappointment, along with many others, in the moral strength of women, which had yielded to the pressures of modern ways of life: 'When regulated prostitution was opposed, it was opposed on the grounds that it was wrong to apply a double standard in morality, that is to say to measure men by different standards than women when it came to moral conduct, which amounted to saying that a man could be permitted to engage in conduct that a woman should deny herself. This double standard was condemned in the abolition of regulated prostitution, and those who are well-disposed towards the welfare of the lives of ordinary

people had hoped that the woman would raise the man to her level, and would set him an example. In various respects the opposite has occurred. The woman has taken to allowing herself to behave in ways men once claimed as their own right, and she has descended to his level instead of elevating him.'

Hijmans (1934:12-4) regarded the increase in immorality among women as a consequence of the complete change in relations between the sexes, to which no one had yet become accustomed, and hoped that this type of conduct would prove to be a transitional phenomenon. Van der Hoog (1930:33-4) explained the looser behaviour of girls in terms of an increase in freedom rather than an increase in immorality; he ascribed the many mistakes made in the realm of sexuality to ignorance.

100.   Van der Hoog [1930]:32-3.

3

Promiscuous Girls (1920–1955)

After the First World War, the debate on venereal disease underwent a subtle shift of tone. The hum of consternation that had become audible in the 1920s about a perceived slackening of moral values had grown steadily louder until for a short time in the late 1940s it reached a crescendo of panic. Promiscuity among girls and young women was the keynote of this concern; between 1930 and 1950, the promiscuous girl in all her manifestations was by far the most important character in the tales of woe related by the narrators of the Dutch Anti-Venereal Disease Society. This chapter will describe the development of this emphasis and relate it to the content and organizational structure of the fight against venereal disease. The chapter will conclude with a consideration of the years immediately after the Second World War, the second period – over fifty years after the *fin-de-siècle* abolitionist offensive – in which the problem of venereal disease aroused especial alarm.

The amateur

As the 1930s progressed, it became an accepted view that professional prostitutes were playing a far less crucial role in the spread of venereal disease than in the past. Time and again this opinion was presented – without much in the way of evidence or explanation – and hailed as a salutary turn of events. Yet satisfaction on this score was soon tempered by a new bugbear, namely what was described as a shocking increase in unpaid extra-marital sexual intercourse. This turned the spotlight on a new source of infection: young women who had sex with a variety of men on a non-professional basis, and who were known variously as occasional prostitutes, pick-up girls or 'amateurs'.[1]

The term 'amateur' bears witness to the fact that extra-marital female sexuality had always been defined, in the debate on venereal disease, in terms of prostitution. The concept reflects something of society's difficulty in seeing women in any position between that of prostitute and source of infection at one end of the scale, and the innocent victim of male desire at the other. Other terms too – 'semi-' and 'pseudo-' prostitutes – show just how hard it was to conceive of an active female sexuality that was separate from prostitution. It was the ways in which the amateur differed from her professional counterpart, rather than the correspondences between them, that occasioned such uneasiness in those who struggled to grasp the new trend.[2] This distinction had three main features.

In the first place, of course, there was the question of payment. The dermatologist Muller emphasized this aspect:

> A prostitute is someone who makes it her profession, from considerations of a financial or material nature, to fulfil the sexual desires of others, exerting little if any selectivity. An amateur, on the other hand, is someone who makes a habit of fulfilling the sexual desires of others, whether for material (or even culinary!) motives or as driven by her libido, and who *is* selective in her actions.[3]

Whereas the professional prostitute had the decency, or sense of tradition, to request payment for the services she provided, the amateur broke with this tradition and contented herself with compensation of a different order, such as an evening out or a new piece of clothing. At least, this was how most people pictured these young women. There was some confusion of terminology, however, as those who occasionally received money were also sometimes defined as 'amateurs', if this did not provide them with a regular source of income. This is how the social worker and Nurse Kuypers described the difference between amateur and professional prostitutes:

> The former – well-known as a source of infection – are girls who engage in a variety of sexual liaisons, but are also in employment. They are found in all classes of society, i.e. among servants, shop-girls, office clerks etc. Their recompense consists less of money than of gifts, visits to the cinema or the public house, fur coats and the like, and differ from professional prostitutes solely in that they do not, as the latter, make their living entirely from prostitution.[4]

In some cases, there was no material compensation whatsoever. The amateur's promiscuity could stem from real enjoyment or it might be, as in the quotation from Muller, 'driven by her libido'.[5]

The second difference was one of social class, or to put it more precisely, of social integration. Every article that appeared on the subject singled out one trait for special attention: amateurs had jobs. They did not work in prostitution but were ordinary wage-earners, and as such were far more part of the regular life of society than prostitutes had ever been. Some were servants, but the majority were factory workers, shop assistants or office clerks. Where social origins were concerned, opinions varied: while some thought the phenomenon was confined to girls of relatively high social standing and others maintained that all ranks of society were concerned, the most common reference was to the lower middle classes.[6] All agreed, however, in identifying a respectable family background as a common denominator. The dermatologist Van der Hoog gave the following description of the girls who were turning up at specialists' surgeries with increasing frequency:

> However, an exceedingly large number of young girls are presently coming to see us, particularly from the middle classes. I am referring to all those thousands of young girls who used to stay at home helping their mothers around the house, but these days work in shops or offices, earn some money there and thus contribute towards the cost of their upkeep, but who have more freedom because of this, and towards whom parents no longer dare to act as resolutely, perhaps, as in the past. Part of this freedom is celebrated in the streets, where new acquaintances are made, and errors in the realm of sex are the inevitable result.[7]

One last point in which amateurs distinguished themselves from professionals concerned safety. In the 1930s, anti-venereal disease campaigners regularly described professional prostitution as far safer than the irregular practices of the amateur and those like her. In 1939, Muller observed, surprisingly, that most prostitutes insisted on their clients using condoms, and

> moreover, prostitutes frequently examine their clients for symptoms of venereal disease, and are in the end frequently able to manipulate them to such an extent as to prevent penetration.[8]

Descriptions of such practices had not been heard before: until recently, safety had not exactly been thought of as the most salient feature of prostitution; witness the efforts described in the previous chapter for the benefit of its victims. But even without the manipulative practices to which Muller referred, professional prostitution appeared to be safer, precisely because the risks involved

126

were so well known. Whereas men would always be to some extent suspicious of a prostitute, they tended to have 'an almost childish faith', in the words of Muller, in the amateur.[9] The medical practitioner Voorhoeve likewise stressed that the embraces of a 'girl-friend' all too frequently conferred a false sense of security:

> For when the brothel was the only place where extra-marital relations were possible, anyone who visited such a place knew the dangers to which he was exposing himself and would be anxiously on the look-out for any visible signs of danger. The red lamp that generally provided some indifferent lighting for the dark rooms served as a danger signal that warned visitors to practise constant vigilance. The girl-friend has no such red danger light in her room. She is more likely to have a cosy table lamp or some soft, indirect lighting that is pleasing to the eye; the colour red is banished altogether. This means there is no warning, no danger signal. The man may become infected by one girl-friend and then infect another, without being aware of what is happening. As this relationship seems so much more innocent than a visit to a brothel, little sores are overlooked.[10]

Men were relatively blind to the risk of venereal disease with their companionable (and less businesslike) girl-friends, while the risks were in fact greater: naïve girls were themselves less alive to the dangers, and took no more account of it than did the men. Where the spread of venereal disease was concerned, a visit to the brothel might be actually the lesser of two evils.

But these arguments are purely theoretical. In order to understand why the promiscuous working girl became such a prominent character in the fight against venereal disease, we must first find the basis on which she was deemed to pose a grave threat. Had there been a definite increase in infections, for instance, that could be traced to these girls? As in earlier periods, we are hampered by a lack of clear data, but something can be said on this score all the same. The decline in incidence of venereal disease that set in shortly after the end of the First World War was reversed in the late 1920s. Numerous doctors working at outpatient clinics reported an increase in the number of patients, but said nothing whatsoever about a strikingly high proportion of promiscuous girls.[11] True, remarks of this kind became quite common in the 1930s, but this was at a time when incidence was falling again.[12] In 1935, the Society conducted a questionnaire among dermatologists and medical practitioners at clinics. The chief fact to emerge from this exercise was that the Netherlands had a conspicuously low incidence of venereal disease in comparison with other countries. The number of new syphilis, gonorrhoea or soft chancre infections per 1,000 inhabitants was 74 in the Netherlands, as against an annual rate of 292, 300 and 298 in Germany, France and Denmark respectively.[13] These figures cannot unfortunately be compared with any for previous years, nor do they include any breakdown into male vs. female cases. But even if we assume that the proportion of a new category of girls had risen sharply, it remains the case that the incidence of new infections in the Netherlands had seldom been so low. Anti-venereal disease campaigners would later look back nostalgically to the relative calm of the 1930s.[14]

This lack of documentation for the advance of the amateur applies equally at local level. Medical practitioners and social workers who discussed the increasing significance of the amateur seldom presented any figures to support their case. The occasional social worker might produce something from her own records, but in general there was a complete lack of evidence for the development described.[15] What statistics we do have fail to corroborate the belief in the advance of the disease-ridden amateur. The records kept by Rotterdam municipal outpatient clinic show that in the mid-1930s, most female patients belonged to the categories of 'housewife' and 'prostitute', who accounted for 56% and 19% respectively of the female patient population. These are followed, but at considerable distance, by the categories of 'servant' (5%), 'waitress' (3%) and 'charwoman' (3%). Among male patients, the majority were seafarers, men who worked in the street (merchants, haulers, milkmen) and factory workers. In 1935, 25% of these men had become infected through paid sexual favours, while the figure for 1937 was 37%.[16] All told, these figures neither bear out nor disprove the story related with so much confidence at this time. The patient population considered here is too unrepresentative to be used in either way.

In short, although the true state of affairs is impossible to reconstruct, the growing public concern about the amateur as a source of infection at least until the Second World War, cannot be explained by the available data. So even if the promiscuous girl had become as widespread as commentators suggested, the perils of associating with her were at any rate exaggerated. To understand the narrators' tales, we need to look beyond mere statistics.

The problem can perhaps best be approached by recalling that the amateur was a girl with a job. Girls who went out to work were not of course a new phenomenon in the 1920s and 1930s. Even so, this trend was blamed for much of the decline in moral standards – also in contexts unconnected with the debate on venereal disease – that was so bemoaned in this period. Religious groups in particular were horrified by the depravity of modern times, and launched a vigorous offensive to ward off a further degeneration.[17] Working girls were not the sole target of this offensive, but certain contemporary problems were undeniably projected onto them.

In the working classes, the notion that factory work for girls was tied in with moral decay had been common currency since the late 19th century. In the mood of moral anxiety that set in during the 1920s and 1930s, attention focused on female factory workers once again. Part of the concern was related to the wretched conditions under which many girls worked and the soul-destroying monotony of their duties, but many other features attracted opprobrium: the girls' vile and suggestive language, their uninhibited sexuality, the youthful age at which dating began, a blunting of moral sensitivity and habits such as drinking, going out on the town, flirtatiousness and the use of make-up. Factory girls were associated with such a range of evils that several campaigns were set up with a view to their edification. Classes were organized in subjects ranging from cooking and needlework to religious instruction, the girls were given decent rooms to sit in during their breaks, and they were prepared for their prospective duties as housewives and mothers. Most of these activities took place under the banner of Catholic campaigns such as the Eucharistic Crusade for Factory Girls.[18] This is not so surprising when one recalls that the modern industries had established themselves chiefly in the Catholic south of the country with its large families, where cheap female labour was easiest to find. Furthermore, Catholic disquiet was fed by an 'indifference to religion' among the girls that attracted much comment, and by the magnetism that 'the utopias of socialism' were said to exert on the young employees of industry.[19]

In the 1920s and 1930s, this concern about a laxity of moral standards moved beyond the factory gates to include other working girls such as shop assistants, office clerks and public servants. In his *Rotterdam sketches of manners* the journalist Brusse observed in the early 1920s that the participation of women in the world of work was having far-reaching consequences on relations between the sexes.[20] Now that girls were increasingly abandoning their traditional environment – the family – and spending their days in factories, workshops, shops and offices, in Brusse's view, their feminine characteristics were being increasingly undermined by the hard businesslike attitudes of industry, with the result that men and women found themselves on a different footing. For what did women have with which to defend themselves from this businesslike manner? How could they keep afloat in the competitive world outside except by exercising the 'power of their charms'? They used their salaries largely to spruce themselves up; to be elegantly dressed in the latest fashion had long ceased to be the prerogative of a few privileged ladies. Hence class differences became increasingly blurred, and at the same time, seduction became an increasingly important element of professional relations between the sexes:

> And the factory girls, together with the young shop assistants, short-hand typists, ironing girls and seamstresses, the maidservants and female officials at the counters all make use of those enticements, with their short skirts and see-through stockings, low necks, paper-thin blouses and dresses which display their figures so flatteringly, their provocative hairdos, naughty lace embroidery and silk bows just peeping out, their powder and parfumes. And early each morning they leave home for work in this way, dressed as people used to dress when they were going to a ball or an evening party, in flimsy outfits that sometimes look more like bathing suits – nothing but a seductive covering – and the employers and the supervisors, the bosses and the foremen and the menservants and male workers and officials all have to preserve their composure in these circumstances in an unflinchingly businesslike manner.[21]

The same desire for pleasure that was expressed in their clothing, according to Brusse, meant that working girls were no longer satisfied with the simple atmosphere of their parental home, were little inclined, if at all, to obey their mother and father, and increasingly preferred to seek their amusement elsewhere: in the street, at the cinema, on the dance floor or in the company of men with status and money. And 'as for what all this leads to', Brusse concludes, 'the physicians, the general practitioners, and above all the gynaecologists could tell you in volumes of sad tales'.[22]

The concern expressed by the girls' contemporaries focused particularly on the external forms of pleasure that Brusse referred to as popular among working girls. After the First World War, the growing popularity of dancing halls and cinemas provoked a wave of indignation. Alongside the protests of religious groups (again largely Catholic) came fierce opposition to these new forms of recreation from the social democrats. 'Where there is diversion without any mental exertion, that is where the girls will be found', the female lawyer Ribbius Peletier, secretary of the Association of Social Democrat Women's Clubs, told her audience in a conference on the family held in 1937:

> [you will find her] in the cinema and in the dancing hall – which establishments also, moreover, satisfy her desire to make contact with the opposite sex. Our profit-minded entertainment industry responds to demand. No-one asks whether what is being offered is good and responsible; public demand and the best ways of making a profit are all that counts. Hence girls' inclinations and the desire of the entertainment industry to make money point in the same direction, both tending to ensure that girls spend their leisure time in idle amusement.[23]

Of all the forms of vulgar amusement to which working girls dedicated themselves, modern dancing, in the eyes of their censorious contemporaries, constituted the most serious threat to morality. The sexual nature of dancing itself, the primitive stimulation it generated and the frivolous behaviour between men and women in the dance halls caused many to regard the prevailing 'dance craze' as an unacceptable fad.[24] A frequent visitor to these vile surroundings, not unexpectedly, was the amateur. In 1928, the committee on popular amusement published a report on the new dance halls, observing that:

> In general there is a tendency for dance halls to become meeting-places for men and women, and assignations are a frequent result. In many cases amateurs are involved, that is to say girls of the better social classes who engage in sexual intercourse without deriving any financial benefit.[25]

The self-appointed arbiters of moral standards in society became more and more firmly convinced, in the 1920s and 1930s, that the immorality long associated with factory girls was spreading to working girls of other classes. In trying to understand this concern, it would be well to begin by finding out, firstly, whether there had been a great increase in the number of girls with paid employment. A casual glance reveals nothing of the kind. When we look at the working population, the invariable proportion of female workers is striking: between 1900 and 1960, the percentage of women in the total working population remained at more or less the same level, at around 23%.[26] A closer look at the figures, however, reveals a different picture. Although women made up a constant proportion of the total workforce, their absolute numbers almost doubled simply because of the overall growth of the working population. In 1909 there were some 540,000 working women, by 1930 there were over 760,000 and by 1947 there were over 940,000.[27]

Another significant change was in the kind of women who were taking paid employment. Single women had always worked more than those who were married, but this imbalance was becoming even more skewed. Increasingly, single young women worked, but gave up their jobs after marriage.[28] The reduction in the number of working married women was partly due to the greater responsibility of women within the family, which was increasingly difficult to combine with paid employment, and was also a consequence of the fact that government policies were making it increasingly difficult for married women to work in the first few decades of this century. In 1924 it was even decided to release female government employees from public service on their wedding day.[29] Because of this, girls from a wide range of social backgrounds who had paid employment prior to marriage were becoming an increasingly large majority. There is nothing to suggest that they were driven out of the labour market during the 1930s depression.[30]

One final change relates to jobs that were done mainly by women. There was a striking fall in the number of women employed in domestic positions. Since the end of the 19th century, more and more girls had opted for factory work rather than entering domestic service because it offered more independence, higher wages, more acceptable working hours and contact with other girls. The percentage of women performing factory work remained approximately constant until 1930, while in absolute terms there was a substantial increase. Finally, another significant increase, after 1930 even in proportional terms, was visible in the service sector – government, education and medical services – and in clerical positions.[31] The increase in the number of female office staff was particularly striking: between 1910 and 1930, their numbers rose from some 4,000 to about 48,000, and by 1947 they exceeded 84,000. Indeed, it was these young women who largely accounted for the expansion of the new middle classes between the wars.[32]

These three trends, which first set in around 1900 and gathered steam after the First World War – the absolute increase in numbers of working women, the proportional increase of single young women as wage-earners and the shift in the type of employment done largely by women – play a significant role in the background to the debate on standards of morality. To contemporary commentators on morality, the consequences were clearly visible in the emergence of a new category of working girls. They were 'new' partly in the sense that the army of female workers was larger, more youthful and more diversified than ever before: they were not just factory workers and shop assistants but office and counter clerks, telephonists, short-hand typists and secretaries, they were hairdressers, carers and nurses.

But modern working girls contrasted with their predecessors in other ways. Young and single female wage-earners had a stronger position in relation to their parents partly because they contributed to the family income, and this independence – far greater than girls had had in the past – also gave them more freedom outside the home.[33] Brusse too pinpoints this connection, as he ponders what happens when a daughter finally returns home after 'a night out':

> And when she comes home, her father is beside himself with fury – but her mother will try to calm things down, and sometimes she succeeds in subduing the tempest ... partly because a girl of 18 to 20, say, a short-hand typist with a salary of 120 or 150 guilders a month, has after all become an indispensable wage-earner in the home. And if her parents make life too unpleasant, what is there to keep her there? With wages like this, she can always go and find rooms of her own – especially if, for the time being, she enjoys the favours of a 'smart gentleman'.[34]

The favours of a 'smart gentleman' were indeed a necessity, as the average girl's wages were not enough to live on.[35] Most of them continued to live with their parents. But their independence as wage-earners combined with two other long-term economic advances that had been effected at the same time – higher standards of living and the shorter working day – making it possible for their leisure time to acquire a special character of its own. Increasing numbers of people had money to spend over and above their essential expenses and more time for sport and recreation. The development of an urban industrial society created the conditions for the rise of a commercial amusement and entertainment industry. After the First World War, the transformation and commercialization of traditional forms of amusement moved into top gear. Large old theatres made way for cheaper cinemas, and the traditional dancing establishments for soldiers, sailors and lower-class girls were swiftly replaced by bars and dancing halls with new kinds of music and modern types of dancing. An indulgence in leisure pursuits, once the province of a small elite, was suddenly within the reach of far more people, and this included more and more single working girls.

Dancing was certainly a favourite pastime of working girls. Anxious onlookers of both religious and secular persuasions shook their heads at the tango, the charleston and the shimmy that had captured young people's imaginations. These dances had been introduced into the Netherlands around the turn of the century, but at first only certain young men and women from the urban upper middle classes had come into contact with them.[36] After the First World War, the dance craze moved beyond the scope of an elite, with dance halls mushrooming and the new dances rapidly sweeping the country, starting with the cities and then conquering the provinces. For young people from the middle classes, dance schools were set up which taught respectable adaptations of the new dances. Those who preferred the unexpurgated version went to one of the many new bars or dance halls. These public establishments were frequented mainly by young working people, with girls in the majority.[37] We have already seen the widespread consternation that was generated as working girls flocked to the dance hall, but none of the efforts to halt or deflect the onward march of this new popular culture, whether with dance licences or stern admonitions and menacing sermons, had any noticeable impact.

We are now in a position to answer the question put at the opening of this section, that is to say, where the public commotion about amateurs, and by extension about the conduct of other groups of working girls, came from. First and foremost it had to do with the advent of the new category of working girls just described. Some may choose to emphasize that girls' wages often became an indispensable supplement to their parents' income, that most of their free time was still consumed by household duties, and that in many cases their work was too monotonous and tiring, and too poorly paid to allow for a busy night life. But this is not the whole story. The fact that these young girls had an income of their own, whatever the drawbacks, was also a source of potential emancipation. They were young, there were thousands of them and they had money, however little it may have been in some cases, to spend outside their working hours as they saw fit, which also gave them a measure of economic power. Where their own wages or pocket money did not suffice, new kinds of relationships between boys and girls grew to fill the gap. The relatively low wages of girls tended to foster many infernal new-fangled conventions such as casual boy–girl relationships and dates.[38]

These changes in the position of girls and young women may be regarded as one aspect of a wide-ranging process of modernization of women's lives that took place between the wars. 'The result of this complex and under-researched process', writes the historian Marjan Schwegman, 'was the birth of a new kind of woman.'[39] The particular variant of the new woman that we are considering here, the young single wage-earner, made her entry into a number of arenas. Aside from her role as the villain of the piece in debates on venereal disease and other moral polemics, she also became a regular feature of the worlds of fashion, advertising and literature. The rise of a new generation of women was recorded clearly in novels such as *De Opstandigen* (*The Rebels*, 1926) by Jo van Ammers-Küller and *De Klop op de Deur* (*The Knock on the Door*, 1930) by Ina Boudier-Bakker, although the image reproduced in these books is not devoid of caricature.[40]

The amateur certainly has humbler origins than her literary counterparts. But she does have certain features in common with them: like the office clerk and the dancing girl, she is a prototype of the modern working girl, and we are therefore justified in linking her position at the centre of controversy to the social trends that made the rise of a new kind of girl possible and to the anxiety this new apparition generated in establishment circles. Their concern coloured the new interpretation that these groups gave to what they saw changing around them. Girls were indeed changing, but that is not to say that they were turning into amateurs. In fact the amateur as a separate category seems largely to have been a figment of the imagination concocted by the worried and preoccupied minds of medical practitioners, anti-venereal disease campaigners, Catholic educators and others who thought they were witnessing the collapse of public morality. They were driven by a deeply entrenched opposition to all post-war modernization, and the slacker morals becoming accepted by the 'decent' classes particularly horrified them.[41] It is my contention that, as a result of this revulsion, they adopted a specific moralistic approach to the changes they witnessed, and interpreted them purely in terms of moral degeneration.

In their concern about the slackening of moral standards in 'decent' circles, the moral reformers certainly appear also to have been partly driven by a fear of 'social contamination'.[42] They saw the threat to high moral standards as originating in the contact between 'higher' and 'lower' social classes, given that the latter had an age-old reputation for licentiousness. In this light their central obsession with working girls is far from coincidental. The employment found by modern working girls was no longer dictated along traditional lines by their social origins. In the past, the majority of working women came from the working classes, performed factory work and was clearly marked off from a far smaller group of women from higher social classes who worked in the 'civilized professions'. But from the 1920s onwards, these lines became increasingly blurred, as the daughters of skilled workers succeeded more and more frequently in finding jobs as teachers, nurses, short-hand typists, telephonists or secretaries, all of which had previously been reserved for the respectable daughters of the middle classes.[43] At the same time, unskilled working-class girls entered the job market in poorly paid positions operating punch card readers or counting machines, as many banks and major trade companies mechanized their accounting around 1930.[44] On the other hand, the 1930s economic slump made it a good deal harder for middle-class girls to attend expensive courses, so that they often ended up in jobs their predecessors would have sniffed at as beneath their dignity. Although class barriers were not exactly dismantled – there was no question of a free intermingling between all layers of society – the working life of modern girls nevertheless developed into a fairly mixed phenomenon. In the 1920s and 1930s, girls from a variety of social backgrounds were more likely to meet at work than those of previous generations. They might also meet each other at the dance halls, for here too, the public was more mixed than in the traditional amusements that had been popular before the First World War.[45] In these surroundings, the contacts between boys and girls 'of every social class' prompted grave concern, as is clear from the spate of articles devoted to the new 'dance craze'.[46]

With the wisdom of hindsight, it is easy to see that the effect of this feared amalgam was considerably less explosive than it appeared to the somewhat overheated imaginations of contemporary moralists. Most girls simply did their jobs, wearing suitable clothes, and sometimes went dancing at a safe distance from the 'abyss of sins' that worried observers associated with the subject of modern dance.[47] But while we should not take the highly sexualized impact described by anxious commentators at face value, it was certainly true that times were changing. The power acquired by girls and the onward march of a modern, organized popular culture that crossed class lines did indeed have an effect on prevailing morality.

The changes witnessed by these observers may be viewed as the first hesitant steps towards a free sexual market, if we may call it that, enabling a further differentiation of female sexuality. While in the past there were only two extremes, sex within marriage and prostitution, in the 1920s and 1930s large groups of girls developed sexual practices that resisted classification according to this traditional dichotomy.[48] Because of the new convention of 'going steady', it was no longer the case that every expression of sexuality prior to marriage was necessarily pernicious. Furthermore, the acceptance of an evening out or a gift instead of money severed the traditional association with prostitution, though some observers – at any rate anti-venereal disease campaigners, as we have already seen – regularly insisted on it. The appearance of the amateur in the debate on venereal disease is linked to the emergence of a pre-marital female sexuality that could no longer be automatically situated within the lower classes or described as prostitution.

Social work

The appearance of the amateur affected the organization and practices of the anti-venereal disease movement. Essentially, this new character marked the demise of the traditional link between prostitution and venereal disease. Although, as we have seen, most observers were loath to let this connection go, promiscuity gradually replaced prostitution as the key concept. This meant abandoning the traditional epidemiological model, which had been schematized as clusters of infection, each in the form of a spoke with wheels, with the source of disease at the hub. A model of this kind presented the number of infections in each cluster as limited: the old story went that the prostitute, as the source, infected her clients, after which a second and possibly a third case of infection (wife, offspring) might follow. Tragic though this tale was, the end of every spoke remained visible. Once the focus shifted to promiscuity, this epidemiological model had to be discarded; in theory, promiscuous sexual relations allowed for an endless series of infections.

Venereal disease campaigners did not change their perspective overnight; it was not until the 1940s that the wheel model was finally replaced by a new construction. But even in the 1930s the fight against venereal disease acquired a somewhat more dynamic character; with the appearance of the amateur, the existence of freer sexual liaisons was acknowledged, and contact tracing became a central issue.

In the age of the amateur, 'social modes of control' became popular. The man chiefly responsible for its introduction was the dermatologist E.H. Hermans, who had been involved in the establishment of the clinic for the port of Rotterdam in 1925, and had promoted the follow-up system there. This system was based on the two principles of case-finding and case-holding: the detection of VD sufferers and ensuring their continued treatment. Hermans had a great deal of success with this approach in Rotterdam. As people outside the port clinic gravitated more and more to an epidemiological model with a wider range than the wheel, the need for a more active and investigative approach was felt more urgently there too. The old system of advice centres, however, was inadequately equipped to work along the lines of case-finding and case-holding. The organization of the anti-venereal disease effort was ripe for renewal.

In the early 1930s, the Dutch Anti-Venereal Disease Society, which had hitherto borne responsibility for this organization, handed over many of its tasks to the district nursing services, such as the Green and White Cross. These services had long possessed a far-flung network of outpatient clinics, social work and district nursing services, which the anti-venereal disease campaigners would be able to use. Provincial committees were appointed to this end, their members drawn from the Government Health Inspectorate as well as the district nursing services and the Anti-Venereal Disease Society. Each provincial committee ran one or more VD advice centres, headed by a dermatologist and backed up by one or more social workers. These advice centres – like those set up in the 1920s – were emphatically not meant to provide much in the way of medical treatment. GPs had to feel free to send their patients there for advice and social assistance without being apprehensive that they might lose them. In this way, a new system of venereal disease control gradually took shape. By about 1940 over 30 advice centres were active,[49] all of which operated according to the guidelines set down in a special pamphlet.[50]

The government's role in controlling venereal disease was gradually increasing, partly through the influence of the Health Inspectors in the provincial committees, but also through the state subsidies that these committees received to run their advice centres. The Society was less and less involved in direct intervention to curb venereal disease. With much of its work having been taken over by the district nursing associations, it was able to concentrate all its energies on what it had always seen as its main activity: 'inculcating proper attitudes to sexual hygiene and sexual morality'.[51] To underscore this change of direction, the Society briefly changed its name, in 1933, to the Dutch Society for Moral Hygiene, and again a year later, to the Dutch Society for Moral Public Health. Its role in direct VD control was increasingly confined to the unflagging efforts of Hermans, the Society's secretary.

Organization aside, the actual content of the work was also changing, as the advice centres focused increasingly on social work. Although the older centres too had provided such facilities – ensuring that patients continued their treatment by properly informing them, applying persuasion or providing financial assistance – the painstaking work associated with case-finding did not get under way until the 1930s, with Hermans as its passionate advocate. He was personally responsible for training the first generation of women social workers in the province of South Holland, and believed 'that this social work is of greater value than all the treatment we can give'.[52] The social workers' main tasks were persuading reluctant patients to go on with their treatment and tracing sources of infection and sexual contacts, but they were often obliged to delve into other fields. Associating with uncooperative patients – with home visits a frequent necessity – confronted the social workers head on with a host of social ills. Contrary to the theories that stressed the amateur's leading role in the spread of venereal disease, much of what they encountered was reminiscent of the traditional range of problems: housing shortage, alcoholism, unemployment, prostitution and abuse. Their work thus rapidly broadened in scope: prostitutes had to be urged to turn over a new leaf, women needed help in arranging a divorce or finding accommodation and suitable employment, children often had to be cared 'for when a patient was admitted to hospital, and young girls had to be kept off the street and away from the dance halls and encouraged to join respectable clubs. For all these problems, consultations with other bodies were needed, or people had to be referred elsewhere; at any rate, social workers could not simply ignore them. J. Muizebelt, a nurse speaking to an assembly of medical practitioners and social workers in 1937, declared:

> Dr Hermans has taught us that we should concern ourselves with social conditions as little as possible. Our task is to track down sources and to ensure that patients continue to follow treatment. Having worked in this field for about a year, I would be so bold as to question – with all due respect to the views of my teacher – the practical applicability of this view. It is simply not possible to ignore all the attendant circumstances. It is not possible, because in the course of this search you stumble on conditions that you had not expected. Close your eyes to them? Your *whole feminine being* revolts against such an approach. Hands are reaching out to you for help.[53]

With this appeal to her feminine being, Nurse Muizebelt must have touched a sensitive spot in her audience; that social work was real women's work was something about which all parties agreed. It could not be sufficiently emphasized that tact, patience and dedication were the prime requirements in social work, and women irrefutably possessed these qualities to a greater extent than men. But this did not mean, according to Hermans, that all women were equally suited to this work:

> Candidates must be exceedingly tactful, patient, modest and cultivated. They must demonstrate a capacity to sympathize with the views and beliefs of others, and their work must not be driven by curiosity about the events taking place in the sexual sphere.[54]

Only women who were themselves mature and cultivated would be capable of steering girls – and homes – that had gone astray back on course, of gaining people's confidence and giving them moral support without their authority being undermined. Social work was a job that required women who, in the words of dermatologist J.J. Zoon, 'with great compassion for the human being afflicted with venereal disease, do their work with knowledge and conviction. To perform this task, mature women are needed, women who have a positive attitude and a broad general education.'[55]

The specific feminine slant given to the profession stemmed in part from relations between medical practitioners and social workers at the advice centres, and may be regarded as a compromise acceptable to both parties. For social workers, the typically feminine nature of the work helped procure recognition for their profession. It made their work easily distinguishable from that of GPs or doctors attached to advice centres, and underscored the fact that these men would not necessarily be able, if called upon to do so, to do their work.[56] Medical practitioners had different duties, wrote Nurse A.M. van der Meijden, while her own work

> is purely a social task and a specific care task. It is very time-consuming and requires much tact. A doctor with a busy practice has no time for such things.[57]

While the emphasis on their womanly qualities enabled social workers to define their profession more precisely and to forestall any male incursions into their territory, it also enabled male medical practitioners to leave a significant amount of work to another group without it affecting their position. Precisely by emphasizing the typically feminine aspects of the work, it became easier to separate the two areas, and that the doctor's work was at the top of the hierarchy was deemed self-evident. At the 1937 conference for social workers and medical practitioners already referred to, Zoon also emphasized the 'tact, dedication and patience' that social work required. The doctor's busy duties left him insufficient time for this, and experience had shown that women were far better suited to the task of social worker:

> It is not up to the medical practitioner to try to solve these problems; even if he had the time, he is not the appropriate person to do so ... . This is where the social worker is needed; if she acts tactfully, she can win people's confidence more easily and help the persons concerned to achieve a proper understanding of the situation.[58]

In the prevailing hierarchy, commented Zoon, the social worker thus constituted 'the vital link between doctor and patient'.[59] Hermans' introduction struck the same note. While he expressed his admiration for what social workers achieved, he left the audience in no doubt as to his views on the balance of power that should be preserved:

> The nature of the problem is such that, at all advice centres, the chief medical practitioner should be in charge, something that the social workers should never forget; for although the nurses are undoubtedly responsible for most of the practical tasks, all the centre's work nevertheless takes place under the supervision and responsibility of the chief medical staff.[60]

The fact that this distinction in professional status corresponded to a gender difference made it appear more logical, and undoubtedly helped to maintain it.

All the investigative work, assistance, admonitions, advice and wise words with which social workers surrounded their clients, and all the intimate confessions that they procured along the way, placed the social workers in a long tradition of the middle-class work of civilizing society, in which the poor, the sick and the needy were visited, helped and edified by women of the more civilized classes. Aside from alleviating distress, initiatives of this kind in areas, for instance, such as poor relief, housing assistance and child protection, were partly intended to be educational and uplifting for the lower classes.[61] Although the amateur did not belong to the poorest sections of society, the same was basically true of the social work in venereal disease control. The chasm between her and the social worker remained wide in this case too, if not always on the social scale, certainly in terms of age and moral prestige.

In one respect, however, social work in venereal disease control differed from many middle-class activities in other areas: while elsewhere, the combination of help and moral elevation, of care and coercion, of support and supervision, would often be reinforced with certain sanctions, no such possibility existed where venereal disease control was concerned. Against what was often viewed as laziness, truculence and misconduct, others could take action such as stopping welfare payments, eviction, taking away parental authority or suchlike measures. But when faced with a prostitute who refused to listen to her, a patient who objected to having his movements recorded, or a girl who broke off a course of treatment halfway through, a social worker in venereal disease control was ultimately helpless. All she had were her powers of persuasion.

The possibility, and desirability, of introducing coercive measures regularly came up for discussion. The Scandinavian countries had the longest tradition in this area, but Germany too had introduced sanctions in 1927, both for medical practitioners – in the form of a reporting obligation – and for VD sufferers. The debate in the Netherlands focused on the latter, in other words on introducing a legal obligation for the persons affected to undergo medical treatment, and defining the wilful infection of another person as a criminal offence. Before the Second World War, most of those involved in venereal disease control rejected the introduction of coercive measures. Especially within the Dutch Anti-Venereal Disease Society, where people like De Graaf and Van Leeuwen still held sway, there was a tendency to see such measures as regulated prostitution in a new guise – coercion was even referred to as 'neo-regulation' – and to dismiss it out of hand.[62]

An occasional voice was raised in support of coercion, however, and it often came from the ranks of social workers. Given the passivity with which they were forced to watch obstinate patients frustrating their fine professional intentions, it is not surprising that they, more than anyone else, sometimes bemoaned the lack of sanctions. But before the war very little notice was taken of their views.

We can be sure that many people were unwilling to entertain the idea of statutory measures because they objected on grounds of principle. But another explanation for the lack of interest, and one at least as important, was that the incidence of venereal disease in the Netherlands was extremely low in the 1930s. In these favourable circumstances, fundamental objections scarcely came under pressure, and the disadvantages of coercive measures were deemed to outweigh the potential benefit. During the next few years, however, this situation changed dramatically.

The war: coercion and new modes of treatment

The Second World War called an abrupt halt to the low incidence of venereal disease that had prevailed in the Netherlands in the 1930s. In the latter half of the years of occupation, in particular, the number of cases soared, but even after liberation they continued to rise, attaining 'a frightening peak' in 1946 and 1947, after which they rapidly fell again.[63] In all, the increase justified the label of 'epidemic', albeit a short-lived one: the number of syphilis patients registered at advice centres grew, roughly, by a factor of fifteen between 1940 and 1947, but by the early 1950s the situation had returned to normal. The increase in gonorrhoea cases was less dramatic: the number of patients was about five times the pre-war level, and here too, things returned to normal a few years later.[64]

People tried to halt the epidemic in a variety of ways. One significant improvement in treatment had been achieved in 1937, just before the outbreak of war, when sulfa drugs were first introduced for the treatment of gonorrhoea. These preparations appeared at first to be extremely effective: they caused relatively few adverse side-effects, and they cut back the length of treatment from several months to a few days.[65] All this wrought an immense improvement in the existing situation, but after a few years difficulties nevertheless arose, as the gonorrhoea bacteria developed a large measure of resistance to the new drugs. Nevertheless, the sulfa drugs were the first compounds with a powerful action against gonorrhoea. There were no important breakthroughs in the treatment of syphilis before the war, and patients were still given a combination of Salvarsan and bismuth. After the introduction of penicillin, in 1943, this situation would at long last start to change.

Aside from treatment, establishments engaged in venereal disease control during the occupation continued to rely heavily on social work. The growth in numbers of patients served to reinforce the belief that to succeed, medical treatment must be part of a more comprehensive system of social action. Furthermore, social workers had long demanded an expansion in their scope for tracking down sufferers and ensuring that they finished their treatment. Now, during the occupation, this was achieved: one of the decrees promulgated by the German occupying forces for the occupied territory of the Netherlands was the 'Decree containing provisions to prevent the spread of venereal diseases', which entered into effect in October 1940.[66] Pursuant to this decree, which was modelled on a law that existed in Germany, it became possible, where it could be assumed 'on the basis of facts or circumstances' that there was a danger of a particular person spreading venereal disease, to compel him by force to submit to medical treatment, and if necessary to hospitalize him; furthermore, if patients absconded they could be traced with police assistance.

A year later, new ordinances were added on the supervision of prostitutes. In effect, this second series of ordinances amounted to the reintroduction of regulated prostitution: any woman who made her living from immoral acts was obliged to show her identity papers to the police on demand, and to submit to regular medical examinations. This latter provision was in fact never implemented. However, German and Dutch police did on several occasions raid suspicious-looking bars, arrest the women and girls there and examine them for signs of venereal disease.[67] Professional anti-venereal disease workers looked on practices of this kind with undiluted disgust, and were just as fiercely opposed to any effort to reintroduce regulated prostitution into the Netherlands; no more attempts to do so were made after the liberation.

About the ordinances that had been promulgated in 1940, however, opinions were more positive. Although they were of German origin, these coercive measures became fairly popular during the occupation years, and enforced treatment in particular appeared to work quite well. Although the Anti-Venereal Society had initially been opposed to this coercion, after the war members were calling it 'acceptable', 'indispensable' and 'extremely useful'.[68] And social workers were in no doubt whatsoever: coercion, at least for the time being, had to stay. And stay it did: the German ordinances were adopted almost wholesale by the Military Authority and they remained in force until 1952.

For the armed forces themselves – as in the previous war – venereal disease again proved to be an urgent problem. For the Dutch military authorities the situation was different this time, because the army was no longer in action as such after the defeat suffered in May 1940. After the country's liberation, however, the trouble started again: in 1946, 38 out of every thousand re-enlisted men had venereal disease, a figure comparable to that in the Dutch army just after the First World War.[69] The policy pursued by the military authorities had not changed much over the intervening years: the use of prophylactics was still surrounded with difficulties, so that it was once again necessary to resort to the Dutch compromise of 'early treatment'.[70] The allied armies tackled the problem differently. The Americans, for instance, with the disastrous figures from the First World War still engraved vividly on their memories, aside from handing out vast numbers of prophylactic kits, also supplied their men with some 50 million condoms a month, their motto being 'if you can't say no, take a pro'.[71] During the war, this policy appeared to be reasonably successful, and the number of infected men in the US army was considerably lower than in the First World War. After the war ended, however, this preventive policy no longer seemed to work.[72]

Partly because of this, it was an enormous relief to the allied armies when the new drug penicillin became available around the end of the war. Although the anti-bacterial action of the mould that would later become known by this name had been noted by the Scottish microbiologist Alexander Fleming as far back as 1929, it was not until the 1940s that this discovery – under the pressure of wartime – was given a medical application. After an unusually brief experimental period, production and distribution of the new drug started in the United States, and other antibiotics soon followed in its train.[73] Penicillin acted as no other drug against infected wounds and a large number of infectious diseases, including gonorrhoea and syphilis. In the first instance, the drug was intended for military use: from 1944 onwards, increasing quantities of it were given to the US troops. In the Dutch armed forces too, penicillin was administered systematically in 1946 and 1947, with evident success. Even so, we must again ask whether policy measures and drugs can do any more than consolidate an existing trend. There is no conclusive evidence proving that penicillin was the one *decisive* factor that reduced the number of infections: when penicillin was being administered in the army, it was far from routinely prescribed among the civilian population, certainly not for syphilis. Yet the syphilis epidemic rapidly died down after 1947 among civilians too.[74]

The use of penicillin outside the military domain was in fact a post-war development, and as a treatment for syphilis it gained acceptance quite slowly. As far as gonorrhoea was concerned, penicillin soon took the place of the sulfa drugs, which were by then less and less effective, and its properties were so obvious as to sweep aside any incipient doubts. In 1949 Dr J.R. Prakken, professor of dermatology at the University of Amsterdam, exclaimed in sanguine mood that 'with the advent of penicillin, gonorrhoea is now a benign ailment; tracing sources of infection and monitoring the continuation of treatment are in general of little importance'.[75] But in syphilis treatment the same hesitation occurred that had marked the introduction of Salvarsan. It was some time before the Salvarsan-bismuth combination was completely superseded by antibiotics. Although penicillin was superior to the existing drugs in terms of effectiveness and length of treatment, it was accompanied by more problems than in the case of gonorrhoea. For this reason, many medical practitioners were unconvinced that penicillin alone would suffice, if administered in the later stages of the disease. They used it only when certain specific indications were present, or as supplementary to the Salvarsan-bismuth treatment.[76] After 1950, however, penicillin became standard here too. Although penicillin cannot therefore be said to have been instrumental in halting the syphilis epidemic among the civilian population, it did help prevent a large increase in tertiary cases one or more decades later. When we look at deaths from syphilis during the period 1900–1945, we see a fairly constant figure, averaging 400–500 annually. After 1947 fatalities steadily declined.[77]

Drifting ice

In the Introduction it was noted that certain periods in history have witnessed a marked upsurge in public concern about venereal disease, periods in which the debate has become unusually vehement and wide-ranging. At such moments, instead of being a matter for medical practitioners, other workers in the field and their anonymous patients, venereal disease suddenly becomes the subject of lively debate for a variety of interest groups throughout society. One such period was the closing decade of the 19th century, and another – albeit shorter – was the time immediately after the Second World War.

The debate that flared up shortly after the liberation of the Netherlands was in many ways a continuation of controversies from before the war, but the issues were now magnified and intensified. As in the 1930s, venereal disease was placed in the broad context of a decline in moral standards, and the protagonist of the piece was the promiscuous young woman. Some professionals in the field of venereal disease control had been hammering away at these arguments during the occupation years. Hermans, for instance, addressed a conference held in 1942 that was attended by representatives of various organizations involved in the struggle to halt the moral corruption they saw deepening around them. His contribution, which was entitled 'Moral degeneracy: some

146

preliminary observations', is illustrative for the mood of the times. In it, he observed that the dislocating effect of wartime had prompted 'an alarming wave of moral corruption and degeneracy among the Dutch youth, most especially among Dutch girls, but also among a good deal of Dutch women who have left their girlhood behind them'. The struggle against 'unbridled sexuality' and 'shamelessness in the realm of morals' should be aimed primarily, in Hermans' view, at the 'countless "amateurs" who are presently guilty of misconduct; in other words, these are girls and women who are not compelled to engage in a variety of sexual relations, but who actually seek out such activity themselves'.[78] In both tone and content, Hermans' words were a more incisive variation on prevailing themes from before the war, but they also heralded the widespread panic that would set in after the country's liberation.

This post-war mood of panic, as already noted, placed venereal disease firmly within a broader complex of moral corruption. Many were convinced that the war had had a devastating effect on public morality, leaving the country in a moral morass. People had learnt how to lie and cheat, they had become used to cutting corners and they were now motivated solely by blatant materialism and vulgar diversions. The youth no longer possessed any lofty moral values or ideals, and pursued only the most superficial of pleasures. In the area of sexuality too, the wounds inflicted by the war had struck deep. In many cases, family life had been totally disrupted, and traditional sexual inhibitions had been increasingly eroded.

> The war has violently awoken latent sexual instincts and set them loose. Like a wanton icebreaker it has ploughed through the cold surface of our sexual morality, and now the dykes are groaning beneath the weight of the drifting ice.[79]

This description by A. Bouman reflected the apprehensions of the majority. As a lawyer and a zealous campaigner against immorality, he tried to repair the damage done by the war, for instance by establishing a Committee for Moral Recovery in Amsterdam, one month after the liberation of the Netherlands. A variety of bodies active in social care were represented on this Committee, all single-minded and determined to halt the degeneration of moral standards. For all its fervour, it achieved very little, however, and by early 1946 the Committee existed solely on paper.[80]

Aside from Bouman and his Committee (whatever the factual inertia of the latter), there were many others who set out to stem the tide of moral decay. They included social workers, medical practitioners, educationists, police officers, psychiatrists and politicians of all persuasions. A dominant thrust in politics at this time was a two-pronged effort, that crossed traditional party lines, to reorganize the Dutch political system at the same time as consolidating the moral foundations of post-war society. The main emphasis was on the family, which had emerged truly battered from the war, and which it was felt should be first – as the cornerstone of society – to be repaired. Socialists, communists, religious parties and feminists closed ranks for once in a concerted effort to rebuild the family and society itself.[81]

Both the cultural criticism of these innovators and concrete social measures focused on young men when it came to matters such as rowdy or criminal behaviour, but as soon as sexual morality was at issue, attention focused almost exclusively on Dutch girls and women, on whom the war was believed to have inflicted most harm. Many observers saw the venereal disease epidemic, like the increase in divorce rates and illegitimate births, as self-explanatory.[82] The situation was more serious compared to the pre-war years, it was argued, because moral corruption was now no longer confined to certain classes, but had spread to girls in all ranks of society. That this same trend had often attracted comment in the 1930s tended to be ignored. There was however one new element in the articles that appeared after the war: not only promiscuous girls – the 'perpetrators' – were crossing class barriers, but so was the larger population of venereal sufferers as a whole – the 'victims'. This group had scarcely been discussed before the war, but during the occupation years this silence was broken. In his report for the year 1943, the chief inspector of health remarked on the great increase in the number of persons suffering from venereal disease, 'in which connection it should especially be noted that these diseases are also spreading increasingly among what one may call the better classes'.[83] After the end of the war, many people made the same observation. In April 1946, the Institute of Preventive Medicine organized a one-day symposium on the venereal disease epidemic. Almost all speakers held that these diseases were claiming more victims among the more prosperous classes since the war, and that the distinction between towns and rural areas was likewise becoming blurred: characterized before the war as a typically urban evil, venereal disease was now cropping up in the tiniest of villages. The Dutch situation before the war, the dermatologist Prakken assured his audience, was such that:

148

the possibility of a venereal infection would only immediately occur to one if the patient belonged to one of certain particular groups (sailors, people who had been in the tropics or who belonged to certain other circles in which exposure to infection, whether through circumstances or inclination, tended to be commonplace). The epidemiological picture presented by venereal diseases now – quite aside from the staggering growth in incidence – is different than before. ... Venereal disease may occur anywhere now; it may be suspected even in circles in which, in the past, it was scarcely a matter for consideration.[84]

Whether this was indeed as conspicuous a trend as these speakers claimed we cannot say for sure, but it is not implausible that war and the post-war dislocation of society had brought venereal disease to places where it had rarely been seen before. This said, the point was certainly laboured here; in any case, the picture drawn by Prakken of the situation before the war seems decidedly simplistic. The reiterated claim that all classes had been contaminated was therefore probably intended, at least in part, to have some emotional appeal. If someone wishes to initiate debate on a social evil, common sense dictates that one should make the category of persons who might be affected as wide as possible. Problems that occur in all social classes arouse more concern and appear more menacing than classbound suffering. Knowing this, almost every 'moral entrepreneur' who writes with a view to stirring up public interest in a particular cause will at some point remark that the calamity is not confined to a small minority.[85] The anti-venereal disease campaigners after the Second World War, like the opponents of regulated prostitution half a century earlier, displayed a sound command of this fundamental principle of moral entrepreneurship. With their contention that venereal disease was striking at people in every walk of life, they were underscoring the urgency of their cause.

Despite the introduction of this group of 'victims', attention continued to focus chiefly, even after the end of the war, on female 'perpetrators'. Indignation about the conduct of Dutch girls and women came to a head in the short-lived 'moral panic' that surrounded liaisons between Dutch girls and Canadian soldiers in the summer of 1945. The Dutch press squeezed this issue for all it was worth, dwelling salaciously on the role of what was portrayed as a host of amateurs and pick-up girls in the spread of venereal disease. Meanwhile, the vice squad set out on expeditions, entirely within the German tradition, to arrest under-age girls found at hotels and night-clubs in the company of Canadians, and to detain girls under eighteen years of age who were out in the street after 11 p.m. and take them off to the health clinic to be examined for signs of venereal disease.[86] When the last of the Canadian troops departed, in January 1946, the fuss about the 'Canadians' girls' soon died down. True, the moral unease about the licentious behaviour of young women had not worked its way out completely, but the crest of the wave had passed.

We can easily trace a family resemblance between the portrait of loose young womanhood painted by worried observers after the war and the amateur of the 1930s. The narrators who held forth on the Canadian girls were perhaps a little more inclined to see this particular variant – because of all the cigarettes and chocolate that changed hands – as closer to its touchstone, prostitution, but 'occasional' prostitution was the worst they could make of it. Anyone who peruses the post-war issues of *Sexueele Hygiëne* constantly encounters the familiar figure of the amateur, who – as writers never tired of repeating – had increasingly taken the place of the professional prostitute.[87] Divorced and jilted women, well-off young ladies in search of casual sexual relationships, and girls dazzled by uniforms had bolstered the amateurs' ranks, but the hard core of girls who worked in factories, shops or offices – or who should be doing so, at any rate – were still pursuing the same dissolute path as before. C.D. Saal paid particular attention to this group in the questionnaire he conducted among the Dutch youth in 1946–1947. And with good reason, he explained, because:

> we know that it is particularly among shop assistants that many abuses in this area occur. For instance, when the female personnel of a certain department store had to be searched, it appeared that the vast majority of the girls possessed contraceptives. The type of the amateur, the girl who gives herself in a casual relationship with a young man, reaping the reward of abundant evenings out – as distinct from the professional prostitute – is concentrated most densely, in our cities, in the world of shop assistants.[88]

When he took the group of office staff, telephonists and shop assistants and studied them separately, however, he discovered little basis for these girls' bad reputation. This group was just as opposed to sexual relations outside marriage or engagement as members of the other groups. It is true that they displayed the most tolerance of all those questioned to the notion of sex during engagement. But even here, this (at least, inasmuch as the opinions stated truly

150

represented their views) was far from a majority trend: 20% of shop assistants and office girls thought sex during the engagement was acceptable, compared with 14% of the total number of women questioned and, according to a different classification, 31% of non-churchgoing women. Saal's questionnaire also revealed that young men of all religious denominations, professions and age groups were substantially less averse to the idea of sexual intercourse either during or prior to an engagement than were young women.[89]

That this latter finding scarcely gave rise to any concern about the moral standards of Dutch boys and men may be labelled illogical, or unjust, but it was part of a long tradition that saw women and girls as the guardians of morality. Among other things, the late 19th-century abolitionist offensive had been an attempt to imbue men with the moral standards that respectable women took for granted, but at the end of the 1940s the double standard was alive and well; whereas the mere suspicion of a certain kind of behaviour triggered an avalanche of moral dread when women and girls were concerned, in the case of men there was scarcely anything beyond the shrugging of shoulders even when such behaviour had been demonstrated beyond all doubt.

In retrospect, we might dwell for a moment on the significance of society's collective and undifferentiated preoccupation with the morality of young women in the months following the end of the war. When we look at the figures showing the increased incidence of venereal disease in this period (see Appendix II), we might be forgiven for concluding that observers who bemoaned the widespread lack of sexual restraint among women – to borrow their terminology – were absolutely right. In and around 1945, more women than men sought help at VD advice centres, which was highly exceptional. But these figures are misleading, because they relate only to the patient population of advice centres. Not every patient visited such a centre, but whereas in other periods of time we can assume that the resulting distortion of the figures is divided equally between the sexes, around the end of the war, given the unusually high concentration of men in the armed forces, this was not the case. Both the army of occupation and the liberation army had facilities of their own, which were separate from the system of advice centres used by Dutch civilians. In other words, far more men than women with venereal disease are excluded from these figures.

We do not possess any more detailed breakdown of the figures from the advice centres. Detailed information is available, however, concerning one specific group – syphilis sufferers who attended the university clinic in Utrecht between 1940 and 1945. Here too there were more female than male patients during this overall period: 717 women visited the clinic as against 388 men. In line with contemporary custom, the author, E.P. van Steenbergen, classified these patients, among other things, by 'sexual attitude'. He found that promiscuous individuals, both men and women, were in the majority. Among women, the category of 'amateurs' (266 in total) was the largest group, while the related category of 'occasional prostitutes' came fifth (66). In between were professional prostitutes (136), the group of non-promiscuous wives and girls with steady relationships (111), and those with old infections of unknown origin (81).[90] These figures are actually the first to reflect some increase in promiscuity among girls and women, the trend later insisted upon and analysed by so many indignant observers. But once again these figures provide nothing to substantiate the customary association of this phenomenon with certain jobs. Classified by occupation, out of over 700 female patients, fewer than 40 were factory workers, office clerks or shop assistants.[91]

Whether the figure of 266 amateurs and 66 occasional prostitutes in five years was shocking or not by contemporary standards is hard to ascertain, but judging by the rampant spread of venereal disease and the record number of illegitimate births, it seems fair to assume that many Dutch people had more lenient attitudes to sex in the mid-1940s than before. Reflecting on the furore surrounding the 'Canadians' girls', the historian Herman de Liagre Böhl, a seasoned commentator on the post-war struggle against immorality, concludes that 'in all probability ... during the "mad, mad" summer of 1945 there was a brief, but by Dutch standards unprecedented, explosion of extra-marital sex'.[92] He believes however that the behaviour of Dutch women and girls that aroused such passionate condemnation was not only extremely short-lived, but also that it took place on a far smaller scale than had been suggested in moralistic treatises. Nor was there any question of a conscious departure from traditional moral values in the areas of sexuality, marriage and the family, as some radical sexual reformers had suggested.[93] Other studies too indicate that the post-war alarm was something of a storm in a teacup.[94] Saal's questionnaire reveals that young people in the Netherlands were miles apart from their public image; they were markedly conservative in a host of areas, including attitudes to sexual morality.[95]

All this prompts the question of what it was that caused scores of observers to arrive at such a grave diagnosis. According to Böhl, if we are to understand the brief but vehement post-war outcry surrounding venereal disease and female morality, we have to see it as one of a whole series of campaigns, waged simultaneously, in which the morality of the Dutch nation was denounced. Young people running wild, idleness and black market trade were all issues on which tempers ran high. Böhl believes that this indignation – and the resolute campaigns to raise moral standards – should be explained in terms of their *political* significance. Exponents of the 'breakthrough' movement, in particular, propagated a morality of reconstruction, in which the entire Dutch nation, united and free from political or social divisions, would set to work rebuilding society. The necessary consensus could only be achieved and maintained, however, by converting various modes of social and political resistance into problems of morality, thus rendering them harmless. The fight against immorality thus served a largely political function, as the motor of reconstruction.[96]

This theory is not very plausible. Böhl himself acknowledges that the short-lived climate of sexual abandon after the war was quite harmless. To classify it at the same time as a form of social and *political* opposition that had to be defused in the interests of harmony and reconstruction makes little sense. Although some of the problems – a tendency towards lawlessness among young people, a reluctance to work – may have contained elements of opposition, even these had already been arousing concern before the war. The post-war hullaballoo was not about anything new. Rather, the climate was perfect for the eruption of a moral indignation that had been smouldering for many years. Obviously, the chaotic aftermath of the war, with all its attendant social dislocation, presented untold opportunities for those so inclined to wax indignant. But the lament about the disintegration of moral standards in the Netherlands, sung by a chorus of anxious citizens, had been well prepared by the mood of cultural pessimism that had dominated the 1920s and 1930s.[97] The unduly shrill note that sounded through the litany of complaints served as it were to legitimize the recurrent variations on the theme of moral degeneration that had been droning in the background for twenty years or more. The loud lament soon died down, however. Within a year after the end of the war, people were noticing to their relief that the dislocation and demoralization wrought by the war was less severe than they had feared, and their complaints lost their doom-laden tones. Champions of moral elevation turned their attention to new trends in social care.

Venereal disease and public mental health

Although the panic about venereal disease immediately after the end of the war was largely a magnified version of earlier anxieties, after it subsided certain new trends became visible. In particular, venereal disease was adopted along with a broad range of other social issues under the wing of the movement for public mental health. This movement, introduced into the Netherlands in the 1920s, endeavoured to apply views derived from psychology and psychiatry in many areas of private and public life. In the post-war years, it saw itself as having an important task in helping to achieve the moral recovery of society. Few of the problems of the age fell outside its range of concerns, as we can read in the columns of the journal it published during this period, the *Maandblad voor de Geestelijke Volksgezondheid*.[98] Some of the exponents of this movement set themselves up in the years immediately after the war as narrators in the fight against venereal disease.

Two names were particularly prominent: that of Bouman, the lawyer and founder of the Committee for Moral Recovery, and the Catholic psychiatrist J.A.J. Barnhoorn. Bouman was of the same stamp as A. de Graaf; he was a highly committed and tireless Protestant activist who forged ahead into the furthermost outposts of moral improvement. He, like De Graaf, was still caught up in the endless battle against prostitution and all attempts to regulate it, and was an active member of the international federation of abolitionists. He attempted to bring venereal disease, as well as prostitution, within the scope of mental hygiene. He too observed that professional prostitutes were facing increasing competition from amateurs, 'hordes of girls who think nothing of thrusting themselves on boys who had money, to be taken to the cinema, and who offer "sexual favours" in return'.[99]

Venereal diseases were contracted more and more frequently in casual sex, which was mainly practised, according to Bouman, by the 'mentally immature'. VD patients often had a personality structure characterized by inner disharmony and immaturity, which not infrequently pointed to an underlying psychopathy. Bouman felt that those involved in trying to curb venereal disease must take this into account, and he therefore urged that they should acquire a deeper understanding of the psychological aspects of the problem. His plan for achieving this, however, did not extend much further than a plea for sex education. Such instruction could constitute an important link in the battle against 'the mental venereal diseases, which are the cause of the physical ones'.[100]

The psychiatrist Barnhoorn went one step further. He too saw the battle against venereal disease as largely belonging to the realm of social psychiatry. To demonstrate the distinctive personality structure of VD patients, he drew on research conducted in the British army. This research had clearly demonstrated the 'excessive self-centredness, coupled with an exaggerated attachment to the mother and at the same time generally a strong resentment of, and a barely concealed hostility to, the father', which characterized the promiscuous individual.[101] On the basis of these findings, Barnhoorn concluded that psychiatrists had a crucial role to play in combating venereal disease. As head of the Mental Health Branch of the Royal Army Medical Service, Barnhoorn strongly advocated what he called the 'sociatric' approach to venereal disease. Sociatry was a curious concoction that Barnhoorn explained as a branch of mental health care that combined views derived from sociology, social psychology, psychiatry and where necessary from other social sciences. For the psychological cleansing and strengthening of the army, Barnhoorn designed a comprehensive working plan based on sociatric principles.[102] He hoped that the anti-venereal disease campaign could also be refashioned along sociatric lines, by relying on:

> the systematic psychiatric examination of all members of the armed forces, by means of e.g. group discussions, psychotherapy and sociatric recommendations. ... Those in whom acute or chronic neurotic disturbances of equilibrium play a part in fostering promiscuity should receive psychotherapy.[103]

After his appointment as head of the social psychiatry and mental hygiene department of Rotterdam Public Health Service, Barnhoorn also looked at anti-venereal disease work outside the armed forces. As experience demonstrated time and again that promiscuous individuals included 'a large number of mentally disturbed persons', he again advocated the psychotherapeutic correction of personality structure as the most important weapon in the battle against venereal disease. Both 'manifest' and 'latent' promiscuity, he maintained, could be controlled by these means. Aside from promoting classes to help parents in their children's upbringing, Barnhoorn also proposed that:

> every patient who has exposed himself to the risk of infection should undergo psychological and/or psychiatric examination, in order to gain an understanding of his personality structure and the motives that led to to the habitual or incidental promiscuity, and to

discover whether a psychiatric approach offers a better chance of controlling the tendency to indulge in promiscuous behaviour.[104]

Such notions aroused some interest among professional anti-VD workers, but Barnhoorn's psychiatric approach scarcely influenced the practicalities of venereal disease control. The preoccupation with immorality that dominated the public mental health movement for some time gradually abated as the movement underwent a process of modernization and professionalization. The belief that VD patients included a large number of 'mental defectives' and 'sub-normal individuals' was aired quite frequently, but the measures proposed for dealing with them were not, as we shall see, in the realm of psychotherapy. The far more moderate ideas of Bouman were closer to existing traditions; he later joined the Anti-Venereal Disease Society, in which he mainly concentrated on sex education.

Alongside what was ultimately a fairly unsuccessful attempt to define venereal disease as a derivative of individual personality disorders, there was a second point of contact between venereal disease control and public mental health. This was in the area of social care services, which witnessed a brief but intense dalliance between social workers active in venereal disease control and the post-war campaign against antisocial behaviour.

Social workers stepped up their involvement in the problem of venereal disease during the 1930s, but the rage for tracing sources reached its peak in the late 1940s. One reason for this post-war upsurge of activity was the separation of the problem of venereal disease from prostitution, two issues that had once been inextricably interwoven. During the 1920s and 1930s this link had already become less marked: the prostitute had been joined by the amateur, and venereal diseases increasingly outgrew their traditional niche. After 1945 this process of separation was complete. Although the rise of occasional prostitution was a recurrent theme, especially in the summer of 1945, and even though during the 'Canadian era' professional prostitutes were earning sums that Bouman estimated to be 'outstripping ministers' salaries by far'[105], in the longer term, promiscuity upstaged prostitution as the chief factor in the aetiology of venereal disease. This development was eventually reflected in the acceptance of a new epidemiological model: the chain. The wheel model, with its assumption of virulent sources of infection, gave way to a picture of a theoretically endless chain in which each patient constituted a link. 'The only effective way to fight venereal disease', wrote

Hermans in 1946, 'is to see it in terms of a battle against a large number of chains of infections, each of which has to be broken.'[106]

Once people saw that the prime necessity was to 'pursue the chains of infection from one individual to the next',[107] the significance of social work – with its 'case finding' that was so well suited as a method for tracing chains of infection – increased. Capitalizing on this favourable climate, social workers set out, during the latter half of the 1940s, to give their job a more professional image and to enhance its status. They formed a primitive type of trade union, and held meetings on the need to achieve better salaries, more jobs in the field, and wider responsibilities and powers.[108]

This latter point was a popular battle-cry. Social workers, under Hermans' leadership, wanted greater supervisory powers *vis-à-vis* their clientele. At the public meeting that the Dutch Anti-Venereal Disease Society held in January 1947, M.A. Duvekot spelled out the professional ideals that motivated her and her fellow social workers. Reflecting on her past years' experience, it appeared to her:

> that the social work at the advisory bureaux will be increasingly falling short of its task if it continues to be confined to the narrowly defined tasks of ensuring that patients continue their treatment and tracing them, which subjects I do not intend to discuss further. Useful though this work may be, it has proved to be completely inadequate.[109]

What was needed, according to Duvekot, was an expansion in their range of responsibilities. In addition to what they were already doing in direct venereal disease control, social workers should have far more, and clearly defined, duties in areas such as preventive measures and aftercare. In effect, the first step in social work was with the healthy, who should be deflected 'by all possible means' from promiscuity and pre-marital sexual relations. At the other end of the spectrum, mental and moral care for a certain proportion of patients should be maintained long after medical treatment had ceased: 'these people should not be abandoned the moment they have regained their health'.[110] It was essential to maintain contact with their relatives, their employers and their social environment. This was a form of aftercare that could also have a preventive function in the patient's immediate circle, which it was folly to ignore, contended Duvekot. To realize this objective, far more social workers were needed. But this was not enough. The extensive responsibilities that social workers claimed for themselves would call for cooperation with a wide range of institutions: employment exchanges, probation services, poor relief authorities, the Guardianship Board, vice squads and juvenile units within the police, marriage and family counselling agencies, youth organizations, reform schools and so forth. The result envisaged was a close-knit network of social care with frequent referrals within the circuit.[111]

Social workers were also eager to expand their powers. This related chiefly to the more troublesome aspects of their work. For it was not embarrassed youths and shame-faced girls that made their work difficult, as they repeatedly made clear. They claimed to have constant dealings with a hard core of 'antisocial' and 'feckless' elements from the lowest classes of society. They therefore sought to place their encounters with these groups within the context of the wider-ranging theme of the fight against antisocial behaviour in society.

After the Second World War the issue of 'antisocial behaviour' was very much in the limelight. While not new, this interest was charged with a different emphasis than before the war. Ali de Regt has shown that the rise of 'antisocial elements' as a category in society, at the beginning of the 20th century, was directly linked to changes in the lifestyles of workers in industry.[112] From about the end of the previous century, stricter work discipline and an increase in standards of living resulted in large numbers of workers carving out for themselves a more disciplined and orderly mode of life. But as this was not a universal development, the dividing-line between 'decent' and 'uncouth' workers became sharper than before. The groups fighting their way up the social ladder acquired new standards of propriety and decency, and developed greater sensitivity in these areas. They became increasingly intolerant of the undisciplined behaviour of those who had 'lagged behind'. As a result of this differentiation, and under the influence of action taken by landlords, housing associations and municipal authorities, this class of 'stragglers' crystallized, shortly after the First World War, into what were known as 'unacceptable' families. What was unacceptable was the way they lived: they vandalized or neglected their homes, were a nuisance to their neighbours, frequently allowed their rent to lapse into arrears, and displayed a host of related features such as alcoholism, child neglect and mentally 'subnormal' development. The solution to the problem of unacceptable families was sought in the construction of separate houses or complexes in which they were expected to stay for varying periods of time under the watchful eye of female superintendents. This not only saved 'decent' workers' families from having to endure such neighbours, but was also intended as a step towards educating these groups to become respectable members of society.

While in the 1920s the problem of unacceptable families – later increasingly referred to as 'antisocial' elements – was seen primarily as a housing problem, this emphasis gradually changed. After the Second World War, these families attracted more attention, but unacceptable lifestyles disappeared into the footnotes of the problem definition. The antisocial family was increasingly defined in terms of mental abnormality and psychological disorders. An undesirable lifestyle could be symptomatic of this, as could criminal behaviour, idleness, a lack of order and failure to develop regular habits, an uninhibited sexuality and a general tendency to live as a parasite upon society. But these too were merely symptoms: the post-war generation of battlers against antisocial elements were ultimately concerned to identify and eliminate the deeper-rooted causes. To their minds, the antisocial family was diseased, an entity that had become dysfunctional through a variety of related factors. This meant that in the late 1940s 'antisocial elements' were dealt with as a problem of public mental health, and it was mainly psychiatrists, social workers, pastors and family counsellors who set about tending this 'wound in our society'.

These professionals thrashed out the issue of the antisocial family at seminars, in committees and in numerous articles. This problem had now become such a menace to the spiritual well-being of our nation, according to one of the reports on this issue, that no one could afford to ignore it. Although the extent of the problem was relatively limited, its significance far outweighed the number of persons involved, given the existence of 'sources of infection spreading moral degeneracy'.[113] This insistence on the infectiousness of antisocial attitudes underpinned the belief that to isolate the family concerned, providing supervision, resocialization and therapeutic assistance, was the best way forward. To put it more strongly, one had an obligation to society as a whole to remove this 'rotten apple' from its surroundings while the latter were still healthy. Detached from their former circles and placed under expert guidance, antisocial families could be helped back on the right path. To expand the scope for this approach, a variety of interested parties called for statutory measures to enable antisocial families to be placed under supervision orders. No such measures ever materialized, but countless residential family units – originally they

159

had been evacuation camps for antisocial families from Rotterdam during the Second World War – were still in use in the provinces of Drenthe and Overijssel well into the 1950s. Local projects for socially maladjusted families, later called deprived or problem families, went on functioning even longer than this.[114]

Social workers active in venereal disease control were visibly impressed by post-war measures to curb antisocial behaviour. Although their concerns focused on individuals rather than entire families, they too were eager to expand their scope to act when faced with antisocial groups. Such scope was already much greater than before the war, as the coercive measures introduced in 1940 were still in force. And this met with general approval, as anyone involved in venereal disease control in those years could see that coercion was indispensable. Even Van Leeuwen took this view, despite his obvious aversion to the measure.[115] In 1949 a questionnaire was held among social workers and medical practitioners attached to advice centres, which revealed that all but a handful still favoured the continuation of the existing ordinances.[116] Indeed, the problem was rather that the ordinances did not go far enough. This, at least, was the opinion expressed by Hermans, the great champion of social work. He wrote that VD patients frequently included such antisocial elements that even coercive treatment was futile, and certainly made no contribution to the 're-education of such individuals to become better members of society'.[117] In cases of this kind, other solutions were called for:

> You can take a horse to the water but you cannot make him drink; this will surely apply to forced admissions. Sometimes we encounter such antisocial elements, cleaving to the seamy side of society, that even a hospital admission can achieve nothing. For cases of this kind, resocialization and treatment in labour camps are the only way in which to limit the problem as much as possible.[118]

Some people objected to camps on the grounds that it was wrong to concentrate so many bad elements in one place. But, as Hermans continued, 'let us not forget that evil elements of this kind can also have a profoundly negative effect on the atmosphere in a hospital ward'. To him, it was clear:

> For these antisocial elements, a labour camp is the best solution. They are not sent there as a punitive measure, because they are ill, but merely because their sub-standard, antisocial behaviour constitutes a serious menace to society.[119]

Hermans' solution to the problem of antisocial elements was popular among social workers, who claimed that they constantly had to deal with antisocial, uncooperative and untraceable patients, and regarded them as the greatest obstacle to their work. They already made frequent use of the existing coercive treatment when confronting 'the group consisting of antisocial or ignorant individuals, who don't give a fig about anything and who thus constitute a menace to their surroundings', wrote the social worker C.M. van der Fliert. But this did not go far enough:

> When we come to this particular group of antisocial elements, I would also wish to urge the introduction of labour camps for *adult* antisocial elements, who, being too idle to work, live from the profits of indecency. It must be possible to remove such individuals from society and to place them in institutions with a professional staff.[120]

Admission to hospital and internment in labour camps, or, as Nurse Duvekot called it, 'the possibility of internment with employment'[121] were in fact indispensable measures for the most serious cases, in the view of social workers. So it is scarcely surprising that the first speaker at the first national assembly of their trade union in 1947 was A. Diemers. Diemers had been appointed commanding officer of the evacuation camps in Drenthe during the occupation years – the camps that had been converted after the war into residential complexes for socially maladjusted families – and hence could speak from the vantage-point of many years of experience with 'antisocial camps'.[122] With his inspiring address on the 'wonderful but so difficult work among the antisocial members of society', he must surely have bolstered the social workers' convictions.[123] At any rate, a few months later Nurse Duvekot, speaking on behalf of social workers, heartily praised the merits of the 'coercive measures for antisocial elements in the form of internment in resocialization centres' and went on to advocate increased scope for placing adults under supervision orders. She was referring especially to persons she classified as 'individuals who are backward, mental defectives or psychopaths, and who presently vanish from a sheltered institutional life at 21 years of age, often finding themselves in the midst of society without any form of protection. And it is terrible to see where they so often end up.'[124]

In expressing these various aspirations – none of which was in fact realized – social workers were following a characteristic trend in the post-war years, one that favoured a tough line on socially deviant and undesirable behaviour.[125] The popularity of this approach – which eventually proved short-lived – derived from the specific nature of post-war society. Like the rise of 'antisocial elements' as a category in the first decade of the century, the tough clampdown on such behaviour after the war was the expression of a heightened sensitivity to groups of 'stragglers' under the influence of the continuing emancipation of the working classes and a fervent belief in progress. Illustrative of this underlying confidence in development, modernization and progress is *De proletarische Achterhoede* (*The Proletarian Remainder*, 1954) by the sociologist J.A.A. van Doorn. In this book, Van Doorn criticized at length the dissertation published two years earlier by J. Haveman, who had contended that there was a sharp division within the working class between skilled and unskilled workers. The latter, in Haveman's view, were ensconced in their own neighbourhoods, making up a sub-culture that was completely cut off from the middle-class culture of the rest of society. There was an unbridgeable gap between these worlds, he claimed. Van Doorn, on the other hand, emphasized the continuing process of economic, political, social and cultural emancipation that embraced the vast majority of the working class. In a modern society, maintained Van Doorn, most unskilled labourers too would be absorbed by the process of civilization as described by Elias. It was entirely possible that a certain group of people would remain permanently outside this development, but it was wrong to equate them *en bloc* with unskilled workers. Such a group could best be called, simply, an 'unconvertible remainder', who would continue to live in the margins of society without steady employment, and who would be impervious to any process of emancipation.[126]

It was this 'proletarian remainder' that was the target of the post-war clampdown on antisocial elements. Precisely at this time of reconstruction, industrialization and modernization, in which discipline and asceticism set the tone and the population had to be made 'ripe for industry' by means of specially directed efforts, the presence of this group aroused immense resentment. Antisocial individuals were an obstacle to the onward march of social development, and their way of life was a menace to the rest of society. For a brief space of time, it was believed that when it came to combating what was seen as the resistance, on the part of these groups, to integration into industrialized society and middle-class culture, no action could be harsh enough.[127]

Within the Dutch Anti-Venereal Disease Society, not everyone was happy with the uncompromising course – linked to this more comprehensive development – that was briefly pursued in venereal disease control. After the war, the divisions between two opposing schools of thought became increasingly clear. While secretary Hermans toiled away at what he called his medical and social hygiene programme, the new chairman Van Leeuwen continued in the moral and religious tradition of the first chairman, De Graaf. The two barely concealed their animosity towards each other's points of view. The controversy was not new; Hermans had long complained that the moral approach of De Graaf and Van Leeuwen had unnecessarily held up and undermined the social and medical work to be done.[128] Nor was he alone in this view: as early as 1929 the dermatologist Van der Hoog had written an open letter to De Graaf railing against the latter's leadership. 'As Chairman, you have changed the Dutch Anti-Venereal Disease Society into a species of "Pure Life Movement" or an "Association for the Elevation of Moral Self-awareness" ... and this transformation has sealed its doom.'[129] He accused the Society of a complete inability to take decisive action.

Whereas this more pragmatic school of thought, based on principles of social hygiene, initially took the form of marginal jibes at the mainstream approach, it had gradually acquired more support – partly thanks to the indefatigable Hermans – and in the 1930s it was part of the mainstream itself. With the dramatic increase in the number of VD sufferers during and after the occupation, the two camps clashed more openly and more frequently. Both parties were equally convinced of the seriousness and urgency of the problem, yet they developed in two opposing directions, almost to the extent of caricature. Cooperation was not easy in such circumstances, as is clear from some of the very few minutes of Society meetings that have been preserved. During a meeting in 1944, Van Leeuwen underscored the importance of reaching 'a certain measure of consensus', but the rival points of view were irreconcilable. For instance, Hermans, advocating labour camps for antisocial elements, had referred approvingly to 'certain German measures', and during a meeting with social workers he had disparaged the moral side of the venereal disease control movement. All this had antagonized the new chairman Van Leeuwen, for whom 'religious and moral factors' still prevailed: 'The Chairman wishes to lead the Society along the path it has followed over the past 35 years. If the Society changes course, he will step down.'[130]

After the end of the war, the differences of opinion continued undiminished, and the Board decided on a parting of the ways. One branch, led by Hermans with Zoon as second in command, would do its best to promote venereal disease control on medical and social hygiene principles. The other, under the leadership of Van Leeuwen and supported by Bouman, would promote proper sexual hygiene and sexual morality. Parallel to this division, the Society's periodical *Sexueele Hygiëne* appeared in two series from 1946 onwards: series A for venereal disease control and series B for public morality.[131] From the outset it was Hermans' branch that gained the ascendancy and planned its campaign; clearly, in the post-war climate of opinion, his ideas fared considerably better than did those of Van Leeuwen. The sex education and moral improvement in which Van Leeuwen placed his reliance, with their doubtful long-term impact, had had their day, and the main positions he defended – he was first and foremost against regulated prostitution, and against prophylactics – had lost much, if not all, of their topical relevance. Van Leeuwen himself left the Society in 1947, and was followed by Zoon. His vision was represented for a while by Bouman, who had been appointed second secretary alongside Hermans, but with the advance of penicillin its perceived relevance diminished still further. Hermans' victory also proved a temporary one, however. With the restoration of the social order, the end of the epidemic and an increasing mood of optimism engendered by the wondrous workings of penicillin, his extensive social programme was soon seen as obsolete.

Intermezzo: narrators and characters

On the basis of the material discussed in the last three chapters, I would like to dwell for a moment on a few points that have emerged concerning the relations between narrators and characters, a recurrent aspect of the debate on venereal disease. It has become clear from the previous chapters that both roles were played at various times by a variety of different actors. While hygienists cast prostitutes in the leading role, for instance, feminists, together with other abolitionists, turned the spotlight on the prostitute's male client and his innocent victims. Worried men, after the First World War, staged a long performance featuring the amateur and other promiscuous girls. And these are only the barest outlines of the story. With this changing cast on both sides, relations between the two groups changed time and again. Nevertheless, certain aspects of more general power differences recur in these relations. We can express the relations between narrators and characters in terms of three fundamental binary oppositions. These oppositions should not be considered mutually exclusive, and each was topical at a different moment in time.

164

The first relationship expressed in the narrator–character couple is that between the 'higher' and the 'lower' classes. The history of venereal disease and its control is best described, from the vantage-point of social classes, as a lopsided dialogue. Lopsided because one of the voices has scarcely been recorded in the course of history: narrators do not come from the lower classes, and as characters they have not been given the opportunity, by their creators, to answer back. What remains is a protracted complaint by 'higher' groups about 'lower' ones, supplemented with serious admonitions or well-meaning help, but one searches in vain for any rejoinder from the other side. In the description of the relations between social classes, this systematic distortion constitutes a handicap which is obviously not confined to the historical study of the problem of venereal disease.

In a completely different context, the anthropologist James Scott has discussed this point and noted the limited significance of the study of public interaction to descriptions of topical class and power relations in anthropological research.[132] The encounters between more and less powerful persons which are played out in public life provide what Scott calls a 'public transcript' that only records a partial reflection of the power relations existing between them. The knowledge, experience and opinions of the weaker party systematically fail to appear, or at least appear only in a veiled and adapted form. It is therefore important, Scott goes on, to also take note of what he calls the 'hidden transcript':

> If subordinate discourse in the presence of the dominant is a public transcript, I shall use the term 'hidden transcript' to characterize discourse that takes place 'offstage', beyond direct observation by powerholders. The hidden transcript is thus derivative in the sense that it consists of those offstage speeches, gestures, and practices that confirm, contradict, or inflect what appears in the public transcript.

The distortions of the public transcript that Scott refers to appear in a magnified form in a good deal of historical research: the confrontation between different social classes is actually impossible to observe directly, but can only be known to the extent that it has been recorded in writing, which is to say, in almost all cases, as seen through the eyes of the more powerful groups. This constitutes an additional limitation. All this does not mean that the fragments of the venereal disease debate that are now available to us are of no value, but we must bear in mind that they reveal more about these narrators and their backgrounds than about the objects of their irritation or care: persons with a lower social status.

In the second place, relations between narrators and characters were a particular variant of those between men and women. The debate on venereal disease as it has been dealt with up to this point may be viewed as an ongoing dialogue, or rather, an ongoing exchange of views between the sexes. It was no true discourse, but two voices could be clearly distinguished: both men and women at times adopted the narrator's role, and in that capacity held forth on the defining traits, and more especially the shortcomings, of the opposite sex. The casting was far from evenly balanced: men tended to be narrators and most of the characters were women. Viewed as an exchange between the sexes, which chiefly assumed the form of a steady stream of accusations from both sides, the debate on venereal disease is one of the areas in which knowledge about the difference between the sexes, and its significance, is both expressed and generated. This links up with current research on the meanings attached to the differences between men and women in different places and at different times, and which have been encapsulated, in the latter part of the 20th century, in the word 'gender'.

The American historian Joan Scott has studied the analytical possibilities of this concept at length.[133] She distinguishes several levels at which differences between the sexes take on form and significance: *cultural symbolism*, in which images of femininity and masculinity are evoked using symbols and myths of purification and pollution, innocence and corruption; that of *normative concepts*, which are often based on these symbolic representations and are generally expressed in the form of binary oppositions grafted onto the male/female dichotomy in religious, scientific and political doctrines; *social institutions*, ranging from the family to the labour market and from school to politics; and finally the *construction of subjective identity*. Of greatest relevance to the study at hand is the domain of normative concepts. As narrators, men and women focused on their mutual differences and brought their views to life in the form of characters in a play. Thus medical practitioners and regulationists contributed to the image of the fallen woman as a source of pollution while endorsing existing views of male sexuality; on the other hand feminists, supported by Protestant opponents of prostitution and some medics, attacked the notion of the uncontrollability of the male sex drive; then again, army surgeons reaffirmed traditional views of masculine nature; and finally, the view that the preservation of good morals was pre-eminently women's responsibility found its way into almost every treatise, with the result that a majority of narrators during this entire period, apparently without noticing any incongruity in what they were saying, bemoaned the collapse of moral standards and the rise of promiscuity, but only among women. The debate on venereal disease thus alternately created, confirmed and questioned ideas about men and women, and about masculinity and femininity.

Aside from these differences of social class and gender, there is a third distinction which divided narrators and characters: that of experts and laypeople, and in particular, that of doctors and patients. The debate on venereal disease can be construed in part as a series of pronouncements by medical practitioners about characters who, again, were condemned to silence and anonymity. But this interpretation does not figure very prominently in the period under discussion; until 1950 the other two binary oppositions were dominant. Then, as we shall see, the situation changed.

Notes

1. See Van der Hoog n.d. [1930]:32-3; Hermans n.d. [1934]:26, 53-4; L. Heyermans, 'Bestrijding der geslachtsziekten', *NTvG* 80 (1936) IV:5392-9; the reference here is to 5394; Voorhoeve 1951:206; the journal *Sexueele Hygiëne* also includes regular references to the important role that amateur prostitutes had come to play in the spread of venereal diseases; see e.g. *SH* fourth series, no. 2/3 (1937):47; fourth series, no. 4 (1937):141; fifth series, no. 1 (1938):56. The shift of attention from prostitutes to promiscuous young women was not of course a specifically Dutch phenomenon: for England, see Weeks 1981:207-8; Bland 1982; Bland 1985; Mort 1987:190 for the United States: Brandt 1987:168.
2. See also Bland 1982:380-1; Bland 1985:201-4.
3. Muller 1939:48.
4. J. Kuypers, 'De taak van de sociale werkster in een adviesbureau', *SH*, fifth series, no. 1 (1938):56. See also A. Renkema, 'Het opsporen der infectiebronnen in Den Haag. Bijeenkomst te Utrecht der artsen en sociale werksters' (16 April 1937), *SH*, fourth series, no. 2/3 (1937):47; and Hermans (1934:26): 'It would be quite mistaken to believe that she [a social worker seeking to identify sources of infection] should pursue her task exclusively or even mainly among prostitutes. If social work is to achieve its full beneficial effect, it must be capable of penetrating to all layers of society, and where women are concerned, it is of the utmost importance that the social worker should also make contact with shop assistants, visitors to dancing halls and the like, among whom infections are very frequent.'

5. See the description of the amateur prostitute in Van Steenbergen 1950:9-10.
6. In *SH*, fourth series, no. 2/3 (1937), amateur prostitutes were described as 'shop assistants, factory workers or girls with housekeeping duties' (47); in a different edition later that year there was a reference to 'girls from ordinary homes' (*idem*:141); *SH*, fifth series, no. 1 (1938) referred to girls from all classes, who were defined more precisely as 'servants, shop assistants, office clerks etc.' (56). Lewandowski & Van Dranen (1933:160) discussed 'pseudo-prostitutes' known as the 'girls from the Vondelpark'; in his opinion, this category consisted largely of middle-class daughters with jobs in shops or factories. Muller (1939:16) also referred to shop assistants, but observed that these girls often came from the 'less prosperous sections of society'.
7. Van der Hoog [1930]:33.
8. Muller 1939:24.
9. Muller 1939:24.
10. Voorhoeve 1951, 208-9.
11. See Schokking, Beintema & Zoon, 'Voorkomen en uitbreiding van geslachtsziekten in het gebied, bestreken door de dermatologische klinieken in Leiden, Groningen en Utrecht', *SH*, fifth series, no. 1 (1938):16-31. As far as syphilis was concerned, the upward turn of the graph after 1925, according to these authors, was duplicated throughout Europe (21-2 and 26).
12. See Hermans [1934]:2, 70.
13. T.M. Van Leeuwen & E.H. Hermans, 'De frequentie der geslachtsziekten in Nederland', *SH*, fourth series, no. 1 (1937):3-12; also reproduced in *NTvG* 80 (1936) IV:4741-7.
14. See e.g. E.H. Hermans, 'Vrijheid of dwang bij de geslachtsziektenbestrijding', *SH* 1946, no. 2:1; M.H.E. Nolthenius de Man, 'De verijdeling van de volledige uitvoering der prostitutie-reglementeering in Nederland', *SH*, 1946, no. 4:23.
15. Nurse A. Renkema (*SH*, fourth series, no. 2-3 (1937):47) reported, for instance, that some 70% of the infections recorded at the office in The Hague were caused by amateur prostitutes, but gave no comparative data. Hermans (*SH*, fifth series, no. 2 (1939):87-107) stated, without giving the slightest indication of the basis for his assertion, that where in the past about 75% of new infections had been caused by prostitutes, the proportion at present was only 25% (92). Both authors omitted to mention, incidentally, that they were referring only to infections contracted by men.
16. See Muller 1939:64-9.

17. As far as Protestant groups are concerned, see Van Kaam 1964:13-4; 29-31; 73-5; 104-9; 118-23; 140-1; 145-8; 185-7.
18. See esp. two issues of the Catholic periodical *Dux. Tijdschrift voor priesters*, that discuss the upbringing of young people from Roman Catholic backgrounds: 2 (1928/29) and 3 (1929/30). For the worries about factory girls, see De Regt 1985:122-5; Van Drenth 1991.
19. See G. Lamers, 'Het fabrieksmeisje', *Dux* 2 (1928-199):121-4.
20. Brusse 1921:47-62 (VIII. 'Veranderde zeden'; IX. 'De vrouwen in het bedrijfsleven'; X. 'De omgang van de geslachten').
21. Brusse 1921:57.
22. Brusse 1921:62. The dermatologist Muller (1939:16) likewise pointed to the dangers that threatened when working girls outgrew their home surroundings: 'This danger is greatest in the case of the shop assistant who often comes from a less prosperous background: in the daytime she acts the lady, and in the evening she returns to a completely different environment. This girl soon decides to leave the parental home and give herself up to worldly pleasures, thus exposing herself to all manner of dangers.'
23. Ribbius Peletier 1937:45.
24. Cf. Wouters 1990:152-9; Derks 1991.
25. Report by the committee on popular amusement concerning the question of dance halls and fairs (1928), *Rapport der regeerings-commissie inzake het dansvraagstuk* 1931:85-92; this quotation from 91.
26. *Sociale Atlas van de Vrouw*, Rijswijk, Sociaal en Cultureel Planbureau 1983:189-90; Blok 1978:56.
27. 'Vijfentachtig jaren statistiek in tijdreeksen', 1899-1984, CBS 1984:76.
28. Cf Morée & Schwegman 1981:138 ff.; De Regt 1985:54-5; Van Drenth 1991:24-5. Examining the number of employment cards issued in municipalities clearly shows a change in the ratio of unmarried to married women: in 1915 the ratio of the number of cards given to girls (14-17 years) as compared to married women was about 3:1; by 1935 it was 8:1. See *Centraal verslag der Arbeidsinspectie in het Koninkrijk der Nederlanden van de jaren 1915-1939*.
29. See in this context Posthumus-Van der Goot & De Waal (eds.) [1968]:270-81; Blok, 1978:118-24.
30. *Sociale Atlas van de Vrouw* 1983:189.
31. For these developments, see Posthumus-Van der Goot & De Waal (eds.) [1968]:267-9; Blok 1978:57-8, 66; Morée & Schwegman 1981: 125-6; *Vijfentachtig jaren statistiek in tijdreeksen* 1899-1984, CBS 1984:76. Although women's share in factory work remained constant, the nature of industry – and therefore of their duties –

changed considerably. On this subject, see Caljé & Den Hollander 1990:70-81; Glucksmann 1990.

32. Cf. Wijmans 1987:149-50; De Haan 1992:209, 399.

33. See De Regt 1990, esp. 35-6.

34. Brusse 1921:62; see also Heertje 1934:48.

35. Ribbius Peletier 1937:46.

36. Derks 1991:388.

37. See Derks 1991. A good deal of research has been done in other countries, especially in the United States (far more than in the Netherlands) on the rise and heyday of popular forms of night-life and their significance to working girls; see Peiss 1984; Peiss 1986; Meyerowitz [1988].

38. See Peiss 1986:108-14.

39. On other aspects of this process, see Schwegman 1989a (this quotation from 44).

40. Annie Romein-Verschoor, in her familiar disdainful tone, refers to the appearance of a new type of women in the work of middle-class female writers after the First World War. Authors such as Emmy van Lokhorst, Jo de Wit and Julia Frank, in describing this new woman, emphasized above all their frankness in the erotic sphere. See Romein-Verschoor [1935]:133-40. For portrayals of the office-clerk in literature and films, see De Haan 1991:152-6.

41. See Röling 1991.

42. The term originates from Wouters 1990, Chapter 2.

43. Morée & Schwegman 1981:126-7;140.

44. Blok 1978:58.

45. See Klöters 1987, Chapter 3.

46. See 'Rapport van de commissie inzake volksvermaken ten aanzien van het vraagstuk der dansgelegenheden en kermissen' (1928) in *Rapport der regeerings-commissie inzake het dansvraagstuk* 1931:85-92. See also Wouters 1990:155-9.

47. See the pastoral writings by the Dutch bishops in 1928, quoted in Van Ussel [1968]:337.

48. For the development of these more differentiated sexual practices among working girls, see Peiss 1984.

49. For these figures, see *SH*, fifth series, no. 3 (1939):158-64; sixth series, no. 3 (1942):33-43.

50. The pamphlet was entitled *Tien richtlijnen voor de sociale bestrijding van geslachtsziekten*. For the new organization and guidelines, see 'Kort verslag van de jaarvergadering', *SH*, first series, no. 1 (1932):1-3; 'Richtlijnen', *SH*, fourth series, no. 2/3 (1937):78-80; C.P. Schokking, 'De organisatie van de sociaal-hygiënische bestrijding der

geslachtsziekten in Nederland', *NTvG* 81 (1937), IV:5471-6; Van Steenbergen 1950:82-5 and 131-3.

51. 'Verslag van de openbare bijeenkomst der Nederlandsche Vereeniging voor zedelijke volksgezondheid' (22-9-1934), *SH*, third series, no. 1 (1935):1-36; this quotation from 8-9.

52. E.H. Hermans, 'De mobilisatie en het geslachtsziekteneuvel', *SH*, fifth series, no. 3 (1939):111-23; this quotation from 120.

53. 'Bijeenkomst te Utrecht der artsen en sociale werksters (16 april 1937)', *SH*, fourth series, no. 2/3 (1937):43-77; this quotation is from 63.

54. Hermans 1934:24. When asked whether it would not be better for men to do this work, he replied that 'although that theoretically might be the case, experience has shown that the female social worker acts with more tact and patience than her male counterpart, and that in this respect too a woman can exert more influence on patients than a man' (24).

55. J.J. Zoon, in *De bestrijding van de thans heerschende epidemie* 1946:5.

56. This development quite transcended activities related to venereal disease, and characterized the tradition of social work in general. When social work came into existence in or around 1900, the accentuation of the difference between the sexes served among other things to reserve an important place for women within this work; see Bervoets 1988.

57. A.M. van der Meijden, 'Uit de practijk der geslachtsziektenbestrijding' 1, 2 and 3. *SH*, sixth series, no. 2 (1942):19-25; no. 3:44-7; no. 4:53-5; this quotation is from 20.

58. 'Bijeenkomst te Utrecht der artsen en sociale werksters (16 april 1937)', *SH*, fourth series, no. 2/3 (1937):68, 72.

59. 'Bijeenkomst te Utrecht der artsen en sociale werksters (16 april 1937)', *SH*, fourth series, no. 2/3 (1937):73.

60. 'Bijeenkomst te Utrecht der artsen en sociale werksters (16 april 1937)', *SH*, fourth series, no. 2/3 (1937):46. See also Hermans 1934:24.

61. For initiatives in the realm of poor relief and housing assistance, see De Regt 1985, Chapters VI and VII; for a history of social work described far more in terms of force, control and discipline, see Michielse 1989.

62. See e.g. De Graaf 1929; T.M. van Leeuwen, 'Is het wenschelijk, in de wet een bepaling op te nemen tot strafbaarstelling van het opzettelijk blootstellen van anderen aan gevaar voor besmetting met een geslachtsziekte?', *SH*, vol. VII, no. 1 (1930):93-103; E.H. Hermans, 'Geslachtsziektenbestrijding en dwangmaatregelen', *SH*, fourth series, no. 4 (1937):135-48. For an overview of the Dutch debates on

coercive measures, see Van Steenbergen 1950, Chapter VII. The positions concerning the question of coercive treatment in venereal disease control were distributed among the various countries in more or less the same way as those relating to eugenic coercive measures, in particular eugenic sterilization. Here too, it was the Scandinavian countries and Germany that went furthest. See Noordman 1989:198-201.

63. Records were kept of the post-war venereal disease epidemic in the province of Utrecht for several successive years; see G.D. Hemmes, 'De omvang der geslachtsziektenepidemie en haar bestrijding', *NTvG* 90 (1946) IV:1518-24, 91 (1947) IV:3014-6, 92 (1948) IV:3331-2, 93 (1949) IV:3578-9, 94 (1950) IV:3334-6.

64. For the precise figures, see Bijkerk 1969 II:33 and Appendix II. Bijkerk was responsible for compiling the first longitudinal statistics on venereal disease. He collected his data from all the advice centres around the country, and produced a table showing annual numbers of patients registered as having syphilis or gonorrhoea between 1940 and 1967. Not all VD sufferers ended up at advice centres, so that the figures do not present a reliable impression of the true number of VD sufferers in the Netherlands. The series does however reflect the trends in the incidence of venereal diseases in the Netherlands.

65. See J.J. Zoon, 'Over de gonorrhoe bij de vrouw', *SH*, sixth series, no. 6 (1943):75-8. For further observations on sulfa drugs, see also Dowling 1977, Chapter 8; Spink 1978, Chapter 5.

66. For the literal text of these ordinances, see *Verordeningenblad voor het bezette Nederlandsche gebied*, document 30. Published 5 October 1940. This text is also included in Prakken 1948:267-70; Van Steenbergen 1950:134-7.

67. On prostitution and regulation during the years of occupation, see [anon.], 'De prostitutie-bestrijding in Nederland sinds 1940', *SH* 1946, no. 4:17-22; M.H.E. Nolthenius de Man, 'De verijdeling van de volledige uitvoering der prostitutie-reglementeering in Nederland', *SH* 1946, no. 4:22-5.

68. See T.M. van Leeuwen, 'De geslachtsziekten na den oorlog', *Tijdschrift voor Sociale Geneeskunde* 23 (1945):35-6, 90-1, 101-2 (these quotations are from 102); [editorial], 'De bestrijding der geslachtsziekten in Nederland van mei 1940 – mei 1945', *SH* 1946, no. 1:3-5; E.H. Hermans, 'Vrijheid of dwang bij de geslachtsziektenbestrijding', *SH* 1946, no. 2:1-4.

69. See J. van der Veen, 'De venerische ziekten in het leger', *NTvG* 92 (1948) I:1135. One year later, this figure of 38 out of every thousand

men had already fallen to 22 (1140). In 1919 the number of infected men in the Dutch army had been 34 out of every thousand men (see Haustein 1927:665).

70. See B.J.W. Beunders, 'Enkele aspecten van het vraagstuk der geslachtsziekten in het leger', *Tijdschrift voor sociale geneeskunde* 26 (1948):420-2; P.J.A. van Voorst Vader, 'De locale "vroege behandeling" van geslachtsziekten', *Nederlands Militair Geneeskundig Tijdschrift* 3 (1949), no. 1:7-11.

71. Brandt 1987:164.

72. See B.J.W. Beunders, 'Enkele aspecten van het vraagstuk der geslachtsziekten in het leger', *Tijdschrift voor Sociale Geneeskunde* 26 (1948):421. Beunders therefore ascribed the favourable results achieved during wartime not to the large-scale distribution of prophylactics, but to other factors: 'The fact that during this past war the figures for venereal disease were far lower than during the 1914–1918 war should be attributed to a large extent to the circumstance that this war, much more than the previous one, has been a war of movement. The physical effort and the constant concentration of each man was probably many times greater, and at the same time, the individual as such also acquired greater significance. Add to this the far greater interest of the average soldier in the military operations that lay ahead and the policy of a general such as Montgomery of ensuring that every man felt that he was part of the team, and we see all the various factors that contributed towards limiting the number of venereal infections.'

73. For a description of the developments surrounding the introduction of penicillin, see Voorhoeve 1951:155-78; Spink 1978, Chapter 6.

74. See E.P. van Steenbergen, 'Iets over de organisatie van de geslachtsziektenbestrijding in deze tijd', *Nederlands Militair Geneeskundig Tijdschrift* 9 (1956), no. 8:250-2. Another argument advanced by Van Steenbergen for not ascribing too dominant a role to penicillin in the abating of the post-war epidemic is the fact that the fall in the number of syphilis cases was so much more dramatic than in the case of gonorrhoea. (In 1955 the number of syphilis patients had fallen to 5% of the 1947 figures, while the number of gonorrhoea patients was still 20% of that in 1947. See Bijkerk 1969 II:33. This is striking, as gonorrhoea responds far better and more rapidly to penicillin than syphilis.)

75. J.R. Prakken, 'Enige opmerkingen over de geslachtsziektenbestrijding in Nederland', *Tijdschrift voor Sociale Geneeskunde* 27 (1949):351-4; this quotation is from 353.

76. See Gerda Kjellberg, 'De behandeling van syphilis door penicilline

en arsenicumpraeparaten in verschillende landen', *SH* 1948, no. 4:5-8; J.J. Zoon & E.P. van Steenbergen, 'De penicillinebehandeling der syphilis', *Geneeskundige Bladen* 43 (1949):99-156; Vinks 1954, Chapter III.

77. See Bijkerk 1969, I:20-1; II:36-7. These mortality rates (400-500 deaths per annum) have not been corrected to allow for the increase in population. Expressed as a percentage of the population, therefore, syphilis mortality rates show a steady decline since the beginning of the century.

78. E.H. Hermans, 'Inleiding over de zedelijke verwording', *SH*, sixth series, no. 1 (1942):8-16; see also Romeyn, 'De amatrice', *SH*, sixth series, no. 6 (1943):91-4.

79. A. Bouman, 'Welke uitwerking had de oorlog op de sexueele moraliteit van ons volk?', *Maandblad voor de Geestelijke Volksgezondheid* 1 (1946):98-104; this quotation is from 98.

80. De Liagre Böhl & Meershoek 1989:88-9, 146.

81. For more detailed accounts of the campaign to halt the decline in moral standards after the Second World War, see De Liagre Böhl 1985; De Liagre Böhl [1987]; De Liagre Böhl & Meershoek 1989.

82. See De Liagre Böhl & Meershoek 1989:85 (illegitimate births) and 142 (divorces).

83. 'Verslag over het jaar 1943 van den Geneeskundig Hoofdinspecteur van de Volksgezondheid', *SH* 1947, no. 4:14-15; this quotation is from 14.

84. *Bestrijding van de thans heerschende epidemie* [1946]:16. For similar views expressed by other speakers, see 12, 27 and 34. See also T.M. van Leeuwen, 'De geslachtsziektenbestrijding na den oorlog', *Tijdschrift voor Sociale Geneeskunde* 23 (1945):35-6; 90-1; 101-2; the reference here is to 101; and E.H. Hermans, 'Ons programma ter bestrijding der geslachtsziekten', *SH* 1946, no. 5/6:6-9.

85. For a discussion of the 'moral entrepreneur', see Becker [1963], Chapter 8.

86. On the panic surrounding liaisons between Dutch girls and Canadian men, see De Liagre Böhl 1985 and De Liagre Böhl & Meershoek 1989, esp. 83-90.

87. See E.H. Hermans, 'Vrijheid of dwang bij de geslachtsziektenbestrijding', *SH* 1946, no. 2:2; [anon.], 'De prostitutie-bestrijding in Nederland sinds 1940', *SH* 1946, no. 4:19-20; A. Bouman, 'Welke uitwerking had de oorlog op de sexueele moraliteit van ons volk?', *SH* 1946, no. 4:27; M.A. Duvekot, 'Contact tussen directe en indirecte geslachtsziektenbestrijding', *SH* 1947, no. 2/3:32.

88. Saal 1950:62. The same groups were identified as the chief culprits in discussions of 'Canadian girls'. One complaint that was often made, for instance, was that the Canadians were stopping the girls from going in search of jobs in factories or sewing workshops or as domestic servants; see De Liagre Böhl & Meershoek:118.
89. Saal 1950, Chapter III.
90. See Van Steenbergen 1950, Chapter II.
91. Van Steenbergen 1950:32.
92. De Liagre Böhl 1985:245. The same view is propounded in Kooy 1980:41.
93. De Liagre Böhl 1985:254. Here too he concurs with Kooy 1980:41-3.
94. Cf. e.g. Vinks (1954) for the return of Utrecht's syphilis patient population to normal levels in the period 1945 to 1950.
95. For this questionnaire, see Saal 1950; on the discrepancy between contemporary views on youth and the results of the questionnaire, see Poortstra [1987].
96. On this theory, see esp. De Liagre Böhl [1987]; see also De Liagre Böhl 1985.
97. Cf. De Rooy 1991:236-41.
98. See Van Lieshout 1985. For a more detailed discussion of the movement for public mental health, see Van der Grinten 1987.
99. A. Bouman, 'Welke uitwerking had de oorlog op de sexueele moraliteit van ons volk?', *Maandblad voor de Geestelijke Volksgezondheid* 1 (1946):100.
100. A. Bouman, 'Sexuele voorlichting en geslachtsziektenbestrijding', *SH* 1947, no. 2/3:12-20.
101. J.A.J. Barnhoorn, 'De bestrijding der geslachtsziekten in het leger', *SH* 1947, no. 2/3:21-9; this reference is to 25.
102. See J.A.J. Barnhoorn, 'Sociatrie in het leger', *Nederlands Militair Geneeskundig Tijdschrift* 4 (1951), no. 2:33-50.
103. J.A.J. Barnhoorn, 'De bestrijding der geslachtsziekten in het leger', *SH* 1947, no. 2/3:21-9; this quotation is from 26-7.
104. J.A.J. Barnhoorn, 'Psychiatrische en sociaal-psychiatrische beschouwingen over geslachtsziektenbestrijding, prostitutie en promiscuïteit', *Maandblad voor de Geestelijke Volksgezondheid* 9 (1954):138-51; this quotation is from 149.
105. A. Bouman, 'Welke uitwerking had de oorlog op de sexueele moraliteit van ons volk?', *Maandblad voor de Geestelijke Volksgezondheid* 1 (1946):100.
106. E.H. Hermans, 'Vrijheid of dwang tijdens de geslachtsziektenbestrijding?', *SH* 1946, no. 3:1-6 (this quotation is from 1). He had made this point before: 'Unfortunately it is still

insufficiently understood', he wrote, commenting on the clear
increase in the number of VD patients during the occupation years,
'that each case of venereal disease which presents for treatment is
merely a link in a chain of infections, and that a constant effort must
be made to break this chain.' See E.H. Hermans, 'De beteekenis der
geslachtsziekten als oorlogs-infectieziekten', *SH* sixth series, no. 5
(1943):62-72; this quotation is from 69.

107. E.H. Hermans, 'Vrijheid of dwang bij de geslachtsziektenbestrijding?'
3. *SH* 1946, no. 4/5:4.

108. See 'Voorloopig programma van de contactorganisatie voor de sociale
werksters van de geslachtsziektenbestrijding in Nederland', *SH* 1946,
no. 5/6:10; 'Verslag van de landelijke bijeenkomst van de
contactorganisatie der sociale werksters', *SH* 1947, no. 1:8-11.

109. M.A. Duvekot, 'Contact tussen directe en indirecte
geslachtsziektenbestrijding', *SH* 1947, no. 2/3:30-4; this quotation is
from 34.

110. M.A. Duvekot, 'Contact tussen directe en indirecte
geslachtsziektenbestrijding', *SH* 1947, no. 2/3:30.

111. On these plans for cooperation, see M.A. Duvekot, 'Het sociale werk
der adviesbureaux', *SH* 1946, no. 5/6:13-18; 'Contact tussen directe
en indirecte geslachtsziektenbestrijding', *SH* 1947, no. 2/3:30-4;
'Sociaal werk bij de geslachtsziektenbestrijding', *NTvG* 92 (1948),
III:2688-95.

112. On the following section, see De Regt 1981; De Regt [1984],
Chapter VIII. See also Dercksen & Verplanke 1987, Chapter 1.

113. *Rapport van de studie-commissie Querido.* Quoted in M.J. Hoytink,
'De zorg voor het onmaatschappelijke gezin in nieuwe banen?',
Tijdschrift voor Maatschappelijk Werk 2 (1948), no. 24:374-5.

114. For a survey of the history of the fight against antisocial conduct, see
Dercksen & Verplanke 1987; cf. also Van Dongen 1968, a historical
study, esp. 32-9. Van Dongen gives a survey of all research on
antisocial conduct that was done between 1945 and 1966. For
contemporary views on the antisocial family, see the special issue of
the *Tijdschrift voor Maatschappelijk Werk* 2 (1948), no. 24 and the
Maandblad voor de Geestelijke Volksgezondheid in the years 1945–1950.
See also Mol & Van Lieshout 1989:91-5. De Regt 1986 gives an
account of the disappearance of the category of the antisocial family.

115. Van Leeuwen did indeed consider coercive provisions to be
indispensable, but added the proviso 'as little coercion as is absolutely
essential, and as much voluntary cooperation achieved through
persuasion as is possible'. See Van Leeuwen, in *De bestrijding van de
thans heerschende epidemie* [1946]:29-30.

116. For the approval of coercive measures after the Second World War, see e.g. *Bestrijding van de thans heerschende epidemie* [1946]; and *SH* 1949, no. 3/4, which include the results of the questionnaire.
117. *Bestrijding van de thans heerschende epidemie* [1946]:45.
118. Hermans, 'Vrijheid of dwang bij de geslachtsziektenbestrijding', *SH* 1946, no. 5/6:2-6; this quotation is from 5.
119. Hermans, 'Vrijheid of dwang bij de geslachtsziektenbestrijding', *SH* 1946, no. 5/6:2-6; this quotation is from 5.
120. C.M. van der Fliert, 'Naar aanleiding van de praeventiedag te Leiden', *SH* 1946, no. 5/6:10-13; this quotation is from 11.
121. M.A. Duvekot, 'Het sociale werk der adviesbureaux', *SH* 1946, no. 5/6:15.
122. See Dercksen & Verplanke 1987:78 ff.
123. 'Verslag van de landelijke bijeenkomst', *SH* 1947, no. 1:8-11.
124. M.A. Duvekot, 'Contact tussen directe en indirecte geslachtsziektenbestrijding', *SH* 1947, no. 2/3:32, 33.
125. The repressive tendencies in post-war attitudes to the tackling of social abuses tempt us to concur with theorists such as Foucault [1975;1976] and Donzelot [1977] in pointing to the disciplinary and normalizing character of social work in this period. In their theories they place particular emphasis on the force exerted by interest groups in society, and at a somewhat later stage by care institutions, in deliberate contacts with the lower classes in which they set out to subjugate these persons by, among other things, imposing middle-class lifestyles on them. As I do not, for the rest, adhere closely to the views of these theorists of the 'disciplinary' process, I shall not embark on a more detailed discussion of this incidental interpretation in their terms.
126. See Van Doorn 1954, esp. 81-90. See also Gastelaars 1985, Chapter 4.
127. See De Liagre Böhl, Nekkers & Slot (eds) 1981; De Rooy 1986:122-3.
128. See e.g. E.H. Hermans, 'Geslachtsziektenbestrijding en dwangmaatregelen', *SH*, fourth series, no. 4 (1937):136. Later too, in his memoirs, Hermans bemoaned the fact that venereal disease control had so often become entangled in matters of morality; cf. Hermans 1976:96-7.
129. P.H. van der Hoog, 'Open brief aan den voorzitter van de Ned. Vereeniging tot Bestrijding der Geslachtsziekten', *NTvG* 73 (1929) II:5295-7.
130. Minutes of the meeting held on 20 July 1944. Archives of P.G. Bakker, Sexually Transmitted Diseases Foundation (SOA Stichting), Utrecht.
131. It had already been announced in 1942 that *Sexueele Hygiëne* would

appear in two series: one for the 'practical workers' that would be
entirely devoted to venereal disease control, and another that would
focus on the battle against the moral degeneration of the Dutch
youth, and Dutch girls in particular. See editorial 'Bij het begin der
zesde reeks', *SH*, sixth series, no. 1 (1942):1-3. Not many more
editions of the periodical appeared, however, and after early 1943 it
stopped altogether. It was not until 1946 that the split was effected.
Series B was closely attuned, both in its objectives and through the
person of Bouman, to the public mental health movement discussed
above. For a time, there was some talk of including series B in the
Maandblad voor de Geestelijke Volksgezondheid, but this idea was
abandoned. See Minutes of 28 March 1946. Archives of P.G. Bakker,
Sexually Transmitted Diseases Foundation, Utrecht.

132. James Scott 1985:284-9; James Scott 1990.
133. Joan Scott 1988, esp. Chapter 2: 'Gender: a useful category of
      historical analysis'.

4

Calm Before the Storm (1950–1985)

Seldom did it appear quieter on the VD front than in the 1950s. An extensive and well-organized control network routinely traced contacts and ensured that sufferers were referred for medical treatment, while penicillin and other antibiotics had improved treatment immensely and the shrinking patient population was a source of complacency. By 1959, the number of new syphilis patients had dwindled to a mere 2% of the corresponding figure at the height of the epidemic in 1947. In the case of gonorrhoea the drop was less spectacular, but here too, the number of new patients in 1959 was a mere 16% of the number registered for 1947 (see Appendix I). In such circumstances it appeared somewhat exaggerated to maintain facilities at their existing post-war levels: the advice centres' annual reports revealed that some provinces had almost no patients at all.[1] Furthermore, tracing patients and ensuring that they finished their treatment, which was what these centres did, seemed far less urgent than it had in the past, now that penicillin treatment had proved so successful. So it was not long before cuts were made in the subsidies that the diverse establishments received for venereal disease control.[2] Out of the fifty-odd advice centres that had been operational shortly after the war, fewer than 20 remained in the early 1960s; in the provinces of Friesland, Drenthe, Gelderland, Noord-Brabant and Limburg, every single one had been closed.[3] The Anti-Venereal Disease Society, whose journal had appeared for the last time in 1949, lost its subsidy and continued to exist on paper only, with a nominal chairman and secretary presiding over the silence.

Hardly had all these cuts and closures been completed when the optimistic mood began to falter. In 1959, 1963 and 1967, the Chief

179

Health Inspectorate conducted questionnaires among GPs that revealed a steady rise in the incidence of syphilis: per 1,000 inhabitants it grew from 1.8 in 1959 to 3.9 in 1963 and 5.2 in 1967, and this trend continued, bar an occasional deviation, until the early 1980s.[4] The same rise in incidence had been noted – even earlier – in other countries.[5] Some few people directly involved in VD control, most of them health inspectors and dermatologists, followed these foreign developments and reported them in medical journals, but such narrators aroused little broad-ranging concern in society at this time.

This chapter deals with a unique interlude in the history of venereal diseases, a period during which most such ailments, as far as they were identified as such, could be cured rapidly and easily. This situation coincided with certain medical and social trends, producing a mood of unconcern about VD that was historically quite rare. Then, with the advent of herpes genitalis, this cavalier serenity collapsed.

New characters

The annual figures published by the Chief Health Inspectorate for visitors to advice centres show that it was not only the size of the patient population that changed in the first few decades after the war, but also its composition. Patients tended to be younger than before, and they were more likely to be single. This trend was especially pronounced among men: between 1946 and 1965, the percentage of married men out of the total number of male VD sufferers dropped from 45% to 18%. The same trend was visible among women, though to a lesser extent. From a comparable initial position in 1946, the proportion of married women declined to 36% in 1965.[6] This shift towards a more youthful, single patient population aroused little comment, and did not prompt the introduction of any new characters in VD scenarios. The modest number of sufferers and the effective ways of dealing with them made venereal disease something of a non-issue.

In the 1960s, however, a few alarm bells started to ring. Three new characters were hesitantly brought onto the stage, apparently linked to the single young person who was now the standard VD sufferer. The amateur who had played such a prominent role in the preceding period no longer figured in the cast. This is easy to explain: the rise of amateurs as a special category had signalled the emergence of an extra-marital female sexuality that could no longer be confidently placed within the context of prostitution. The very

180

word 'amateur' inevitably evoked an association with the 'professional' from which, as a concept, it was derived. As female sexuality started to take on an independent existence outside marriage, the association with prostitution came to seem misplaced, and the amateur disappeared into the wings. In the 1960s, however, a new and younger variety of promiscuous girl made her entrance – the *teenager*. Anxious commentators cited developments in England, the United States and Scandinavia in support of their plea for heightened vigilance in relation to teenagers. It was feared that in the Netherlands too, more and more teenage girls would be exposed to venereal diseases.[7] The same fears were expressed, albeit in more muted tones, in relation to teenage boys.

There were two other new characters. The first was the *foreigner*, a term that included sailors and tourists, but that was used primarily to refer to foreign employees in the Netherlands. In 1964 the *Nederlands Tijdschrift voor Geneeskunde* published a letter to the editor alleging a connection between foreign employees and the rising incidence of venereal disease. The author, the intrepid E.H. Hermans, was not the type of man to mince words:

> In the first place, I would point out that venereal diseases are rampant in some of the regions from which these persons hail. But even if they enter our country untainted, these dark-skinned foreign workers have a southern air about them that evidently exudes a certain fascination, which plays an important role in the sexual contacts that these warm-blooded men, who, living as they do here in an unmarried state, will naturally seek out. As a rule they have little difficulty going from one sexual liaison to the next, which will obviously increase the risk of the rapid radial spread of any treponema or gonococcal infection that is contracted along the way.[8]

Again, evidence from abroad was used in support of these allegations. Research findings from countries that included England and Germany evidently fuelled the belief that foreign workers in the Netherlands, too, were much to blame for the spread of venereal diseases.

The third new character that appeared in the 1960s was the *homosexual*. Curiously enough, this character had been completely ignored in all the previous debates on venereal disease. Even in discussions of the all-male worlds of army and navy, there was no allusion whatsoever to the possible existence of homosexuality. It was not until the mid-1950s that the homosexual stepped out onto the stage; research (most of it from London and Paris) demonstrated an increasing number of infections contracted through male homosexual contacts.[9] These research findings were regularly cited in and around 1960 – the *Nederlands Tijdschrift voor Geneeskunde* published them, for instance – but comparable data for the Netherlands were unavailable. Reference was simply made to the prevalence of promiscuity among male homosexuals, another foreign research finding, after which it would be concluded that the situation in the Netherlands was presumably much the same.[10]

Thus the teenager, the foreigner and the homosexual were the main characters in the VD plots produced by a small group of narrators in the 1960s. They made up a tightly-knit threesome, as it was even rumoured – also on the basis of foreign reports – that teenage girls tended to be infected by immigrants, while teenage boys often contracted the diseases from older homosexuals.[11] The dermatologist Suurmond commented as follows:

> It has clearly emerged from foreign publications that the increase in lues and gonorrhoea chiefly manifests itself in certain population groups and occupations, viz. homosexuals, foreigners (sailors, foreign workers and tourists) and teenagers.[12]

There was in fact no reason to assume, on the strength of these foreign publications, that the pattern they revealed could also be applied to the Netherlands. And we are now in a position to examine the truth of these alleged connections: for the 1960s and 1970s, unlike previous periods, we can draw on a certain amount of statistical information.

Before delving into these statistics, however, I wish to comment briefly on the link between promiscuity and venereal diseases. As emerged in the previous chapter, casual sexual liaisons, later simply called promiscuity, acquired an increasingly prominent position in the aetiology of venereal disease from the 1930s onwards. After the Second World War, this strong link between promiscuity and venereal diseases was expressed in the new chain epidemiological model. This link was retained in the 1960s. The amateur and the three new characters had in common their supposedly promiscuous sex lives, a pattern of behaviour that contemporary commentators assumed to be directly related to the graph showing the incidence of venereal disease. Other circumstances – indifference among medical practitioners, public authorities and society at large, and the inadequacies of medical students' training – though not dismissed altogether, were believed to be of secondary importance. Despite the continued identification of promiscuity as the main aetiological factor, however, it was placed in a wider context. During the 1960s, the causal relationship between promiscuity and venereal disease was 'sociologized': narrators increasingly highlighted the sociological factors underlying promiscuity, and hence linked a broad spectrum of changes in society to the new increase in cases of venereal disease.

Where previous generations had insisted on the need to fight against moral degeneracy and the loss of religious faith, now the emphasis was all on social and cultural change, a theme less likely to polarize public opinion. Such change included secularization and freer attitudes to sex, but it also embraced matters as diverse as higher standards of living and the increase in tourism. The onward march of urbanization and industrialization, too, were seen as having influenced people's way of life.[13] This widening of outlook altered the causal relationship between promiscuity and venereal disease, hushing somewhat the accusatory note of the past; what had once been a moral indictment was now merely a sociological correlation. Rather than pointing to a defect in someone's character, a failure to uphold moral standards, during the 1960s promiscuity increasingly came to be seen as a phenomenon influenced by diverse social, economic and cultural developments.

This widening of outlook leaves unanswered, however, the question of whether the central assumption – that promiscuity was directly linked to the incidence of infection – was actually true. In general, to state that promiscuity leads to the spread of venereal disease is a truism, but the converse does not necessarily follow. If it can be shown that the three groups referred to (or indeed quite different groups) contracted more cases of venereal disease after 1960, we cannot immediately conclude that they became more promiscuous. In specific cases, other, or additional, explanations may be at hand. For instance, the increased incidence of venereal disease in the 1960s and 1970s may have been partly – or even primarily – caused not by any increase in promiscuity but by the large-scale rejection of the condom, the only contraceptive that also protects against venereal disease, in favour of new methods of contraception.

In specific situations there are almost always attenuating factors where a direct link is posited between promiscuity and the frequency of venereal disease. The particular significance of an increase in incidence – and in the case at hand, an increase among specific population groups – therefore has to be investigated each time afresh.

If we wish to focus on the characters highlighted in the literature on venereal disease in the 1960s, we can use three syphilis questionnaires that the Chief Health Inspectorate conducted among GPs in 1959, 1963 and 1967, and the questionnaire on the incidence of syphilis and gonorrhoea that Bijkerk conducted among dermatologists in 1967. Aside from these sources, there are also the advice centres' figures for 1940 and afterwards. Finally, in 1976 the compulsory registration of syphilis and gonorrhoea was introduced, so that national figures were compiled, and for the year 1980 detailed statistics were published on the basis of the registration figures and the figures reported by outpatient clinics. On the whole, the figures for the period 1960–1980 lack uniformity; any comparative analysis calls for a certain flexibility in the methodological approach, but there is no reason to doubt the trends they indicate.[15] It would be a pity not to take the opportunity to test the robustness of the new characters against the backdrop of the statistics, although the following analysis should not be accorded too much weight.

The role of the *teenager* tended if anything to diminish between 1959 and 1980. Although the number of cases per 10,000 persons rose slightly, the increase was less than the total rise in the incidence of venereal disease in this period.[16] In percentage terms, teenagers accounted for a small proportion of VD from 1960 onwards. It is however striking that girls accounted for more than twice the percentage of total female VD patients relative to the equivalent figures for boys among male sufferers, both at the beginning of this period and in 1980: the percentage of teenage girls (interpreted here as the 15–19 age group) among women with syphilis fell from 14% in 1959 to 10% in 1980, with occasional deviations from this trend in between. During this same period, the percentage of teenage boys fell from 7% to 4%. For gonorrhoea the percentage of girls declined less markedly, from 17% to 15%, with the percentage of teenage boys remaining stable between 1967 and 1980 at 5.5%. Viewed from this vantage-point, it would indeed appear that it was mainly young girls that were becoming infected, but because of the numerical preponderance of male patients, in absolute terms teenage boys were in the majority.

Turning to consider the proportion of *foreigners* among VD sufferers – and foreign workers in particular – we discover a declining trend, belying the assumptions of contemporary observers, from about 30% in the mid-1960s to about 20% in the early 1980s. In both cases, almost all were men.[17] The figure of 30%, which derives from the 1963 questionnaire, was entirely undifferentiated: it lumped seamen, foreign workers and tourists under a single heading, so that – as expressly stated in the conclusion – 'the questionnaire does not provide any basis for finding a correlation between the relatively large number of foreign syphilis patients and the foreign workers employed in this country'.[18]

That immigrants and foreign workers continued to be labelled as a high-risk group, despite the actual drop in the percentage of foreign patients, is not impossible to explain. Firstly, the figure of 30% from the 1963 questionnaire suggests that the number of foreigners with venereal disease had always been large or that it had risen sharply in the 1950s.[19] As this was the precise period during which foreign workers started coming to the Netherlands, the suspicions that came to the fore may be seen as expressions of a mixture of personal experience, observation and xenophobic sentiments.

Another fact that may have associated foreigners with venereal disease in people's minds was the large number of Dutch people who contracted VD in another country. In 1963, over one-fourth of Dutch nationals with syphilis had been infected abroad. The corresponding figure for 1967 was over 20%; for gonorrhoea it was 10%. After 1967 records were no longer kept on the country of infection. Nevertheless, the expansion of international contacts of all kinds probably played a key role in the increased incidence of venereal disease in the 1960s and 1970s. Two long-term trends are involved here, both of which accelerated tremendously after the Second World War: the enormous growth in international trade and mass tourism, and the development of ever faster means of transport. The combination of these two trends had significant epidemiological consequences.[20] Contacts between people from various parts of the world now occurred with unprecedented frequency, and at the same time it had become possible for infections to travel half-way across the world while the person carrying the disease remained entirely oblivious of it. Although there was of course nothing new about germs crossing borders – and in previous chapters we have already noted the awareness of the problem and willingness to act internationally to curb it – the rapid expansion of contacts had outpaced all such measures. In the past, international infections mainly reared their head in wartime or during periods of mass migration, but by the second half of the 20th century all such qualifications of time and place had become diluted.[21]

Finally, the concern about the number of *homosexual infections* – in contrast to those singling out teenagers and foreigners – appears to be supported by statistics. The percentage of gay men among the total VD patient population increased rapidly after 1959. An initial indication of this change is the male:female ratio. While men had always been in the majority, the ratio became considerably more lopsided in the 1960s: in 1959 men with syphilis outnumbered women by 2:1; in 1963 the ratio was 4:1 and in 1967 5.5:1. By 1977 it had reached 6:1. A different trend was visible in respect of gonorrhoea: a ratio of 4:1 in 1967 declined to 2:1 in 1976, at which level it has since remained stable. This accords with the fact that gay men accounted for a far higher proportion of syphilis than of gonorrhoea patients: in 1963, 11% of men with syphilis were homosexual, in 1967 this percentage had risen to 26% and by 1980 it was almost 60%.[22] Where gonorrhoea was concerned, the percentage rise was from 8% in 1967 to approximately 25% in 1980.[23] The increasing proportion of gay men among VD sufferers, especially where syphilis was concerned, is one of the most pronounced developments of the 1960s and 1970s.[24] It obviously calls for an explanation. Is it correct, in this case, to interpret this trend as indicating an increase in promiscuity among gay men?

In the first place, the increase in the number of infections in gay men paralleled the increasing openness of society *vis-à-vis* homosexuality, so that the trend outlined here may have been enhanced by a growth in the number of persons 'confessing' to homosexuality. Another possibility is that of a change in sexual practices, perhaps involving a shift towards more anal intercourse. The third conjecture is more general – bearing on homosexuals and heterosexuals alike – and concerns the number of patients presenting with a second or subsequent infection – known in the professional jargon as 'repeaters'. The statistics are generally compiled either from the number of cases or from the number of new diagnoses. Neither of these, it will be appreciated, equals the total number of patients. Someone who presents with a new syphilis infection five times within the space of one year will inflate the statistics for both the number of cases and the number of diagnoses. And someone in whom two separate diagnoses are made during a single visit to the doctor's surgery will have a proportionate effect on the figures for new diagnoses. In other words, it is possible that the statistics were in part made up, year in year out, of the same people.[25] In this case, the increased incidence would be the result, not of promiscuous lifestyles spreading among ever larger groups, but, for instance, of an increasing degree of promiscuity among one or more sub-groups. In other words, a substantial number of homosexual patients registered each year may have belonged to relatively small sub-groups, who indulged in specific sexual practices and were – within their own group – extremely promiscuous. Research on recurring infections demonstrates a high rate of repeaters among VD patients. The 1967 questionnaire revealed that about 35% of sufferers had had venereal disease before,[26] and later studies turned up even higher percentages.[27] When considering the increase in the number of homosexual infections, the fact that there was one disease in particular – syphilis – in which homosexuals accounted for a particularly large proportion of patients also points in the direction of small groups within the homosexual sub-culture whose members were constantly re-infecting one another.

All things told, these three reservations do not appreciably undermine the conclusion that homosexual promiscuity soared during the 1960s and 1970s. It is however likely that a relatively large proportion of the homosexual patient population was accounted for by a small sub-group. The striking increase in the number of homosexual infections from the 1960s onwards is best attributed to a combination of the spread of promiscuity among the gay population as a whole and the development of extremely promiscuous and relatively isolated sub-groups within that population. Sexual practices associated with a high risk of infection probably became more popular in these circles. All this happened against the backdrop of the emerging gay liberation movement, one result of which was the growth of a thriving gay sub-culture with a high concentration of sexual meeting-places. This internationally oriented sub-culture created ideal conditions for the development of a close-knit network of sexual relations. As will be shown, later research, conducted after the advent of AIDS, confirmed the belief that gay men, on average, have far more sexual partners than heterosexuals.[28]

Thus far we have checked the extent to which the naming of new characters in the early 1960s corresponded to the picture presented by the statistics. The beliefs popularly held and expressed were in fact borne out only in the case of gay men.[29] Neither the teenagers nor the foreigners contributed appreciably to the increased incidence of venereal disease in the 1960s and 1970s, and they soon vanished from the stage. The gay man remained, but his shoulders were surely not broad enough to carry the weight of two decades of venereal afflictions. So who was actually contributing in the wings? In fact, the group mainly responsible for the growth of VD infections was almost too obvious to be noticed: the heterosexual population in the 20–30 age group. Not a single narrator troubled to create a new character out of this category, yet for both sexes it was the 20–30 age group that provided most patients, and in which the incidence was several times higher than in the population as a whole, and so it remained over the years.[30] The increase of homosexual patients in this age group explains at most a part of this discrepancy, and even then only, in the main, among men with syphilis. The lion's share of the increased incidence of VD was attributable to heterosexual men and women in their twenties.

New diseases

People active in venereal disease control in the 1960s and 1970s had more on their minds than the growing group of syphilis and gonorrhoea sufferers. Their attention was increasingly claimed by 'new' diseases. Different types of venereal disease existed alongside one another, each representing, as it were, a different generation.[31] Syphilis and gonorrhoea belonged to the oldest generation, and acquired more and more the status of 'classical' ailments. Effective treatment had removed their most alarming features, without however preventing their resurgence, after a lull in the late 1950s. In 1976 the Netherlands introduced a compulsory obligation to register cases of syphilis and gonorrhoea. From that point on, gonorrhoea has topped the frequency list of diseases liable for registration; around 1980 it was also, worldwide, the most common infectious disease. Syphilis and gonorrhoea both peaked in the early 1980s, with incidences of about 8 and 100, respectively, per 100,000 inhabitants.[32]

The second generation consisted of a cluster of bacterial venereal diseases, most of which are curable, but which are often asymptomatic or accompanied by few, vague complaints, so that they often go unnoticed. What is more, these disorders do not attract much attention. The public has little awareness of trichomoniasis or non-gonorrhoeal urethritis, for instance, although both became quite common after the Second World War.[33] Nor do these diseases dazzle medical minds with their complexity: they merely call for better public information and routine screening, which is not the stuff of sensational research discoveries. Infections caused by the micro-organism *Chlamydia trachomatis* loom particularly large in this second generation of diseases.[34] This micro-organism produces a variety of disorders: among other things, it causes most non-gonorrhoeal urethritis, a disease that occurs almost exclusively among men. In women, a chlamydia infection can likewise result in a variety of complaints, some of which are known collectively as pelvic inflammatory disease. A chronic inflammation of the fallopian tubes resulting in permanent infertility is among the possible effects of an undetected chlamydia infection.[35]

Then there is a third generation, comprising incurable viral venereal diseases. Since 1980 genital herpes and hepatitis B have figured at the top of this list, but genital warts and cytomegalovirus infections are also included. Hepatitis B was shown to be a sexually transmitted disease in the early 1970s: as a venereal disease, it proved especially prevalent among homosexual men. A study conducted in 1980 on a large group of homosexuals showed that some 60% had had a hepatitis B infection, which was roughly six to ten times the incidence in the Dutch population as a whole.[36] There was a brief flare of publicity surrounding herpes genitalis; we shall return to this in due course. There is as yet no cure for either hepatitis B or genital herpes, although we do have a vaccine for hepatitis. While not life-threatening, these diseases are both unpleasant and persistent. Furthermore, in the case of hepatitis B, serious complications may develop.

Too little material is available to allow us to draw any precise conclusions from the introduction and spread of these new diseases; at best we can hazard a few general comments. One possibility, for instance, is that the apparent increased incidence of these diseases is partly attributable to improvements in diagnostics. A disease such as non-gonococcal urethritis, for instance, did not become visible until after the introduction of penicillin, when it became apparent that certain gonorrhoea-like conditions totally failed to respond to the new drug.[37] There are many other ways in which diagnostics and registration have been improved over the past few decades, some enabling the identification of new types of sexually transmitted diseases and as a result possibly creating a distorted picture of their occurrence. Nevertheless, improved identification cannot completely explain the upsurge in these diseases or the resulting change in the venereal landscape.

In his book *Plagues and Peoples*, William McNeill gives several other possible explanations for the new patterns of disease. In it, he emphasizes the impact of changes in patterns of contact between and within societies on the rise and spread of diseases. In line with this thinking, the rise of an entire collection of apparently new sexually transmitted diseases in the latter half of the 20th century can be seen as an indication – in two different ways – of changes of this kind.

Firstly, the growth of such diseases points to a gradual intensification in sexual relations between people. With the exception of hepatitis B, the modern venereal diseases are first and foremost indices of heterosexual behaviour. Here again, the largest group affected is that of people in their twenties. Among men the 25–30 age group prevails, but those in their thirties are also well represented; the majority of female patients are in their early twenties, with the 15–19 age group more in evidence than in the case of boys.[38]

Secondly, the general changes outlined above were found throughout Western countries, which likewise attests to new patterns of contact – more frequent and on a larger scale – between different parts of the world. More regions than before were now linked through sexual liaisons, multiplying the channels through which venereal diseases could be passed on. AIDS provides the most recent illustration of this, but before this the 'classical' disorders had already acquired an increasingly international character,[39] and 'new' ones had arrived. Among prostitutes and their clientele, for instance, penicillin-resistant gonococcus strains had become particularly entrenched.[40] Hepatitis B and sexually transmitted intestinal parasites, on the other hand, had spread among homosexual men.[41] Herpes, chlamydia and other maladies were being diagnosed with increasing frequency in heterosexuals, and soft chancre – still a native disease in the late 19th century, but now classified as 'tropical' – was being imported from abroad once again from the late 1970s onwards.[42] Other 'tropical' venereal diseases have also been detected in the Netherlands, though on a limited scale, over the past few decades.

All these changes meant that the chain epidemiological model was increasingly found wanting: it was too primitive a model to accommodate the expanding range and complexity of the problem of venereal disease. Although the change-over to a new model was already being prepared in the 1970s, it was with the advent of AIDS that the defects of the chain model became glaringly obvious.

The resurrection of venereal disease control

Despite the clear increase in the number of VD patients, it was not until the 1970s that practical consequences ensued, and the job of venereal disease control was given a new lease of life. The Dutch government took a leading role here. Viewed historically this is interesting, as the government had in the past kept out of this area, leaving it to private organizations to take action. Private initiative was not left out of the new proposals, but it was now upstaged by the government, which insisted to district nursing services and the Dutch Anti-Venereal Disease Society that the work of venereal disease control should be resumed, and which made the necessary resources available. In the 1960s, at the request of the Ministry of Social Affairs and Public Health, two advisory reports were drawn up on the revival of the control system, one by the Public Health Central Council and one by a working party of the Chief Health Inspectorate.[43] These led, in 1970, to a memorandum by State Secretary Kruisinga which was the first step towards the rebuilding of a control apparatus.

This memorandum announced certain organizational changes. For a start, new subsidies were created to enable district nursing and municipal health services to extend the remaining advice centres, which they renamed and incorporated into the new VD Control Services. Like the old centres, these services were intended to focus on non-curative aspects of control, and were hence expressly not involved in the actual business of medical treatment. After 1980, most of them resorted directly under municipal or district health services.

Secondly, Kruisinga's plans jerked the Dutch Anti-Venereal Disease Society, which had been slumbering for some fifteen years, back to life. Its initial movements were sluggish – not surprising as all it had left was a Chairman, ex-secretary Hermans, and the dermatologist Van Steenbergen, who was then the nominal secretary. After reading the State Secretary's announcement, Van Steenbergen proposed to Hermans that a meeting be called. But who should be invited? And what should the agenda look like? 'Don't start talking about the minutes of some previous meeting', warned Van Steenbergen. 'There aren't any, nor is there even a minute book. Or has your secretary perhaps kept something of the kind?'[44] The government had listed seven tasks to be undertaken by the Society, but first the latter had to decide whether it could still justify its existence. When a meeting was called in 1972 to debate this issue, a unanimous decision was reached to keep the Society alive.[45] In the years that followed, the Society took a few hesitant steps forward: it became a foundation and from 1979 onwards it acquired a journal of its own again: *Sexueel Overdraagbare Aandoeningen* (*Sexually Transmitted Diseases*), shortly afterwards renamed the *SOA-Bulletin*. In the Society's name too, 'venereal disease' changed into sexually transmitted diseases, so that the Society began its second childhood in the mid-1980s as the *SOA Stichting*, or Sexually Transmitted Diseases Foundation (referred to hereafter simply as the Foundation).

In the meantime, new provisions had also been put in place in the medical sphere. In 1976, a reporting obligation was introduced for syphilis and gonorrhoea that enabled the authorities to keep track of the incidence of these diseases to a reasonable degree. In the same year, the government provided a subsidy to establish seven new outpatient clinics in Amsterdam, Rotterdam, The Hague and Utrecht, where treatment was free of charge and no referral was required from a GP. A few years later, it became possible in the rest of the country to have venereal disease treated free of charge by a dermatologist with an independent practice. In addition, one could still get treatment (for a fee) at contraception clinics. And as an extra service for persons suffering frequent re-infections, Amsterdam Health Service sent a nurse off once a month, armed with a syringe, to a number of homosexual meeting-places, where those present would be scrutinized for signs of neglected or hitherto unnoticed cases of syphilis and appropriate action taken.[46]

In the 1970s, various curative facilities were created at the government's initiative, to accommodate a growing number of patients. But at the same time, the debate on venereal disease, that had raged more or less continuously until the early 1950s, fell strangely silent. A small group of professionals working in the field monitored the latest developments, but that was all. The menace of venereal disease, once a stock item in almost every treatise on sexual activity, dwindled into the most marginal of concerns in the 1960s and 1970s. Or in the words of C. Wright Mills, while venereal infections probably gave rise to a good deal of 'personal troubles', they certainly did not constitute a 'public issue' in this period.[47]

Against the backdrop of a steadily growing disease rate, all efforts focused on the availability of medical facilities, while pronouncements of moral or religious concern, which had traditionally set the tone of the debate on venereal disease, were heard no more. For a while, cure was easier than prevention. In the 1960s, the emphasis was all on timely treatment, while at the same time brave efforts were made to dispel the atmosphere of drama and sinfulness that had traditionally surrounded the problem of venereal disease and to replace it with a more matter-of-fact approach. The message was loud and clear: venereal diseases were normal diseases, and just as in the case of other *normal* diseases, anyone afflicted should go to the doctor as soon as possible. D.J.H. Vermeer, a dermatologist and later chairman of the Foundation, expressed these sentiments, which had a no-nonsense ring about them that was characteristic of their day, when he said he hoped that venereal disease could be discussed 'without all those emotions'. He was irritated by the lingering sense of mystery and guilt that still obscured a clear view of the problem, and regarded the sense of sinfulness that continued to oppress many patients as completely unnecessary; these diseases were quite simply ordinary infections. People burdened by such feelings should emulate the attitude of sailors, who were streets ahead in this area: 'A sailor simply turns up at the clinic and says: Doctor, I've got the clap. Right, we say, let's do something about it. And no bullshit.'[48]

People writing public information leaflets also made every effort to avoid striking a dramatic note: the message was 'simply to keep your eyes open a bit and go to the doctor'. In retrospect, these publications have an air of almost forced breeziness about them:

> But there is no need to make a fuss about venereal diseases. You should take a sensible view of them however, and at the slightest suspicion that you might have one you must simply go to your GP just as you do with any other disease. The plain truth is that anyone who has sex can get venereal disease, and that danger will always be there. If you really wish to eliminate the risk of venereal disease altogether, there is in fact only one way to do so: don't have sex at all. But that is like staying inside all the time to be sure you will never be run over. A better option is simply to keep your eyes open a bit. And if you think you've got something – just go to the doctor. A doctor is someone who tackles diseases. And that includes venereal diseases.[49]

Venereal diseases had been stripped of the aura of seriousness that had always enveloped them in the past, and seemed to have moved quite outside the realm of social problems. The message propagated in the 1970s was that anyone who saw or felt anything suspicious would do well to have it checked out straight away; with any luck it would only be a venereal disease.

Sexual enthusiasm and medical authority

Within a relatively brief space of time, the problem of venereal disease was transformed, losing a large part of its traditional ballast. Two trends in particular helped to work this metamorphosis: one was a change in public attitudes to sexuality, and the other was the tendency for medical science to acquire the status of a moral authority. Although to some extent interconnected, these developments can be followed separately.

The first was triggered by the introduction of penicillin. Diseases that had for centuries been closely associated with sexual intercourse, that had for most of that time been incurable and had only become treatable in this century – and even then only when patients submitted to years of medical intervention – could be dispelled, from 1950 onwards, by a simple course of treatment. Antibiotics must be credited with having largely defused the menace of VD, removing a major constraint on freer sexual relations. But there was another significant turning-point in the 1950s, relating to ideas about birth control.[50] The advent of oral contraception in the early 1960s reinforced the new way of thinking and helped accelerate its general acceptance.

These two innovations occurred on the eve of the changes during the 1960s and 1970s that have acquired the name of a sexual revolution. It is now generally agreed that this 'revolution' largely consisted of a drastic narrowing of the gap that had widened over several generations between words and deeds; in other words, it was largely attitudes that changed, and not so much sexual behaviour, which had been undergoing a gradual liberalization over a much longer period of time, and which the new ideas of the 1960s at most served to accelerate in certain sections of society.[51] But even if the sexual revolution is seen as an ideological 'catching up' with reality, its revolutionary quality appears, in retrospect, to have been greatly exaggerated. The 1950s had paved the way for many of the changes that occurred openly in the 1960s, so that it is inaccurate to speak of a new departure.[52] This is not to say that this period did not witness some essential changes; gradual developments, too, may eventually turn the tide. In this case the cumulative result was the predominance of a different way of thinking and talking about sexuality, the development of a new attitude that has been aptly characterized as 'sexual enthusiasm'.[53] The key element of this attitude is the belief that sexuality is a vital part of human existence, and crucial to each individual's well-being. Besides being of fundamental importance, sexuality is seen by sexual enthusiasts as having a marked salutary influence. They accordingly believe it should be viewed in positive terms, as something in which a person participates voluntarily and for pleasure, not only a means of obtaining physical satisfaction but also a necessary condition for realizing one's full potential, for achieving a harmonious development and for building up successful relationships.[54]

Sexual enthusiasm had long been an undercurrent that occasionally ruffled the surface of conventional attitudes.[55] But what was new in the period following the Second World War was its sudden popularity: within a short space of time, a fundamentally positive view of sexuality ousted the traditional attitude that had

194

seen sex largely as a problem area. So the introduction of penicillin and increased acceptance of birth control, swiftly followed by the advent of the pill, cannot be identified as the root causes of sexual enthusiasm. They did provide the enabling conditions, however, for the new dominance of this view. Penicillin vanquished the perils of venereal disease, and the pill made it possible for sexuality to be seen primarily as an important part of a relationship rather than an act with a reproductive function. The combination of these two sealed the permanent redefinition of sexuality, as Paul Schnabel has put it, as an area 'free of consequences',[56] with the ideals of sexual enthusiasts becoming more attainable than ever before.

This chapter focuses chiefly on the way changing attitudes to sexual morality have helped to transform the problem of venereal disease over the past few decades.[57] One contributory factor was the fundamental optimism encapsulated in the 'enthusiastic' point of view; another was the resulting redefinition of the impediments that hampered people's sex lives. It is not surprising that a climate of sexual enthusiasm should have increased interest in the negative aspects of sexuality. After all, sexual problems and matters such as sexual abuse only become unseemly – are in fact only mentioned – once sex is labelled good, pleasurable and desirable. The 1960s and 1970s were preoccupied with a variety of problems associated with sexual relationships, but the danger of venereal disease was no longer one of them. Schnabel has defined the developments in sexual morality as a transition from a code of control or prohibition, characterized by a handful of strict rules, to a more elastic but far more complex morality of lifestyle. As a consequence, he explained, the problem of transgression had been replaced, in the public mind, by the problem of sexual failure.[58] Venereal diseases had traditionally played a role in regulating sexuality; they were the 'electric fence' that marked out the forbidden area. In the new scheme they had no such role; sexual enthusiasm largely highlighted sexual dysfunctions such as impotence, inhibitions, anorgasm and disorders of sexual arousement. These complaints did not underscore the perplexing and dangerous nature of forbidden sexuality, as venereal disease had always done; instead they were obstacles on the path to the best possible enjoyment of sexuality.[59]

There was another trend that helped to change the problem of venereal disease, namely the rise of medical science as an arbiter of moral issues. As far as venereal disease was concerned, this new role first became apparent in the 1970s, but in a wider context it was rooted in many long-term developments: secularization, rationalization, state building and the establishment of professional regimes. The first three of these constitute the explanatory backdrop for the fourth. Here, what is concerned is the establishment of a medical regime that De Swaan has described as 'the unintended effect of social contradictions which time and again appeared to be solvable by allowing medical people to decide'.[60]

The medicalization of society was not an automatic result of the growth of medical knowledge, nor of an unchecked tendency to imperialism on the part of the medical profession. It came about through the involvement of individual medical practitioners in social conflicts, partly because of personal ambition, and partly because the disputing parties believed that their conflict could be resolved by medical intervention. Eventually this meant that problems that were essentially of a social or moral character were increasingly translated into medical terms. The boundary between medical problems and those of a social or moral nature was thus constantly shifting, and medical science increasingly became the arbiter of issues that had previously belonged to the moral or religious domain. Crime, sexual perversion and alcoholism are just a few of the areas in which this trend has manifested itself.[61]

The Netherlands entered a period of rapid economic growth and unprecedented material prosperity after the Second World War, which accelerated the expansion of professional regimes such as medical science.[62] Medical advances reinforced this trend still further. These developments boosted people's appreciation of good health and their faith in medical science, a subject dealt with at length in the following chapter. The history of venereal disease since the Second World War also shows that medical science has acquired a more authoritative voice over the years in relation to sexual codes of conduct; other points of view have been increasingly marginalized. Moral and religious considerations were dominant in this area during the early decades of this century, and continued to make themselves felt up to the Second World War. From the mid-1950s onwards, however, their importance rapidly diminished. This trend was reflected in the prevailing balance between narrators and characters. While these had previously tended to express relations between men and women, and between social classes, they now increasingly came to express the doctor–patient relationship.

All this does not mean that medical guidelines and considerations were the only ones that counted. A change took place in the realm of sexuality – as in many other areas of social life – that De Swaan has described as a transition from a management by command to a management by negotiation; by mutual agreement and with regard for one another's wishes, and without the use of force, a great deal is now permissible.[63] These ostensibly simple rules of the negotiation regime map out the primary framework of limiting conditions which have been imposed on sexuality, and which determine the moral admissibility of specific sexual practices. In the absence of alternative authorities, medical opinion – within the bounds, it should be emphasized, of the negotiation regime – has become the main source of arguments advanced to explain and justify new sexual codes of conduct.[64] A medically based moral doctrine replaces standards of devoutness and virtue with standards of hygiene and statistical probability; while this makes its precepts less moralistic it does not make them any less compelling. But as long as venereal diseases were still easy to treat, the main sign of the advance of medical science as a moral authority in sexual matters was a negative one: the previous sources of moral inspiration had clearly dried up. In a positive sense, the authority of the medical voice first became clearly apparent with the advent of AIDS.

The development of sexual enthusiasm and the shift away from a sexual code of conduct based on religious and moral precepts to one based on medical science together transformed the significance of venereal disease in society. The triumph of medical morality meant that venereal diseases were above all to be taken seriously as diseases, and not as a punishment for immoral behaviour or degeneracy. While this explains the absence of traditional moral and religious agitation in the 1960s and 1970s, however, it does not altogether explain the absence of any public debate on venereal disease in this period. Even given the primacy of medical science, the development of widespread concern would have been entirely possible. But in an age in which venereal diseases were easy to cure, there were no medical grounds for concern, and sexual enthusiasm could flourish unchecked. This latter trend intensified the rejection of moralistic interference, and also made it less likely for people to think of VD as something that could put a damper on sexual pleasure, as it highlighted other kinds of sexual difficulties that were at the time regarded as more urgent. Viewed in this light, the historically curious lack of concern about venereal disease in the 1960s and 1970s becomes more intelligible. Indeed, this explanation not only clarifies the beginning of the silence, but also points to the two circumstances that could bring it to an end: a decrease in enthusiasm, and the rise of an incurable disease. After 1980, these two developments in turn triggered the revival of the debate on venereal disease.

Waning enthusiasm: the commotion surrounding herpes genitalis

As already noted, the rise of medical authority was a necessary but not a sufficient condition for the relative absence of comment on the steady increase in the incidence of venereal disease. It is only when combined with the reverse in traditional attitudes to sexuality that this mood of unconcern becomes intelligible. This public silence was first broken around 1980. It was not however the growing incidence of syphilis and gonorrhoea that revived public concern – both peaked in the early 1980s, with figures of 8 and 100 per 10,000 inhabitants respectively – as these could still be cured with a minimum of effort. Nor was it the second generation of sexually transmitted diseases, for which medication was also available. It was the disease herpes genitalis that first disturbed the calm waters of complacency.

The herpes debate distinguished itself from previous responses to venereal disease in a variety of ways. Firstly, American views were dominant in a way unknown in the past. Much of the preoccupation with herpes genitalis originated in the United States, and Dutch articles were virtually without exception a watered-down version of reports published in the United States. The concern about herpes remained mild in contrast to the American hype, but the subject nevertheless commanded a great deal of attention in the early 1980s. Another new feature was the importance of popular magazines and newspapers. Special pamphlets were a thing of the past, and the broad surveys and critical articles that once filled medical journals had dwindled into a bald presentation of medical facts; the social context of herpes was now discussed in daily newspapers and popular weeklies. The third difference had to do with the relationship between narrators and characters in the herpes scare; I shall return to this point later on.

The quantity and tone of the articles that appeared about herpes made it clear that the disease was taken very seriously. Headlines told a grisly tale. At one point half the population of the United States was reported to be infected with the virus. More cautious estimates put the infected population at 10–20%. *De Volkskrant* daily newspaper uncritically reproduced these figures, and on 25 September 1982 it reported that one out of seven adults in the Netherlands was infected with herpes genitalis. Moreover, the article went on, this figure was bound to rise in the near future, as no vaccine existed to prevent the disease nor had any medicine been found to cure it. 'Once you've been infected with the virus, it remains in your system'[65] was the dire American message.

This brief moment of renewed panic on the venereal front raises certain questions. Firstly, was herpes a new disease? Commentators were in complete agreement on this point: no, it was not. Descriptions of it had appeared, as writers never tired of pointing out, in the writings of Hippocrates in the 5th century B.C. The Emperor Tiberius was also confronted with the existence of herpes, and displayed considerable knowledge of the means by which the virus was transmitted. His promulgation of a decree forbidding kissing during public ceremonies, we are told, was prompted by concern about the high incidence of cold sores, a malady closely related to herpes genitalis.

The herpes family includes the Epstein-Barr virus (the agent that causes mononucleosis, also known as glandular fever or 'kissing disease'), cytomegalovirus (which causes a variety of infections) and herpes simplex (HSV), the virus that is at issue here. The latter has two variants: HSV-1, which generally causes cold sores, and HSV-2, which generally gives rise to genital herpes. We have to add 'generally', as cross-infections have been shown to exist, but HSV-2 is found in the vast majority of cases of genital herpes. This variant too was known in the past: in the late 19th century it was described as a fairly innocuous disorder.[66]

Since the disease was clearly not a new one, the next question to ask is whether its incidence had sharply increased. This was certainly the impression that was created. In the late 1970s a spectacular rise in the number of herpes sufferers was reported, and these numbers peaked in the early 1980s. Public concern increased in due proportion. Those wishing to acquaint themselves with all the ramifications of this problem had a wide range of books to choose from: *The Herpes Book*; *The Truth about Herpes*; *Herpes: the Facts*; *Herpes, Coping with a New Epidemic*; *Living with Herpes*; *Herpes, What to Do when you Have it* and so the list continues. An estimated 20 million Americans had been infected with the disease by 1982, a figure said to be increasing at the rate of 250,000 to 500,000 annually.[67] US medical practitioners are under no obligation to register cases of herpes, however, so that all these figures are estimates that may have been somewhat inflated at the height of the herpes scare.

The Netherlands also has no registration obligation, which means that no national figures are available. Aside from the estimate in *De Volkskrant* already referred to, however, certain statistics were compiled. First of all there are the records kept by the venereal disease control units of Amsterdam Health Service, which show a clear rise in incidence during the first half of the 1980s. The number of patients presenting with genital herpes rose from 218 to 517 between 1981 and 1985, but fell back to 284 in 1988.[68]

The National Institute for Public Health and Environment also has some useful statistics. From 1981 to 1988 it kept records on HSV-2 diagnoses from a number of cities – including Amsterdam and Rotterdam, where figures were highest. These show the same trend as in Amsterdam: a rise from 1981 to 1985 followed by a decline in incidence.[69] So figures covering a larger area also demonstrate a clear increase in the number of diagnoses of herpes genitalis.

Finally, several incidence studies were conducted using questionnaires. The results of one retrospective questionnaire on the presence of venereal disease, completed by treating physicians, showed that in 1985 – the peak year for herpes – an estimated 9,000 new cases of herpes genitalis were diagnosed. For syphilis and gonorrhoea the corresponding figures were about 1,400 and 36,500 respectively.[70]

That the number of registered herpes cases rose during the early 1980s is beyond dispute. But this is not necessarily a direct reflection of an actual rise in incidence. The great strides made in diagnostics played a role here, for instance, strengthening the impression that a new epidemic of an old disease had suddenly broken out.[71] One contemporary observer commented judiciously: 'Much uncertainty clouds the epidemiology of genital herpes infections. The current alleged rise in incidence is not proven: it is not impossible that identification and diagnostics have improved.' He accordingly concluded that 'there is apparently no foundation in the Netherlands for the alarmist tone characterizing recent articles in the daily press'.[72] We should therefore exercise a little caution when interpreting the registered increase in cases of herpes genitalis. Besides improvements in diagnostics, other factors may have also played a role. For instance, the introduction of acyclovir (which inhibits herpes but does not cure it) combined with the panicky reports on herpes in the media may have prompted numerous patients with recurrent infections to seek medical advice.[73]

But even when we leave all these considerations aside, and look at the bald statistics, the rise in the number of herpes patients – at any rate in the Netherlands – was scarcely as spectacular as the media suggested. This brings us to a third question: was herpes in fact a very serious disease? In the beginning it certainly appeared to be. Firstly it was nasty and painful, a venereal disease that marked you for life, coming back to haunt you whenever it chose after the primary infection had subsided. Secondly, there were two medical complications that heightened the aura of dread surrounding herpes. Both related to female sufferers: HSV was said to play a role in the aetiology of cervical cancer, and presented special dangers during pregnancy and childbirth. Early reports on both these additional risks were decidedly pessimistic.

The carcinogenic aspects of the herpes virus were discussed regularly from the late 1970s onwards. As antibodies against HSV-2 were found more frequently in patients with cervical carcinoma than in healthy women, a causal relationship was posited between the two. As early as 1978, the *Nederlands Tijdschrift voor Geneeskunde* carried a critical article on this suggested link. The writers exposed weaknesses in the evidence allegedly identifying HSV-2 as the cause of cervical carcinoma, and went on to remark that 'one sometimes gets the impression that for some authors, the notion of HSV-2 as the sole oncogenic agent for cervical carcinoma is wishful thinking'.[74] Despite this refutation, the alleged carcinogenic properties of HSV-2 were referred to constantly at the peak of the herpes scare, with some reports stating that herpes sufferers were five to eight times as likely to develop cervical cancer as others. This reverberation of the initial furore gradually died away along with the rest of the media hype on herpes. Since then, the idea of HSV-2 as a key element in the aetiology of cervical carcinoma has been discredited, with other factors – both virological and behavioural – taking its place.

The second complication concerns the consequences of a herpes infection during pregnancy. Infection with HSV-2 was reported to present such a serious risk to the unborn child and newborn that it could even prove fatal. Childbirth itself was considered the most hazardous moment, and in the 1970s it became customary to give women who had previously had a herpes infection regular HSV tests in the last few weeks of pregnancy. If a test result showed up positive within five weeks of the expected date of delivery, a Caesarean section would be decided upon. Later, this measure was deemed to have been unduly drastic. In 1987 the policy of testing for HSV on a weekly basis came under close scrutiny, and by the end of the year the controversy was resolved: the figures showed that routine screening for HSV at the end of pregnancy was pointless. Caesarean section was indicated only in the case of women with a primary infection of herpes genitalis in the last two weeks of pregnancy.

It is clear that alongside an exaggeration of the rise in incidence of herpes, the medical complications associated with it were also overstated. This is not, of course, to dismiss the entire issue as a fuss about nothing. Herpes genitalis could be a prime example of what William McNeill has called 'diseases of cleanliness' – diseases that flourish best in good conditions of hygiene.[75] As long as everyday life is scarcely, if at all, governed by principles of hygiene, children encounter germs at an early age, developing relatively mild reactions that confer immunity. When hygiene improves beyond a certain level this no longer occurs. If these same germs are then encountered later in life, the repercussions on incidence and on the severity of the disease are a good deal more serious. HSV-1 is a particularly common virus, against which a large proportion of the population has antibodies. Present medical evidence suggests that HSV-1 and HSV-2 antibodies provide mutual protection, which means that the drop in casual exposure to HSV-1 in childhood in Western countries could be related both to the recent increased incidence of herpes genitalis in these countries, and to the possibly more virulent form in which this virus began to occur around 1980.[76]

The herpes scare remains a strange phenomenon. The inflated reports of both the extent and seriousness of the disease were avidly consumed for several years. Both the disease and its possible complications were known in the 1970s without causing much of a stir, and meanwhile the rising incidence of gonorrhoea and syphilis since the 1960s was scarcely commanding any attention at all. What was it that suddenly made herpes genitalis so special?

Several studies focusing on sexuality and related issues have reached a high level of consensus on the significance of the herpes scare. Herpes was brought to life, they contend, by interest groups set upon rehabilitating the traditional moral curatorship of sexuality. In their campaigns to restore a restrictive sexual morality such people pounced on a disease that to their minds demonstrated beyond any doubt the pernicious consequences of free sex, and stressed the prevalence and seriousness of the disease out of all proportion. Jeffrey Weeks refers to herpes in connection with 'the new moralism' and discusses the moral panic that surrounded it,

Frank Mort speaks of shrewd moralists who skilfully exploited the increased incidence of herpes to serve their own purposes, and Dennis Altman believes that the disease was used as a puritanical warning against promiscuity.[77] Historian Allan Brandt, reflecting on the herpes epidemic, sees the recurrence of three dominant themes in the history of venereal disease: firstly, the interpretation of venereal disease as a disease of behaviour, a punishment for people who take risks; secondly, the use of venereal diseases as an argument in favour of a more restrictive sexuality; and thirdly the concept of venereal diseases as symptomatic of an underlying malady – a fundamental 'sociosexual maladjustment'.[78] Brandt views herpes as no different from other venereal diseases: they are all easy to exploit as instruments of sexual repression, and are thus transformed from medical syndromes to symptoms of social and moral degeneracy. And with herpes, as in the case of other sexually transmitted diseases, it was this metamorphosis – from sickness to sin – which prevented a rational approach to the disease and which made the disease so terrifying in the public eye.

Viewed in this light, herpes – or rather, the construction of herpes as a horrifying disease – was the work of a kind of morality brigade. This was described as a rather diffuse assembly, its members ranging from medical practitioners and ministers to worried parents, and sometimes referred to as the moral majority; none of the authors referred to above knows exactly who they are, these people so determined to police the highroads of sexual activity, people for whom the presence of herpes proved so convenient. Two things make this conspiracy theory less than convincing: firstly, it is hard to reconcile the vague definitions of the instigators of this morality drive and the interests they served with an allegedly purposeful campaign, and secondly, this theory fails to account for their success. After all, why should the rest of society have taken any notice, in the early 1980s, of a collection of horror stories designed to restrict the newly acquired freedom in the domain of sexual relations? In retrospect, it would seem that an explanation of the herpes scare should be sought elsewhere.

One striking feature of the herpes scare was the fertile soil that apparently existed for rumours, fact and fiction – the public's hunger for everything printed on this topic. Along with this came a confessionalism that attested to a great willingness – at least a professed willingness – to change or renounce certain sexual habits. Although the presence of herpes may well have been seized upon by shrewd moral entrepreneurs in their efforts to turn the tide and to extol the virtues of monogamy once more, the general public was so receptive to this message, so willing to entertain the advisability of temperance in sexual matters, that one is inclined to conclude that the new restraint was mainly self-imposed.

In the countless personal confessions that the herpes epidemic in the United States brought forth, the emphasis was not so much on the shibboleths of traditional moralism as it was on the frustrations of a sexually liberated generation. Herpes, it was said, would bring 'an era of mindless promiscuity'[79] to an end, as a good many participants had long anticipated ('This promiscuity thing is just too unhealthy – both physically and emotionally'[80]) or hoped for ('Herpes might bring about the emotional revolution that should have happened with the sexual revolution'[81]). No moral authorities uttering menacing predictions here, but instead the followers of the sexual revolution themselves who had apparently changed their minds, and who were using herpes to provide an 'objective' basis for their growing sense of unease. The comments 'I don't just hop into bed with anybody. I have to go out a while and see if it feels right. ... I'm not going to get that. It's a bad disease'[82] were typical of responses to the 'new' menace.

Dutch reactions were a pale reflection of their American counterpart. Statements such as 'I don't go to bed with strangers any more'[83] turned up in newspaper headings here too, but they were fewer in number and less fired with the convert's zeal. Even so, a brief survey of the Dutch press reveals a similar mechanism at work in the Netherlands to that in the United States. This survey reveals some interesting findings. Firstly, the herpes scare was dealt with quite differently in different daily newspapers: the dailies that contributed most to the panic were those with a largely young, progressive, urban readership. The most spectacular articles on the new disease appeared in the progressive *Volkskrant*, which not only applied American statistics unblinkingly to the situation in the Netherlands, but in other respects too displayed little inclination to adopt a critical distance to the furore raging on the other side of the Atlantic. Readers of *De Volkskrant* were informed, without further comment, of 'the as yet quite incurable disease of herpes, a viral disease that is highly infectious and can be transmitted not only in bed but even by a handshake, and which has been related to a certain kind of cancer'.[84] This article magnifies the little blisters that are symptomatic of this disease into 'swellings between the legs with blisters' which may even prevent the person so afflicted from sitting down. Nor does *De Volkskrant* hold out to the unfortunate herpes sufferer any prospect of alleviation: no cure existed, and none was expected in the near future.

Compared to this, the more conservative daily newspapers *De Telegraaf* and the *Algemeen Dagblad* were paragons of sober journalism. The *Algemeen Dagblad* told its readers that herpes was 'not a serious ailment' and that its symptoms were 'fairly minor'; the frequently aired suggestion of a causal connection between herpes and cervical cancer, it went on, had 'never been proved'. Only a herpes infection in the case of approaching childbirth was referred to as a dangerous situation.[85] *De Telegraaf* likewise distanced itself from the American reports. There were no grounds for the 'fearful expectations' that had been expressed in a variety of 'panicky articles' prompted by the alarming noises emanating from the United States, this newspaper concluded; herpes would not spread so dramatically in this country. The disease did not appear to be serious, with some guidance the symptoms could be controlled quite well, and as for the relationship between herpes and cervical cancer, this was a claim lacking any basis in scientific fact.[86] *De Telegraaf* even went as far as to try to understand the curious herpes commotion that had arisen in the United States. It pointed out, for instance, that American GPs had improved their methods of examination, hence increasing the number of herpes diagnoses. The paper even hazarded a modest sociological analysis: 'Certain conservative/religious groups in the United States are striking hard, confronting public opinion with the divine punishment meted out to the spread of free love in their lewd society. AIDS and herpes are perfect ammunition for those who wage war on sin.'[87] Although this analysis has been questioned in the above paragraphs, the fact that *De Telegraaf* and the *Algemeen Dagblad* adopted considerably more distance than *De Volkskrant* to the herpes threat supports the proposition that it was the progressive and sexually liberated public who were most interested in the terrifying presence of herpes. If indeed a moral panic can be said to have broken out, it was in a different section of society than Jeffrey Weeks and company would have us believe.

Other sources confirm that this disease was a useful focal point for sexual dissatisfaction in these circles. Previous discussions among feminists had already brought out the fact that it was women who, making up the balance after years of sexual enthusiasm, were most dissatisfied. A few years later this was still the case: the confessional literature surrounding herpes was a genre chiefly practised by women. They of course had most reason for concern, as the complications of the disease that had been described only affected women. But this was not the aspect that dominated the confessional literature. In such writings, which were again strongly influenced by American precedent, herpes was mainly related to a lack of satisfaction in relationships and to the unpleasant aspects of a sexually liberated lifestyle. One characteristic of herpes made it especially liable to interpretation – the recurrent attacks. Not everyone who had a primary HSV infection suffered a recurrence, but many did. These seldom occurred at anything like regular intervals; the only thing that was clear was that the risk of a recurrence was greatest at times of reduced resistance. Whenever you felt unwell or tired, or were suffering from nervous tension, that was when herpes tended to strike. This description was vague enough to give those concerned an opportunity to imbue recurrent attacks with a significance of their own, a significance sought chiefly in the realm of friction in sexual relationships. Sufferers discussing their experiences with herpes, most of them women, used the disease as a medical argument to reinforce their dissatisfaction with the sexual codes they had previously embraced. Herpes came in handy when one wished to escape from the unwritten laws of the 1970s: 'In January a man I knew came to stay at my house for a week', one American reader wrote to the *Nieuwe Revu* weekly magazine, 'But I wasn't too keen. I immediately got herpes, and it stayed the whole time he was there. So I couldn't sleep with him. The truth is, I didn't want to. I had a perfect excuse.'[88]

Herpes attacks were sometimes held to shed new light on a relationship. The women's magazine *Viva* carried the following story related by a woman named Ellen. Ellen appeared to have accepted her herpes quite well when she started a relationship with Robert. They talked about it and all seemed to be going fine. But soon after this discussion Ellen had an attack, the first after a long remission, and after this her herpes started coming back more and more frequently. Ellen had considered resigning herself to a life without sex. 'But because things had been going badly between Robert and me for some time, I also started to wonder whether the herpes attacks might have something to do with a dissatisfaction about our relationship.'[89] Shortly afterwards, the couple split up.

Finally, herpes could itself sometimes oil the wheels of friendship and emotional intimacy between men and women that had been neglected somewhat in all the sexual enthusiasm, and for which there was apparently a definite need in the early 1980s. The herpes sufferer who described her experiences for the monthly magazine *Cosmopolitan* ended her story on a hopeful note with a new and promising encounter on a skiing vacation. She wrote: 'After a few days I felt the time had come to break the news. When I told him "I have herpes", he just laughed and said "I sometimes have that too". My first reaction was to feel incredibly happy. Anyone with herpes will understand that sense of relief. But I soon realized that it also scared me. "When would you have told *me*?" I asked. He was taken aback, but once we talked about it, it brought us really close for the first time. The end result was a very special friendship.'[90]

Popular magazines thus presented the following picture of the typical herpes sufferer: a young city-dweller, educated and reasonably well off, someone who had taken advantage of the new climate of sexual freedom. Leaving aside the question of whether this picture corresponded at all to reality, it may be assumed that herpes evidently struck a particular chord in these circles, a small, tone-setting élite, a sexual and moral vanguard that was able to make herpes into what it became: a media spectacle with a star role for the 'worried well'. The incidence of herpes started to rise at a moment when the developments described above as sexual enthusiasm had produced some less than delightful consequences that had not been envisaged beforehand.[91] In feminist circles such dissatisfaction had been expressed some ten years earlier, but now other sections of society were finding in herpes a new justification for their complaints. Herpes was an ideal issue around which to crystallize their sense of unease, as it enabled the sexual vanguard to change course and adjust their ideals without having to suffer an *ideological* defeat. The shortcomings of medical science were to blame; unfortunately, there was no cure.

Whether herpes did in fact influence sexual behaviour remains unclear, but it would be wrong to say that the disease was exploited by fanatical guardians of monogamy and the family; it seems clear that the risk of contracting a venereal disease was not without its uses for the disenchanted sexual enthusiasts themselves. Of course, the way they used it was not likely to win the approval of their conservative contemporaries, as herpes by no means occasioned a fundamental reappraisal, merely a little reflection – a change of pace rather than direction. Thus it proved possible for a venereal disease to be used, without religious conviction or moralistic admonitions, to shape a mode of sexual discipline. Shorn of its traditional association with guilt, immorality and moral decay, the presence of herpes constituted a medical argument, for certain groups that wanted to change the pattern of their sex lives, that prevented an ideological loss of face.

We have seen that the resulting preoccupation with herpes distinguished itself from previous peaks of unrest surrounding venereal disease by its American character and the role of the popular press. Looking at the narrators and characters involved, we find yet a third distinguishing feature. It was not the themes they discussed that were new, as narrators and characters of the herpes era clarified an aspect of the relations between the sexes just as some of their predecessors had done. The novel feature was that for the first time, there was a considerable overlap between the two groups. In the herpes scare, the social gap that had previously separated narrators from their characters was bridged completely for the first time. Many of those who commented on herpes were speaking of their own experiences: a party that had been excluded from VD debates in the past – the patient – finally acquired a voice. This was partly because the 'typical' herpes sufferer clearly had a higher social status than earlier characters. Whereas previous characters had been created by narrators who felt eminently superior to them in terms of status and potential power, this new patient group consisting of an influential, well-educated, left-wing and sexually liberated section of the population succeeded in attracting the public's attention to its own plight: these characters came to life and told their own story. Another factor that helped bring narrator and character closer together was the increased dominance of medical authority. Now that venereal disease was no longer inextricably bound up with moral degeneracy, patients were less burdened with feelings of shame and guilt, and less likely to suffer moral condemnation.

The preoccupation with herpes blazed briefly and spectacularly, and then died away. Its sudden disappearance was of course closely related to the advent of a new disease, in comparison to which herpes paled into insignificance. But the herpes debate itself marked a transitional phase in which sexually transmitted diseases were once again in the forefront of public attention. A flagging of sexual enthusiasm was at the root of this, but in spite of all the reports to the contrary, there was no question of traditional moralistic authority regaining control of sexuality.

Notes

1. Bekker 1960:5.
2. The subsidy fell from fl. 287,000 in 1951 to fl. 117,000 in 1961. See P. Muntendam, 'Geslachtsziekten nog steeds een bedreiging voor de volksgezondheid', *NTvG* 108 (1964) II:1389-93; this quotation is from 1391. See also the notices in the *Tijdschrift voor Sociale*

Geneeskunde 37 (1959):324; 38 (1960):324.

3. See S. Santema, 'Geslachtsziektenbestrijding', *Medisch Contact* 21 (1966): 953-4; 'Rapport van de commissie consultatiebureau-wezen: Het adviesbureau geslachtsziektenbestrijding', *Medisch Contact* 22 (1967):671-3; D. Suurmond, 'De frequentie van geslachtsziekten in en buiten Nederland', *Tijdschrift voor Sociale Geneeskunde* 46 (1968):141-5.

4. See e.g. Bekker 1960; Bijkerk 1966; Bijkerk 1969. According to the figures supplied by the advice centres, this rise was somewhat indefinite and changeable for the first ten years, but from 1970 onwards it became more marked. The number of syphilis diagnoses increased between 1960 and 1980 from approx. 100 to approx. 1,000 annually. For gonorrhoea the same period witnessed an increase from 1,200 to about 9,000. These figures mainly reflect a trend, and provide only an indication of the true number of VD sufferers in the Netherlands, since many sufferers had no contact with an advice centre.

5. WHO research reveals an increased incidence of syphilis, during the late 1950s, in over 70% of those countries that had registration in some form or other. The corresponding figure for gonorrhoea was almost 50%. In Europe almost 95% and 80% of countries witnessed a growth in syphilis and gonorrhoea rates, respectively, during this period. See Bijkerk 1969 I:12-3.

6. For these figures see the *Verslagen en Mededelingen betreffende de Volksgezondheid* for the years 1946–1965, available e.g. in the library of the Ministry of Health, Welfare and Sport. On the basis of these figures, Bijkerk later compiled a longitudinal survey of the number of patients registered at advice centres in this period (see Bijkerk 1969 II:33 and Appendix 2 of this book), but he did not include statistics on age and marital status.

7. See e.g. P. Muntendam, 'Geslachtsziekten nog steeds een bedreiging voor de volksgezondheid', *NTvG* 108 (1964) II:1389-93; A.P. Roodvoets, 'Toenemende promiscuïteit een bedreiging voor de volksgezondheid', *Medisch Contact* 20 (1965):83-7; D. Suurmond, 'De frequentie van geslachtsziekten in en buiten Nederland', *Tijdschrift voor Sociale Geneeskunde* 46 (1968):141-5.

8. E.H. Hermans, 'Buitenlandse arbeiders en besmettelijke ziektenbestrijding', *NTvG* 108 (1964) II:2188.

9. The role of homosexual women is mentioned occasionally, but to date lesbian practices are regarded as having very little significance to the spread of venereal diseases. Other references in this book to homosexuality should therefore be understood as referring exclusively to male homosexuality.

10. See e.g. E.H. Hermans, 'Problemen betreffende de bestrijding van geslachtsziekten', *NTvG* 103 (1959) I:963-8; P. de Cock & E.H. Hermans, 'Geslachtsziekten en homoseksualiteit bij mannen', *NTvG* 107 (1963) I: 940-4. H. Musaph, 'Homoseksualiteit bij mannen en venerische infecties', *NTvG* 109 (1965) I:45.

11. Cf. Bijkerk 1969 I:33; D. Suurmond, 'De frequentie van geslachtsziekten in en buiten Nederland', *Tijdschrift voor Sociale Geneeskunde* 46 (1968):143-4.

12. D. Suurmond, 'De frequentie van geslachtsziekten in en buiten Nederland', *Tijdschrift voor Sociale Geneeskunde* 46 (1968):142. See also 'Rapporten van de commissie consultatiebureau-wezen. Het adviesbureau geslachtsziektenbestrijding', *Medisch Contact* 22 (1967):671-3: 'The groups currently under greatest threat of exposure are adolescents and homosexuals. The Commission also regards the growing number of foreign workers in the Netherlands as an increasingly significant factor in the spread of venereal diseases' (672). The extent to which these new characters were defined in other countries, their definition being adopted wholesale, though in diluted form, in the Netherlands, is also apparent from Bijkerk's 'archives', which are open to inspection at the *SOA Stichting* (Foundation for Sexually Transmitted Diseases). Between 1950 and 1975, he collected the most important articles about venereal disease that were published in medical journals. Counting only those that appeared in or after 1960, this collection amounted to over 600 articles, most of which were English-language articles focusing on the teenager, the foreigner and the homosexual.

13. See e.g. E.H. Hermans, 'Problemen betreffende de bestrijding van geslachtsziekten', *NTvG* 103 (1959) I:963-8; P. Muntendam, 'Geslachtsziekten nog steeds een bedreiging voor de volksgezondheid', *NTvG* 108 (1964) II:1389-93; D. Suurmond, 'De frequentie van geslachtsziekten in en buiten Nederland', *Tijdschrift voor Sociale Geneeskunde* 46 (1968):141-5; Bijkerk 1969 I:24-8. Idsoe & Guthe 1967 tackles this subject in greatest detail.

14. Countering the notion that the contraceptive pill superseded the condom is the view that the advent of the pill triggered a general debate on birth control which ultimately led to an increase in *all* means of contraception, including the condom. Cf. Weeks 1981:260. This latter view derives support from the research findings of Fabery de Jonge, who found an increase, between 1968 and 1973, not only in the number of women who used the pill (from 11% to 29% of women in the 15–45 age range), but also in the number of condoms

sold (3 million in 1950, 22 million in 1969 and 32 million in 1972).
See I. Fabery de Jonge, quoted in Kooy 1975:155-6.

15. Appendix I deals with these figures at greater length.

16. The incidence of syphilis among persons in the 15–19 age range rose,
between 1959 and 1980, from 2 to 5 per 100,000 inhabitants, and in
the population as a whole it rose from 2 to 8. Between 1967 and
1980 the incidence of gonorrhoea among teenagers rose from 22 to
85, whereas the corresponding rise in the population as a whole was
from 26 to 87.

17. Bijkerk 1982:38.

18. See Bijkerk 1966:17. The 1967 questionnaire, in contrast, did
distinguish between foreigners whose place of residence was abroad
and those who lived in the Netherlands. At this point, in 1967, 28%
of the total number of patients were foreigners, among whom 30%
resided abroad and 70% in the Netherlands (see Bijkerk 1969 II:20).
The incidence of venereal disease among foreign workers may
therefore be assumed to have exceeded that among Dutch men, at
any rate at this point in time.

19. The 1959 questionnaire does not provide any information on this
point.

20. As an indication: the number of passengers processed annually by
Amsterdam's Schiphol airport grew from 383,000 in 1950 to
5 million in 1970 and over 9 million in 1980. Source: Central
Bureau of Statistics. See also Idsoe & Guthe 1967:238-9.

21. Cf. De Swaan 1987:24.

22. No figures are available for 1959. The 11% for 1963 should be
treated with caution as this syphilis questionnaire did not include any
specific question about homosexuality. The figure of 11%
represented unsolicited information, and we may assume that the
actual percentage was higher. Furthermore, the percentage of gay
men among syphilis sufferers was even more pronounced in the
major cities, and especially in Amsterdam, where it approximated
85% in the early 1980s. See *Jaarverslagen Geslachtsziektenbestrijding*
for 1981–1988, Amsterdam Health Service.

23. The findings of Beek's research too showed an increase of homosexual
infections among single male gonorrhoea patients in Rotterdam.
Whereas in the period 1954–1956 no such infections were recorded,
in the years 1964–1966 18% of the persons concerned were
registered as having contracted the infection through homosexual
contact. See C.H. Beek, 'Vergelijkend onderzoek naar de
samenstelling der groepen lijders aan gonorroe, die in 1954–1956 en
1964–1966 ter behandeling kwamen', *NTvG* 112 (1968) I:989-91.

24. On the increase in the number of homosexual patients and some of the reasons underlying it, see Joop van der Linden, 'Homosexualiteit en de emancipatiestrijd van een culturele minderheidsgroep', *SOA* 2 (1981) no. 4:8-10; Wim van der Plaats, 'Over processen die zich afspelen bij bewustwording en acceptatie van eigen homosexualiteit en de keuze voor een bepaalde levensstijl', *SOA* 3 (1981) no. 1:3-5; Rein van der Leeuw, 'De homosexuele subcultuur: ontstaan, functie en uitingsvormen', *SOA* 3 (1981), no. 2:8-9 and 13; Lode Wigersma, 'Homosexualiteit en soa: kennis van sexuele gewoonten is nodig voor inzicht in gezondheidsrisico's', *SOA* 3 (1982) no. 3:6-7 and 9.

25. On this problem, see also J.B. Luijkx, G.W. Marsman & G.A.J. van der Rijt, 'Problemen rond registratie geslachtsziekten', *Medisch Contact* 41 (1986):517-18. Commenting on the increased incidence of venereal disease, the authors noted that registering the number of cases rather than patients made it impossible to see whether more people were contracting VD or the same people were doing so more often. Hence the fact that only numbers of cases were registered could lead to a substantial exaggeration of the problem of venereal disease.

26. Repeaters are broken down by sex and nationality, but not by sexual preference. Of the Dutch patients, 35% had previously suffered from syphilis and/or gonorrhoea (39% of men and 21% of women). The corresponding figure for foreign patients (men only) was 36%. See Bijkerk 1969 II:128-31.

27. Most of this research dates from the 1980s. Records kept by the Venereal Disease Services (*Diensten voor Geslachtsziektenbestrijding*) for the year 1984 gave a percentage of 47% repeaters; almost half of heterosexuals and almost three-quarters of homosexuals had previously suffered from one or more venereal disease. (I am grateful to Martien Sleutjes of the *SOA Stichting* for making these figures available to me.) A study conducted in 1987 among 855 people from different regions who were known to have, or suspected of having, a venereal disease demonstrated that more than half were repeaters. Broken down by sexual preference, a single recurrence proved equally common among heterosexual and homosexual men (28%), but homosexual men presented relatively more frequently with more than one recurrence (44% compared with 24% of heterosexual men). See Leenaars, De Weert-Van Oene & Schrijvers 1989:71.

28. See e.g. Van Griensven 1989; Van Zessen & Sandfort (eds.) 1991:50-1.

29. Whether the expectation expressed as early as the 1920s, but repeated

constantly after that, that the significance of 'classical' prostitution was sharply diminishing, is hard to ascertain. The study conducted in 1967 revealed that 23% of Dutch men and 42% of foreign men had been infected by a prostitute. There is no historical material with which we can compare these data.

30. In the mid-1960s the incidences of syphilis and gonorrhoea respectively, per 100,000 inhabitants, were 4 and 26; the corresponding figures for the 20–29 age group were 11 and 103 (see Bijkerk 1969 II:102-3). In 1980, the overall incidence of syphilis was 8, and for gonorrhoea 87, per 100,000. In the 20–24 and 25–34 age groups, the respective figures were 19 and 22 for syphilis and 288 and 231 for gonorrhoea (see Bijkerk 1982:37). While it is true that these figures include homosexual men in the relevant age groups, this explains only a limited proportion of the rise in incidence, which, it may be added, also showed up clearly among women.

31. See Waugh 1990.

32. In general the number of cases registered at the Health Inspectorate is assumed to be inaccurate as a measure of the true number of individuals suffering from venereal disease in the Netherlands. For instance, the number of cases registered in 1985 for syphilis and gonorrhoea were only 37% and 34% respectively of those that emerged from a telephone questionnaire conducted that year among medical practitioners: registered cases showed an incidence per 100,000 inhabitants of 4 and 86 for syphilis and gonorrhoea respectively, while the questionnaire turned out figures of 10 and 253. See Miltenburg et al. 1988.

33. See E. Stolz, 'Een nieuwe seksueel overdraagbare aandoening?', *SOA* 1 (1979) no. 1:4-5; K.H. Tjiam, 'Niet-specifieke genitale infecties: een ander beleid?', *SOA* 2 (1981), no. 4:7. There are no national figures for the incidence of this type of disease in the Netherlands. The records kept by Amsterdam Health Service, however, give an indication of the increasing significance of these diseases relative to the classical disorders. In 1981, for instance, there were in total around 5,000 diagnoses of trichomoniasis, candidiasis and non-gonorrhoeal urethritis (NGU). Since the mid-1980s, the latter has overtaken gonorrhoea as the commonest venereal disease. See *Jaarverslagen Geslachtsziektenbestrijding* for 1981–1990, Amsterdam Health Service. At international level, as early as 1960 the WHO reported a growing similarity between the frequency of NGU and that of gonorrhoea (Bijkerk 1969 I:17): in countries keeping detailed records on venereal disease, such as England and Wales, NGU emerges as the more common of the two in the 1970s

(Bijkerk 1982:31).

34. On this subject, see the special issue of the *SOA-Bulletin* 6 (1985), no. 1. Chlamydia has been attracting attention for some time outside the inner circles of experts: see e.g. Anke Manschot, 'Steeds meer vrouwen onvruchtbaar. De harde feiten over een onderschatte geslachtsziekte', *Opzij* 16 (no. 12), 1988:52-4. Bart Meijer van Putten, 'De echte reden voor veilig vrijen', NRC *Handelsblad* 13-6-1989. 'Chlamydia, geslachtsziekte nummer één', *Trouw* 29-3-1990.

35. In a study conducted in Tilburg among women requesting artificial insemination, over half of the cases presenting with blocked fallopian tubes proved to be the result of chlamydia infection. See M.F. Peeters et al., 'Chlamydia trachomatis, infertiliteit en in vitro-fertilisatie', *NTvG* 132 (II) 1988:1438-42. For the past few years, chlamydia has been named as the most common sexually transmitted disease in the Western world. See e.g. Marcia Inhorn Millar, 'Genital chlamydial infection: A role for social scientists', *Social Science and Medicine* 25 1987:1289-99.

36. Coutinho 1984:33-4. This group consisted of 2,946 homosexual men. For the rest, little is known about the frequency of hepatitis B as a sexually transmitted disease. While it is true that an obligation exists to report all cases of this disease, this includes those transmitted by other means. Moreover, only a minority of cases are diagnosed, and even those often go unreported. Around 1980 the number of cases reported was about 700, while Coutinho estimates the real number to have been roughly 10 to 20 times higher (37).

37. Cf. Michael Waugh, 'STDs in the modern world', *Venereology* 3 (1990) no. 4:105.

38. These remarks are based on the records kept by the outpatient clinics run by Amsterdam Health Service.

39. Research done in Amsterdam suggests that this was particularly clear in the case of syphilis; cf. B.R. Franken & S. Belleman, 'Sociaal-psychologisch onderzoek naar patiënten met lues I of II', *Medisch Contact* 35 (1980):1537-40.

40. See E. Stolz, 'Penicillinase producerende gonococcenstammen: een probleem in Nederland?', *SOA* 2 (1980), no. 1:4-5; J.D.A. van Embden & B. van Klingeren, 'Sinds medio 1980 aanzienlijke stijging van het aantal penicilline-resistente gonococcen', *SOA* 2 (1981), no. 4:3 and 10; R.A. Coutinho et al., 'De verspreiding van penicillinase vormende gonokokken in Amsterdam', *NTvG* 126 (1982):221-3; the Chief Health Inspectorate kept records of the import and spread of resistant gonococcus strains. Between 1976 and 1983 the number of registered cases rose from 2 to 1,018. For an overview, see the

Jaarverslag 1983 *van de Geneeskundige Hoofdinspectie*, Ministry of
Welfare, Health and Cultural Affairs 1984:32.

41. H.E. Menke, 'Sexueel overdraagbare darmziekten', *SOA* 1 (1979), no.
2:6-7.

42. See A. Leentvaar-Kuijpers, 'Ulcus molle (chancroid) komt in ons
land steeds meer voor', *SOA* 1 (1979), no. 2:13; E. Stolz,
'Importziekten onder sexueel overdraagbare aandoeningen', *Medisch
Contact* 35 (1980):1576-82; H.E. Menke, 'Ulcus molle' in Stolz &
Suurmond (eds.) 1982:176-8.

43. On this and for the following overview, see Wiebes 1986; Raamplan
1987.

44. Letter from Van Steenbergen to Hermans, 23-11-1970. Archives of
P.G. Bakker, *SOA Stichting*, Utrecht.

45. Minutes of the meeting held on 27-01-1972. Archives of P.G.
Bakker, *SOA Stichting*, Utrecht.

46. See L.H. Lumey, Jeannette Kok & R.A. Coutinho, 'Screening for
syphilis among homosexual men in bars and saunas in Amsterdam',
British Journal of Venereal Diseases 58 (1982):402-4.

47. See Wright Mills [1959].

48. Dick P. J. van Reeuwijk, Interview with D.J.H. Vermeer: 'Geen
paniek over toename', *Verstandig Ouderschap. Maandblad van de
Nederlandse Vereniging voor Sexuele Hervorming*, September
1967:240-1.

49. Jos Bienemann, 'Geslachtsziekten, een beetje uit je doppen kijken (en
naar de dokter gaan)', *Sekstant* July/August 1974; see also the
pamphlet enclosed with *Sekstant*, 'Een geslachtsziekte is een heel
gewone ziekte (waar de dokter je van af helpt)', February 1975.

50. On this subject see De Bruijn 1979, Chapter VIII; even in the group
that held out longest against birth control – Catholic medical
practitioners – there was a notable change of attitudes in the late
1950s. See Van Berkel 1990, Chapter III.

51. In general, what took place was a gradual increase in pre-marital
intercourse at an increasingly early age. See Kooy 1975; Kooy 1980;
Van der Vliet 1990. Van Zessen & Sandfort (eds.) 1991 point out
that women, who had traditionally 'lagged behind' in the realm of
knowledge and sexual experience, caught up quickly in the 1960s
and 1970s; see 14-15 and 41. The main group for whom the sexual
revolution may truly be said to have been revolutionary was probably
that of homosexual men.

52. See Akkerman & Stuurman 1985. Schnabel too (1990) considers
the *public* nature of the debate on sexuality in the 1960s to have
been more revolutionary than its content. This toning-down of the

revolutionary reputation of the 1960s applies not only to changes in the area of sex, but equally to those related to social and political issues. See various articles in *Wederopbouw, welvaart en onrust* 1986; Van Berkel 1990.

53. The term derives from Robinson [1976], who defines it as 'the conviction that sex is a vital and a fulfilling human experience' (vii-viii) and who describes modern sexologists as 'sexual enthusiasts' (2-3).

54. For the first explicit formulation of 'sexual enthusiasm', we may look to the Dutch Society for Sexual Reform (NVSH), which included the following precepts in its statutes as early as 1947 (articles 4a and 4b): 'a. [The Society] considers a healthy sex life to be necessary to the achievement of a harmonious development, mentally as well as physically, of individual personality, of the family and the community, and therefore regards the right to such a sex life as a human right, that may therefore not be violated by the State. It views the deliberate control of conception as an indispensable element of this ... . b. Its definition of a healthy sex life is one that fully provides the harmonious satisfaction that is appropriate to each particular stage of life.' See Nabrink 1978:337-8. This point of view spread beyond NVSH circles; see e.g. the resolution on marriage and sexuality that the National Federation for Public Mental Health submitted to the government and parliament in 1965, which concluded that 'it is of the utmost importance from the point of view of mental health that every section of the Dutch population should learn to appreciate sexuality not only as a driving force and a means of reproduction but also as one of the main factors necessary to developing a relationship between a man and a woman to the fullest possible extent.' *Medisch Contact* 20 (1965):1120.

55. The idea that sex should be aimed less at reproduction and more at pleasure was also expressed at the beginning of this century. In the *Pure Life Movement*, whose adherents certainly thought nothing of the kind, such views were referred to as *the creed of indulgence*; cf. Van der Splinter 1986:63. After the Second World War, the lawyer Bouman discerned a different aspect of sexual enthusiasm – the belief that every person has the right to a sex life – which he characterized as *sexual communism*. See A. Bouman, 'Sexuele voorlichting en geslachtsziektenbestrijding', *SH* 1947, no. 2 and 3:12-8.

56. Schnabel 1980:19.

57. In a wider context, Van Ussel [1968] dwells at length on the roots

and development of the positive appreciation of sexuality. His views are coloured, however, by a somewhat outmoded notion of progress, from repression to liberation. For a critical discussion of his approach and an interesting alternative sociological point of view based on Niklas Luhmann's theory of functional differentiation, see Schnabel 1973.

58. Schnabel 1978; Schnabel 1980.

59. An anthology edited by Frenken, that appeared in 1980, is illustrative of the loss of interest at this time in infectious diseases associated with sexuality. Alongside articles on problems of sexuality and relationships, sexual dysfunction and modes of therapy, a separate item was included on sexuality and disease in medical practice. This article contains not one mention of venereal disease. See M. Moors-Mommers, 'Seksualiteit en ziekte', in Frenken (ed.) 1980:397-409. For an overview of 'new' sexual difficulties, see Frenken 1987.

60. De Swaan 1990:58.

61. See Wootton (1959: esp. 337-9) on the intrusion of medical – in this case psychiatric – theories into ideas on crime; see also Conrad & Schneider 1980.

62. De Swaan 1988:223-44.

63. De Swaan 1990, esp. 150-61. See also Schnabel 1989a:213.

64. Whether this scientific justification is sufficient remains controversial. Theorist Jürgen Habermas thinks it is not. He does not regard science to be functionally equivalent, as an authority that can explain and justify human behaviour, to traditional ideological systems. Habermas believes that the continuous decline of the latter systems, a characteristic feature of late capitalist societies, has resulted in a loss of meaning and significance in personal life, and has produced elements of crisis in the socio-cultural system. See Habermas 1973.

65. Nora Gallagher, 'Fever all through the night', *Mother Jones* VII (November 1982):38.

66. J. Spruijt Landskroon, 'Iets over herpes, vooral met het oog op de diagnose van syphilis', *Geneeskundige Bladen* IV (1897):247-69.

67. The number of herpes patients reported for 1980 varied from 5 to 14 million; see 'Herpes, the new sexual leprosy', *Time,* 28 July 1980:43. By 1982 the number reported had risen to 20 million; see e.g. 'The new scarlet letter', *Time,* 2 August 1982:46; 'Fever all through the night', *Mother Jones* VII, November 1982:38. In spite of the predicted rise in incidence, this figure remained constant until the end of the 1980s; see Brandt 1987:3; Rodway & Wright (eds) 1988:1.

68. The following figures may be useful for the purposes of comparison:

	herpes gen.	gonorrhoea	syphilis
1981	218	4,671	291
1982	359	4,197	278
1983	361	3,898	308
1984	452	3,311	222
1985	517	2,906	150
1986	431	2,374	107
1987	387	1,509	112
1988	284	1,035	111

Source: Amsterdam Health Service venereal disease units annual reports for 1981–1988.

69. The RIVM procured its statistics for the monthly virological surveys used here from laboratories located in the following 15 districts: Amsterdam (2), Bilthoven, Delft, Eindhoven, Enschede, Groningen, Leiden, Maastricht, Nijmegen, Rotterdam (2), Tilburg, Venlo and Zeeland. The figures are therefore not national, and even for the area covered they do not give a completely accurate picture of the total number of cases of herpes genitalis, as the HSV-1 diagnoses, which always account for a small proportion of genital herpes infections, are left out of consideration here. The numbers of HSV-2 cases for the years 1981 to 1988 are as follows: 580, 787, 958, 1,169, 1,413, 1,253, 1,138 and 971.
70. See Miltenburg et al. 1988. As already noted, the figures in this report are a great deal higher than those for cases reported to the Chief Health Inspectorate.
71. The clinical diagnosis of herpes genitalis must be supplemented by culturing the virus or by microscopic analysis. Amsterdam district laboratory, for example, first cultured the herpes simplex virus in 1981. When such an innovation is followed by an increase in the number of herpes diagnoses, this may create the impression of a sudden epidemic out of the blue. See the annual report of Amsterdam Health Service district laboratory for 1981:23.
72. F.B. Lammes, 'Herpes Vulvitis', *Nederlands Tijdschrift voor Geneeskunde* 127 (1983):1562.
73. See J.J.E. van Everdingen, A.M. Dumas & R.A. Coutinho, 'Herpes genitalis', *NTvG* 128 (1984):2271.
74. E.R. te Velde & T.H. The, 'Herpes simplex-virus type 2 en baarmoederhalskanker', *NTvG* 122 (1978):1226-30.

75. McNeill 1976:254.

76. See J.J.E. van Everdingen, A.M. Dumas & R.A. Coutinho, 'Herpes genitalis', *NTvG* 128 (1984):2271.

77. Weeks 1985:44; Mort 1987:214; Altman 1987:141.

78. Brandt 1987:179-82.

79. 'The new scarlet letter', *Time*, 2 August 1982.

80. *New York Times Magazine*, 21 February 1982.

81. *Newsweek*, 12 April 1982.

82. *Washington Post*, 11 October 1982.

83. *De Volkskrant*, 6 December 1982.

84. *De Volkskrant*, 13 April 1982.

85. *Algemeen Dagblad*, 27 August 1980 and 4 October 1982.

86. *De Telegraaf,* 30 August 1983 and 5 May 1984.

87. *De Telegraaf,* 30 August 1983.

88. *Nieuwe Revu* 21, 1982:28.

89. *Viva,* 25 January 1985:45.

90. *Cosmopolitan,* November 1985:86.

91. See Schnabel (1989) on the way in which the joy about the new climate of sexual freedom was toned down after the first sense of euphoria had passed.

5

AIDS and Other Sexually Transmitted Diseases: a Socio–Historical Approach

The preoccupation with herpes genitalis was submerged in the mid-1980s beneath a rising wave of publicity and fearful speculation surrounding the spread of an entirely new disease. Anti-venereal disease workers were forewarned to some extent – reports of an apparently deadly disease in the United States had been appearing in the press for some time – but at a time when the Western world was almost coming to disregard infectious diseases as a serious health hazard, the news was nevertheless a bombshell.

In the United States, 1981 witnessed the first reports of strange and alarming symptoms among growing numbers of previously healthy young men. Those affected had a wide range of non-specific symptoms such as fever, fatigue, general debilitation, diarrhoea and weight loss, added to which their immune system was seriously undermined so that they fell prey to a variety of recognizable but uncommon and as a rule benign maladies. Kaposi's sarcoma, a generally benign form of skin cancer, and Pneumocystis pneumonia figured most prominently in the early reports. The first patients were all homosexual men, and all were associated with the so-called fast-track gay culture. Because of this, two aetiological hypotheses were soon circulating. One was a biomedical theory focusing on an external agent believed to be responsible, whether in the form of a sexually transmitted micro-organism or as a constituent of drugs such as 'poppers', a common stimulant in certain gay circles. The other was a psycho-sexual explanation that blamed the emergence of AIDS on a certain lifestyle, on an imbalance caused by unnatural practices and the excesses of modern life.[1]

Developments since then have bolstered the biomedical approach: the fact that the same symptoms were recorded, shortly after the registration of sick gay men, in haemophiliacs, heroin addicts and recipients of blood transfusions, pointed to the presence of a micro-organism that could be transmitted in blood, at least. One result of this confirmation was that the initial acronym for the disease – GRID (gay related immune deficiency) – was replaced in 1982 by the name by which it has been known ever since – acquired immune deficiency syndrome, or AIDS.

The virus responsible for the disease was isolated in 1983–1984, and a little over a year later a blood test became available, enabling the transmission routes to be verified and described in greater detail. A controversy raged briefly between rival medical teams claiming to have isolated the virus first, and at length the new discovery was named the human immunodeficiency virus, or HIV.[2] It was found, in concentrations capable of transmission, in blood and semen, and could be passed on in three different ways: through sexual contact, in blood, and from mother to child.[3] It could also be demonstrated that HIV had generally entered an individual's system long before he or she was diagnosed as having contracted AIDS. In other words, alongside the population of known AIDS patients there was, and still is, a population of HIV carriers in good health, of whom it was quite unclear – at least at the beginning of the epidemic – whether they would necessarily go on to develop AIDS, and if so, when. It was plain, however, that this 'HIV-positive' group, as they came to be known, was several times as large as that of registered AIDS patients.

As the mode of transmission gradually came to be better understood, so too did the course of the disease. An as yet indeterminate – but constantly rising – percentage of HIV-positive individuals eventually falls prey, usually after an incubation period lasting many years, to an extremely serious weakening of the immune system, exposing them to numerous secondary disorders. In addition to Pneumocystis pneumonia and Kaposi's sarcoma, a variety of other opportunistic infections and cancers also moves in when the immune system breaks down. Furthermore, many AIDS patients suffer brain damage, not only from secondary infections, but in some cases directly from HIV. This produces neurological symptoms such as motor disorders, loss of memory and AIDS-related dementia. Improved diagnostics and treatment, and changes in the diagnostic criteria, have increased average life expectancy after an AIDS diagnosis from a few months to about two years, as far as the Netherlands is concerned.

Since the disease first appeared, it has generated a profusion of literature of almost every kind: alongside a wealth of medical and epidemiological studies there are shelves full of legal, historical, ethical or educational publications, and a good deal of fiction besides. The Netherlands alone has over 20 libraries and other repositories containing thousands of books, articles, reports, collected conference papers and research findings, where the reader can consult the 70-odd journals, bibliographies and newsletters from home and abroad that have a specific bearing on AIDS.[4] I shall not attempt to deal systematically with even part of this material here.[5] Nor shall I give a historical account of the AIDS epidemic in the Netherlands, although aspects of it will be discussed.[6] Instead, this chapter will be structured by the questions that were raised at the beginning of this book. I shall discuss the nature of the recent revival of the venereal disease debate, and the factors leading up to it, and go on to place Dutch reactions to the AIDS epidemic within a historical and sociological perspective. First, however, a few general observations are in order, concerning the conditions that enabled the disease to be identified, and the conditions that have enabled it to spread according to the current pattern.

Sociogenesis and iatrogenesis of an epidemic[7]

Whatever the overwhelming impact of AIDS on society, its emergence is not impossible to explain. The identification and epidemic spread of AIDS are both inextricably bound up with relatively recent events – scientific advances on the one hand, and social and medical developments on the other. In this regard, AIDS may be classified as a distinctly modern epidemic. On the side of science, recent developments in microbiology, virology and immunology have enabled researchers to clarify the relationship between the aetiology of AIDS and its clinical picture. It was not until the late 1970s that it became possible, technologically and conceptually, to isolate a human retrovirus such as HIV and to study its effects. Moreover, a highly specialized barrage of medical apparatus was needed, to compile from the diverse symptoms associated with AIDS – which consist largely of other infectious diseases – a single clinical picture, a coherent syndrome.[8]

Epidemiologically too, AIDS is related to modern conditions. The virus could not have spread so fast were it not for certain recent social, biological and medical developments. Mirko Grmek's interesting historical account of the AIDS epidemic argues persuasively that HIV is not a new virus for humans that originated from an animal virus or from a mutant version of a less pathogenic predecessor.[9] In all probability HIV has long been among us, but in the past its effects were relatively contained. The rapid, epidemic dissemination of the virus only became possible after certain innovations in the latter half of the 20th century. In the realm of social change, the crucial factor was the intensification and expansion of sexual relations, the results of which were discussed in the previous chapter. Various circumstances have contributed to this spread in the different continents of the world. Essential factors in America and Western Europe are the freer attitudes to sex, the formation of highly promiscuous gay subcultures and the explosive growth of tourism. In Africa, migration, urbanization and the accompanying social changes have played a decisive role. Illustrative of this point is the fact that both in the American gay circuit and in African cities, the AIDS epidemic was preceded by a formidable increase in the incidence of other sexually transmitted diseases.

Besides underscoring these social conditions, Grmek dwells on certain paradoxical consequences of the practices and successes of modern medicine, which have made the spread of HIV possible on a hitherto unprecedented scale.[10] The use of the hypodermic needle, for instance, facilitated not only the dissemination of medicine and vaccines, but also the transmission of pathogenic organisms. With the use of Salvarsan to treat syphilis, intravenous injections became an everyday feature of medical practice, but they did not at first play a significant role in transmitting infectious diseases; injections were given on a limited scale, and all the material used was sterile. From the mid-20th century onwards, however, this started to change. Drug-users switched in growing numbers from smoking and swallowing pills to injecting themselves, and in poor countries hypodermic needles became increasingly common in medical and semi-medical contexts in which it was impossible to observe proper procedures. After 1970 the traditional glass and metal needles, which were easy to sterilize, were superseded by plastic disposable ones, which increased the risks still further. Disposable needles are obviously not meant to be sterilized, but in African hospitals and Western drug circuits, the circumstances were such that these precious and scarce commodities were kept for re-use.

Another medical custom that was eventually to take its toll was the administration of blood and blood products. This practice has increased enormously since the Second World War. At the same time, improvements in the preservation of blood and new techniques that enable the extraction of specific constituents have added several stages to what was originally direct transmission from donor to receiver. Present-day blood banks have grown because of this into large-scale facilities, in some countries set up on a commercial basis. This had already substantially increased the risk of infection via blood transfusion, but the situation was more serious still for haemophiliacs, who are dependent on the regular administration of blood clotting factors. Not only do the blood banks in question combine blood from thousands of donors, but an international trade in blood products has now grown up. Within the space of one year, an individual who receives blood products in the Netherlands several times a week will have come into contact with the blood of virtually all the donors in the country. The Netherlands uses only locally obtained blood in preparing the products concerned, a better situation than that in Germany, France and England, say, where blood banks are partly or completely dependent on imported preparations.[11] Once previously separate blood circuits were connected, it created unprecedented scope for iatrogenic infection.

One final factor that enabled the epidemic spread of AIDS is a medical advance that has inadvertently led to a disturbance of what Grmek calls the 'pathocénose', i.e. the balance that exists between the incidences of all the diseases that occur among a particular population. The spread of each individual disease is partly determined by the presence of other diseases. This influence works in three different ways. In the first place, specific competition may arise between related parasites. William McNeill provides several historical examples of this in his book *Plagues and Peoples*. For instance, the decline of leprosy in Europe in the 14th century was probably linked to the increased spread of tuberculosis. The immune responses to the pathogens of these two diseases partly overlap, so that exposure to the TB bacillus increases resistance to leprosy. As TB was the more infectious of the two, it had a major advantage in this struggle for dominance.[12] Secondly, the presence of some bacilli can facilitate the spread of others. The presence of other venereal diseases, for instance, promotes the transmission of HIV, just as an HIV infection in its turn promotes the spread of other infectious diseases. Thirdly, some parasites flourish in the *absence* of others. Hence the AIDS epidemic is closely related to the incidence of other diseases: as some infections vanish, others take their place. HIV, as we have already seen, promotes the development of opportunistic infections, so that the first indication of its spread is an increased incidence of other known disorders. If these infections are already common, the spread of HIV can easily remain concealed, which means that an AIDS epidemic as we are currently experiencing it cannot be identified as such. But it is not only that the effects of HIV only become *visible* once certain other pathogens are absent. The actual course of the HIV infection is itself influenced by other pathogens: these shorten the period of latency during which a subject is merely 'HIV-positive', hence erecting a natural dam against the spread of AIDS. Grmek writes:

> The infectious diseases thus disguise the picture not only because they hide the ill effects of the HIV virus but also, and especially, because they hamper its epidemic diffusion. Introduced into a population in which tuberculosis and other infectious diseases are highly pervasive, the virulent strains of AIDS must have become rapidly eliminated or at least circumscribed. AIDS could only persist in the form of sporadic cases or quite small outbreaks: the preponderance of the infectious diseases reduced patients' survival and hence occasions for the virus to expand. Its dissemination was not possible before modern medicine's successes breached the bulwark that other common infectious diseases had formed against it.[13]

HIV has profited from the recent decline of infectious diseases, a decline increasingly attributable, during the 20th century, to successful medical intervention. In other words, the advent of AIDS must in part be described as an unforeseen consequence of the increased medical control of infectious diseases.

AIDS in the Netherlands

The first AIDS patients in the Netherlands were recorded in 1982, reaching a total of five by the end of the year. Over the following years, their numbers rapidly increased from 19 in 1983 to 64 in 1985 and 239 in 1987.[14] The outlook was alarming, with experts warning that the epidemic would become rampant. One authoritative and much-quoted forecast published in 1987 estimated that 1,900 new AIDS patients would be identified in 1989, bringing the cumulative number to 3,000 by the end of that year. The number of HIV-positive individuals in the Netherlands estimated in the same source was grimmer still: 10,000 to 20,000.[15] The tip-of-the-iceberg metaphor was repeated *ad infinitum*. Notwithstanding all the terrible suffering and fear that AIDS has caused since then, it is a blessing that these predictions were wildly wrong. In 1989 the number of new patients was not 1,900, but about 400, bringing the total number of AIDS patients not to 3,000, but to 1,200. Estimates of the number of HIV-positive individuals have likewise had to be adjusted, but remain to date a matter of extreme uncertainty.[16]

The composition of the patient population in the Netherlands largely followed the pattern that had emerged in the United States. In the period 1982–1990, approximately 1,600 patients were diagnosed as suffering from AIDS, some half of whom have since died. Gay men have been worst hit: over the years the proportion of gay male patients has stabilized at about 80% of registered cases. The figures for drug addicts and heterosexuals are relatively low: of the 1,600 AIDS diagnoses made in the period 1982–1990, these two groups accounted for just over 100 and about 90 of the cases respectively, while over 1,200 were gay men. In addition, there were 50 cases of AIDS contracted by haemophiliacs or by blood transfusion recipients, and AIDS was passed on from mother to child in 7 cases. These figures demonstrate that sexual transmission is by far the most common route of infection for HIV in the Netherlands.

One striking fact to emerge from this brief review is that the current classification of AIDS patients clearly differs from previous structures that have been imposed on the population of VD patients. The age and sex of AIDS patients, of course, may be ascertained without much difficulty, but these are no longer the main parameters. Other traditional modes of classification used in the past – based on social background, occupation or marital status – are not employed. The present classification system is based simply on *mode of infection*, which may be: a) through sex, or – adopting the precise formulation that such classification entails – through blood–semen or blood–blood contact during sexual acts (whether heterosexual or homosexual); b) through non-sexual blood–blood contact; or c) by perinatal transmission.

Thus the different modes of transmission have determined the present categorization of AIDS patients, and have also created a new cast of characters. The hierarchy within this new cast is ruled by statistics: more than ever before, present-day narrators invoke statistics to justify their characters' right to existence. The gay man and the intravenous drug-user have now been cast in the leading roles, but their emergence – unlike that of their predecessors – has been based on figures, and not on any moral dissertation. This is why it has proved impossible, for instance, to make the heroin prostitute into a recognized character. Although her position, midway between an 'infected' enclave and the 'innocent' heterosexual population, made her ideally suited to such a starring role, the efforts that have been made to identify her as a perpetrator-character have foundered, simply, for lack of evidence. In that regard, previous generations of narrators had an easier task.

The authority of statistics, however, is only one way in which the current classification is a new departure. Another is its social breadth. Although it has led to the introduction of the gay man and the intravenous drug-user as characters – members of identifiable groups in society – this statistically-based model differentiates far less fundamentally than did past socially-based models between these groupings and mainstream middle-class society. One used to be able to protect oneself from incursions across the social dividing-line between narrators and characters; the fear of infection struck mainly when these boundaries became blurred, or when they were in danger of shifting. This has changed now: the organizing principle of the mode of transmission theoretically embraces everyone. However small the risk of infection may be in today's reality for most people, there are no *fundamental* barriers to be crossed for the disease to spread among far larger sections of the population. The road that leads in that direction is clear, although actual infection along that route occurs (as yet) on a very small scale. This removes the chief foundation underlying the distinction between narrators and characters.

The main way in which the new classification model differs from previous ones, however, is that it has broken with a time-honoured tradition that associated the risk of contracting a venereal disease with certain elements of society. Although in the early days of the epidemic there was a brief and one-sided concentration on high-risk groups, this soon changed: the danger of infection is now linked not to persons but to behaviour – certain specific acts that are related to the transmission of the virus. Every mode of infection is linked to well-defined acts. These acts, rather than certain sections of society, now represent the danger of infection.

The advent of a new, deadly venereal disease in the Netherlands, and the grim predictions of the course the epidemic would take, prompted a large-scale mobilization of resources. From the outset, it was clear beyond all doubt that national government would have a major role to play. It was immediately agreed that the fight against AIDS should be a government responsibility, whether directly, as in the organization of public information campaigns, or indirectly, through subsidies to specific bodies. This said, the government's actions were often criticized: the slow pace at which it responded was described by some activists as bordering on criminal negligence, the sums eventually set aside were too small, and the content of the public information campaigns was found wanting.[17] But accusations of this kind merely underscored the high-pitched expectations of the government's actions. Whether or not it is right to speak of an unnecessary delay, the fight against AIDS assumed impressive proportions in the second half of the 1980s. At organizational level, a wide range of institutions and committees sprang up within a brief space of time, concerning themselves with advising and coordinating, evaluating and lobbying. Media attention and a series of public information campaigns quickly educated the public about AIDS and instilled the principles of safe sex into large sections of the population,[18] and for high-risk groups there were special facilities and more specific information drives. A new committee was appointed in 1988 to chart and coordinate the proliferation of research on the various aspects of AIDS and to advise on research grants. On the side of the government, the Ministry of Welfare, Health and Cultural Affairs (now the Ministry of Welfare, Health and Sport) bears chief responsibility for developing and implementing AIDS policy; this Ministry's expenditure increased from less than 2 million guilders in 1987 to over 34 million in 1991.[19]

All this means that the period starting in the latter half of the 1980s can be characterized as a third spell – after the time around the turn of the century and the few years following the Second World War – of widespread public anxiety surrounding venereal diseases and related issues. This period needs less explaining than the others. Whereas in the earlier cases an old problem had suddenly given rise to a fresh wave of alarm, the AIDS epidemic is a new phenomenon. Even to ask why the advent of a deadly and infectious disease should have given rise to such a tumult seems a ludicrously redundant question. Yet however understandable the public concern may be, even in these circumstances it is relevant to try to answer this question more precisely.

The kind of explanations presented thus far in this book will not be helpful, however. In the two earlier waves of fear, the consternation had everything to do with society's view of venereal disease as embedded in a wider-ranging set of preoccupations – the narrators themselves made no bones about this. The third period differs in this regard: the official line, at least, eschews such wider implications, thus shielding AIDS from interpretations considered specious and offensive. No one is responsible for the disease; it is neither nature's revenge nor divine retribution. Whatever people may believe in private, the official policy on AIDS takes an explicit stand against such interpretations. AIDS is a disease, and that is all.

This does not mean that the present wave of alarm can be

explained entirely in terms of understandable shock and the newness
and seriousness of the disease. Several added factors play a role, such
as the age and social position of AIDS patients: they are young and
– with the exception of intravenous drug-users – tend to belong to
groups that are at least moderately well integrated into society.
These factors serve to heighten the duration and intensity of public
concern, if only for the simple reason that the groups concerned
have sufficient resources to claim attention in the overburdened
public arena and that they are relatively good at presenting their
problems to the media and political decision-makers. Moreover, in
many ways AIDS is a spectacular disease with plenty of potential for
media exploitation. The connection between AIDS and sexuality, in
particular male homosexuality, exerts a magnetic appeal that no one
should underestimate. Seldom have the sexual habits of a particular
section of the population been exposed to so much public scrutiny as
have those of gay men since the beginning of the AIDS epidemic.
The same cocktail of condemnation and revulsion mixed with
voyeuristic fascination that reared its head in relation to earlier
characters makes the latest venereal disease, too, an engrossing
subject for the present-day general public. Nor has the public been
disappointed: never has an audience been rewarded with so much
detail on techniques, frequency and numbers of sexual partners. This
has produced a situation in which, as Paul Schnabel has put it, AIDS
has become 'a metaphor for the patient's private life', an unwitting
source of information about his past.[20] But this form of openness was
not simply forced upon the persons concerned – it arose in part
because gay men had good reason to believe that complete frankness
would help those fighting the disease, and so ultimately benefit their
own group. The sexual confessions make AIDS a spectacular disease,
and the accompanying clinical picture, with its emaciated patients,
visible signs of decay, and the link that the disease lays between sex
and death, serves to enhance its dramatic nature.

The main factor that has enhanced the current peak of public
concern, however, is the expansion, greater autonomy and
professionalization of the AIDS control circuit since the outbreak of
the epidemic. The research, public information and bureaucracy
have grown, within the space of a few years, into a large and
flourishing industry. Many epidemiologists, virologists and other
medical researchers have dedicated themselves to AIDS research; to
them, the disease represents a scientific challenge and offers new
career prospects. They have been reinforced by a sizeable army of
public information specialists, care workers, journalists, policy

workers, coordinators, committee members, social scientists and others for whom AIDS has likewise become a source of income. In this respect, AIDS is no different from other social and medical problems that arise within the social framework of the welfare state. They are characterized by the professional involvement of groups affected, lobbyists and professionals who, competing with those trying to publicize other problems, are constantly obliged to compete for the public's attention, donations from fund managers and government subsidies.[21] This inevitably means that AIDS experts and professional AIDS workers are little inclined to have the catastrophic nature of the AIDS epidemic and the constant threat it poses to public health put into perspective. The competition compels them to present pessimistic scenarios, and they themselves have a professional interest in the continued existence of AIDS. As Paul Schnabel has put it:

> Researchers, care workers and information officers, as those for whom AIDS prevention work has provided opportunities, have acquired a vested interest – like the pressure groups representing those affected – in the epidemic, the virus and the patients. This interest in part determines their outlook on the problem and its possible development. None of them envisages the imminent disappearance of AIDS, or scarcely even the disease going into a natural decline or the epidemic becoming contained. This is not merely on the basis of scientific evidence. The continuity of their own work and their own research is inevitably also at stake ...[22]

In other words, the concern surrounding AIDS is to some extent self-perpetuating. Relatively positive developments are contrasted with an as yet remote ideal, and seized on largely to underscore the need to undertake fresh activities: the impact of prevention policy is good, but still not as good as it needs to be; the level of public awareness is high, but the risks have still not been impressed upon everyone; many people have changed their behaviour, but information is still failing to reach certain groups; gay men are currently well informed, but too little attention is still paid to the specific risks run by others such as young people, women and migrants. The constant repetition of 'still' in all these observations suggests that more information, more research and sustained efforts on the part of information officers and AIDS prevention workers could eliminate these shortcomings.

Claims of this kind on the part of information officers and AIDS prevention workers characterize the position of groups that are professionally involved in attacking any social problem. Howard

Becker aptly described this type of moral entrepreneur, and the dual task that he sees before him, as early as 1963. As he puts it, on the one hand these professionals have to convince the public of the unrelenting presence and persistent seriousness of the problem in question, and on the other hand they have to make it clear that their solutions are adequate, their activities useful and effective. They have to wield menacing and reassuring language at the same time. 'Therefore', Becker continues:

> enforcement organizations, particularly when they are seeking funds, typically oscillate between two types of claims. First, they say that by reason of their efforts the problem they deal with is nearing a solution. But in the same breath, they say the problem is perhaps worse than ever (though through no fault of their own) and requires renewed and redoubled efforts to keep it under control. Enforcement officials can be more vehement than anyone else in their insistence that the problem they are battling against is still with us, in fact more with us than ever before. In making these claims, enforcement officials provide good reason for the continued existence of their own position.[23]

These remarks are emphatically not intended to impugn the motives of the professionals concerned. Such individuals' efforts are quite possibly, and even very probably, based on a sense of commitment and sincere sympathy with – in this case – AIDS patients, but that is not the point here. Nor is it the intention to imply that the current concern about venereal infections is simply being artificially sustained by these groups, and that when viewed dispassionately, AIDS does not merit all this attention. This, too, is a separate issue. The point being made here is that the autonomous status, institutionalization and professionalization of the various branches of AIDS control, combined with the constant competition with other problems in the struggle for attention and funding, inevitably lead to a situation in which, whatever success may have been achieved, the worst of all possible outcomes will be emphasized. This provides a sociological explanation for what Susan Sontag has called – in relation to AIDS – the 'taste for worst-case scenarios', which may perhaps be more pertinent than her own references to the approaching millennium and the modern Zeitgeist.[24]

It seems, then, that we cannot achieve a complete understanding of the current wave of public concern about venereal infections solely by pointing to the acute threat posed by AIDS and its dramatic effects. Nor can we fully account for the nature of society's reactions to the epidemic without taking other factors into account. The seriousness of the situation does not in itself provide the key to the precise form these reactions have taken.

Before exploring the various determining factors, we first need to define the reactions to the AIDS epidemic more precisely. Dutch commentators have tended to describe them in terms translatable as 'pragmatic', 'liberal', 'down-to-earth', 'undramatic', 'consensual' and 'restrained'.[25] Personal responsibility and voluntary changes in behaviour have taken the place of external supervision and coercive measures, the rights of HIV-positive individuals and AIDS patients have been of crucial importance when deciding measures to be adopted, and the information on safe sex and the safe use of needles is markedly non-judgemental. Indeed, the official policy of the Dutch government is explicitly geared towards restricting undesirable reactions in society – defined as the curbing of anxiety, panic, and the stigmatization of high-risk groups and the avoidance of moralistic standpoints – in addition to preventing the further spread of HIV, ensuring the care of AIDS patients and encouraging research.[26] This choice of policy itself creates certain specific dilemmas. How do you imbue the public with a due sense of alertness without causing panic? And how do you get the message across that AIDS constitutes a serious threat to everyone without strengthening the case for more extreme measures? To date, the firm belief in the need for a liberal and pragmatic approach has triumphed over the notion that a certain amount of panic may be justified in the fight against a deadly infectious disease. This belief has also helped to channel the presentation of gloomy prognoses generated by the compelling and autonomous forces described above. There is no one adopting a hysterical or panicky tone, nor is there a single AIDS professional who urges the use of coercion or the large-scale deployment of repressive measures. The rhetoric contains a restrained warning: *if* certain trends continue and *if* more money, more research and more information do not become available, we may fear the worst.

To a large extent, this low-key policy has resulted from a coincidence of interests between two groups that have been involved in the fight against AIDS from the outset: the medical and paramedical professions and organizations representing gay men. Both sides soon realized that AIDS would not vanish overnight, and that in the circumstances the only option was to revive a tried and tested remedy that had somewhat fallen into disuse: prevention by urging a change of behaviour. The scope and limitations of this remedy were viewed in quite a different light, however, than in the past when this had been the main ingredient of VD prevention. Medics, specialists in VD control and public health information officers were now fully convinced of the vital need to obtain the approval and cooperation of the groups worst affected. This conviction was not plucked from thin air, but derived from a specific sociological theory about behavioural change and the workings of subcultures, in which coercion had no place at all. From the medical point of view, enforcing change – acting without the support of the community concerned – was both counter-productive and dangerous: any subculture that one tries to control through coercion and the enforcement of obligations will simply go 'underground'. Valuable contacts are lost in the process, and confidence in medical authorities and health organizations suffers irreparable harm. When this happens, the situation is out of control.

From this vantage-point, a position informed by sociological insights quite unlike the views propagated in the past, medical practitioners and information officers attached immense value to consulting and maintaining good relations with leaders and spokesmen of the groups to whom this theory was chiefly applied – gay men and drug addicts – and with others representing their interests. Both afflicted groups used the position of power that this attitude suddenly conferred upon them to good advantage, and succeeded in exerting considerable influence on the policies pursued. But this participation and the high priority accorded the suppression of discrimination, stigmatism and judgementalism did not come without a certain *quid pro quo*: leading figures in the gay community must convince their 'rank and file' of the need to change their behaviour – and to do so permanently. In return for participation and protection came an obligation to share responsibility for the measures taken. This situation placed the gay community and individual gay men under social pressure to accept this responsibility and to check the advance of AIDS by changing their behaviour voluntarily.

The coincidence of interests outlined here has coloured the current AIDS policy and suppressed the call for more drastic measures. But even beyond the bounds of official policy, the responses to AIDS have been relatively low-key. Whether or not as a result of this policy, the negative fallout of AIDS on Dutch society has been limited. In defiance of all predictions to the contrary, we have witnessed no mass panic reactions or large-scale discrimination or stigmatization, nor has there been any revival of traditional moralist intervention. Thus, again contrary to expectation, the advent of AIDS has not reversed the process of gay liberation or even retarded its progress.[27] That society's acceptance of homosexuality has proved resilient enough to withstand this blow underscores the successful course of gay liberation, which achieved its major breakthroughs in the previous twenty years.[28] What are generally regarded as the more moderate wings of the gay liberation movement, groups whose main concern is to attain equal rights for gay couples in the areas of marriage, inheritance law and parenthood, appear on balance to have gained ground since the advent of AIDS, while the gay subculture has broadened out to include a variety of consumer services and even a gay ideal homes exhibition.[29] Even the more frivolous aspects of gay life have not been discredited, as is clear from Amsterdam Tourist Office's recent decision to advertise the city as a gay paradise in its tourist brochures.[30]

Given the fairly weak social position of the groups that have been worst affected by AIDS, these reactions to the disease – without wishing to descend into self-congratulation or Dutch complacency – may be viewed in a positive light. It should immediately be added that one significant reason for the low incidence of panic, hostility and ostracism is the limited spread of the epidemic itself. However disastrous the disease undoubtedly is for the patients and those close to them, for the great majority of the population the threat of AIDS is merely academic, and the danger of being involved in a fatal accident or certain other terminal diseases many times greater. Most people are aware of that. It should also be borne in mind that there are certain groups of people – some patients and their friends and relatives, some professionals involved in fighting AIDS, and some AIDS activists – who do not describe the present climate surrounding AIDS in positive terms at all. They instead emphasize the shortcomings in the social acceptance of HIV-positive individuals and AIDS patients, and point to what has not yet been achieved. So the observation that the envisaged wave of AIDS-related judgementalism and discrimination has not materialized should not be taken to imply that such attitudes and behaviour do not exist at all, any more than we can say that the success of gay liberation has put an end to homophobia or gay-bashing. There are strong opposing forces at work in Dutch society, however, and these have prevailed up to now.

This is not only because the epidemic has been contained. Historical factors have also played a role, as will be discussed at length in the next section. One historical reason has been cogently described by Johan Goudsblom. Commenting on the controlled reactions to AIDS, Goudsblom emphasizes the increased authority of the medical establishment, whose strong advocacy of a strictly medical definition of AIDS has done much to check panic and discrimination. Goudsblom attributes the increased influence of medical opinion in part to the great increase in life expectancy in modern industrial societies, because of which

> personal health depends more than ever before on the individual's own efforts, his willingness to 'invest' in it by adopting regular habits, with sufficient physical exercise and rest, and without overeating or indulgence in other excesses. ... The increasing likelihood that the promise of a long and healthy life may be fulfilled has given people a more compelling reason to accept medical authority and to lead their lives in accordance with the precepts of good health.[31]

The conviction that such attitudes – and the behaviour that goes along with them – predominate in present-day society is one of the principles upon which the current fight against AIDS, with its emphasis on individual responsibility, is organized. Whether the conviction can be upheld is another matter, to which we shall return in due course.

One final determining factor has been the relationship between narrators and characters, which has changed in two ways. Firstly, this relationship is far less fixed than in previous venereal scares. In marked contrast to the past, the AIDS characters – with gay men in the vanguard – have helped develop the policies on AIDS, and have played an active role in most of the debates surrounding the epidemic and its consequences.[32] The trend noted in relation to herpes, with characters joining the debate and hence also becoming narrators, has thus been more marked still in this case. There is no doubt whatsoever that this participation has had an effect on society's reactions to the epidemic, on the choice of strategies in the policy on AIDS, and on the content of the information conveyed to the public.

The large amount of overlap between narrators and characters means that they can no longer be classified in terms of a doctor–patient relationship, which was the dominant pattern of the 1970s. But there is another way in which these relations may be characterized now: they may be seen in terms of a relationship among men. In earlier waves of unrest about venereal diseases, sex was one of the categories that could be used to define narrators and characters. Usually – but not always – men were on one side, women on the other. In a previous chapter the VD debate in the armed forces was described as very much an all-male discussion. This led to extremely pragmatic solutions to the problem of venereal infection within the profession concerned: reliable information, prophylactics where necessary, and facilities provided free of charge. Although the AIDS debate is by no means monopolized by male speakers, men nevertheless account for the vast majority of both patients and narrators: of the 1,600 cases registered between 1982 and 1990, 1,500 concerned men. A certain historical parallel may perhaps be discernible here: the commonsensical and relatively non-judgemental approach may in part be attributable to the fact that men have been able to negotiate the necessary decisions among themselves. The accusations and conflicts between the sexes that have so often coloured and polarized the venereal debate in the past have not set the tone in this case. AIDS – in the Netherlands – has impinged too little on the heterosexual community to mobilize forces of this kind.

Midnight mission in the welfare state

Looking back at the history of venereal diseases as outlined in the previous chapters, the differences between the AIDS epidemic and the classical maladies of syphilis and gonorrhoea – that once virtually defied treatment – are more conspicuous than are the similarities. In other words, the AIDS epidemic is 'modern' not only in terms of the *conditions* that allowed it to come about, but also in terms of the *reactions* to it when viewed in a historical perspective. These reactions diverge fundamentally from traditional approaches to the danger of venereal infection. In defiance of the fearful suspicions of some, AIDS has not developed into the syphilis of the 20th century, and the responses to the disease demonstrate a break with the past rather than a reversion to it. This may best be illustrated by three mutually reinforcing developments, the roots and certain implications of which have already been discussed. The first has to do with the range of the venereal debate, the second with the authority of medical science and the third with the distance between narrators and characters. The shifts that have taken place in each of these areas are related to the post-war expansion of the welfare state.

A certain clarification is in order here. Norbert Elias provides a useful basis for an analysis in one of the central concepts of his work: the growing interdependency within and between human societies. As society has become more complex, posits Elias, more and more people have become reliant on one another. Their modes of dependency have gradually multiplied and extended, creating dense and far-flung networks of relationships. As a result, one person's actions have increasingly come to affect others, who are at an increasingly far remove – both geographically and socially – and one person's misfortunes increasingly rebound on others.

In a nutshell, the growth of interdependency in society has given the external effects of circumstances such as sickness, poverty and ignorance a wider range. This provides part of the historical explanation for the eventual willingness of élite groups to exert themselves to alleviate distress which, while it did not directly affect them, might at length rebound indirectly on their lives. Abram de Swaan has convincingly argued this point.[33] Rivalry and coalitions between local, middle-class sections of society and competition between national states were likewise of key significance for the birth and development of collective provisions. We have seen above how these mechanisms worked even in an area as narrow as the fight against venereal disease. Thus the ties between the military authorities and certain groups of medical practitioners led, some hundred and fifty years ago, to the introduction of regulated prostitution, while later a broad-based coalition of moral reformers, feminists and politicians launched an offensive that culminated, among other things, in the establishment of a system of clinics and advice centres. On the other hand it was international competition – whether military or economic – that lay at the root of the efforts to strengthen the fleet in the Dutch East Indies and the merchant navy.

As time went on, collective provisions in the realm of care for the poor, public health and education became more large-scale, more collective, more imperative and increasingly a matter for national governments. After the Second World War, the collectivization of – and state responsibility for – care provisions received an added impulse from the economic growth enjoyed by the Netherlands during the twenty years that followed. Education, health care and social insurance expanded in every direction. In addition to describing the process of collectivization of care that preceded this relatively recent phase of 'hyperbolic expansion', De Swaan also dwells on the deep impact of this accelerated growth on post-war society and on public attitudes.[34] These are the effects that concern us here.

First, the growth of collective arrangements has led to the development of a 'social consciousness'.

In the course of several centuries, the collectivization of health care, education and income maintenance has transformed the relations between people and thus changed their modes of interaction and experience. Where no compulsory and collective arrangements existed, a stranger's adversity and deficiency held an immediate appeal to the beholder's pity and generosity, which he might then heed or reject. But in the course of collectivization of care, such misery was felt to appeal less to personal intervention and was increasingly considered as a matter to be left to specific institutions, which then deserved support. In recent times a 'social consciousness' came to prevail: an awareness of the generalization of interdependence which links all members within a national collectivity, coupled with an abstract sense of responsibility which does not impel to personal action, but requires the needy in general to be taken care of by the state and out of public tax funds.[35]

Thus the consequences of collectivization have been such as to further its expansion. While the collective action resulting from the public's social consciousness has taken the place of charity, in the fight against disease it has replaced an approach that was more small-scale and more judgemental. The recent discussions surrounding AIDS clearly show that the development of the social consciousness has altered the nature of the venereal disease debate in a similar way, making it more anonymous and transferring it to a larger arena. This is the basis for the belief that AIDS is a global issue, for international cooperation and the involvement of the World Health Organization, for aid programmes that rich countries have set up for poorer parts of the world, and for the unquestioned assumption that within each country, the state itself must assume a leading role.

The increasing awareness of people's interdependency is also clear from the discarding of successive epidemiological models. After the long reigns of first the wheel and then the chain, the advent of AIDS precipitated the definite breakthrough of a new model. The chain model, which was already looking rather dilapidated in the late 1970s, eventually collapsed under the cumulative weight of new statistics and fresh insights. What replaced it was the model that became known as the *network*. As reflections of the paths along which venereal infections are believed to travel, the series wheel–chain–network exhibits increasing range and complexity; a sexual network encloses wheels, chains and other configurations, parts of which are linked by 'bridges'. In the most complicated cases, computers are indispensable as an aid to analysis.[36]

It would be wrong to see this succession of models with their ascending size and complexity as a sign that the truth about venereal infections has been slowly but surely laid bare. Each of these patterns of infection reflects the prevailing ideas about venereal disease, and each is bound up with certain specific social conditions under which they are applicable and operative. Furthermore, each of these patterns generates its own solutions to the problem of venereal disease. The wheel led simply to an obsession with the source, hence promoting measures targeting prostitution, whether in the direction of regulation or prohibition. The domino effect suggested by the chain model prompted measures that became popular in the 1930s, aimed at curbing promiscuity: tracing sources and social work. Thus far these epidemiological models and the ideas underlying them centred on certain categories of people, whom we have met in the preceding pages as characters. The network model is too comprehensive and complex to lend itself to any such direct applications; the deliberations on the danger of venereal infections centre neither on individuals nor on specific groups, but on the way in which the patterns are linked together. In terms of the dramatization developed in this book: in previous scenes, each character had a well-defined role. The prostitute was the source of infection, the amateur was the mediating link. In a network, on the other hand, all those involved combine in a form of 'positional play'. A network analysis is not about people but about patterns, frequencies, chances and risks.[37]

The increased awareness of interdependency has thus contributed to making the venereal debate more formal and less attached to particular individuals or groups, and has made it more difficult for traditional moralistic and religious groups to gain a foothold in it.

The development from wheel to chain to network involves an increasing number of people. Along with the increase of scale have come more precise definitions of the modes of viral transmission. Whereas the pathogenic link was once located in prostitution or promiscuity, the present-day venereal debate goes no further than to hold certain well-defined acts and specific 'sexual techniques' responsible for passing on germs, just as specific forms of behaviour associated with drug use rather than drug use itself are seen as hazardous. This enhanced precision, the separation of high-risk behaviour from high-risk groups, was the first step towards dismantling the traditional link between venereal infection and specific characters, a process further hastened by the increasing tendency – for reasons that will be discussed in due course – to reject the concept of a 'high-risk group' as undesirable and unnecessarily stigmatizing.[38] Alongside the official agents of disease – whether these be spirochetes, gonococci or human retroviruses – every epidemiological model is founded on another, more down-to-earth aetiology: the wheel was based on prostitution, the chain was sustained by promiscuity, and within the present-day sexual network, the contraction of disease has become largely a question of technique. The general information campaigns therefore tell the public to avoid high-risk behaviour and high-risk contacts, and not to avoid high-risk groups or homosexuality; the risks have been detached from specific groups and attached instead to certain sexual acts.[39] Aside from the greater range of each successive epidemiological model, the simultaneous specification of risk factors also helped to confer greater anonymity on the venereal disease debate. How many people truly believe in this message, which the majority flawlessly reproduces in opinion polls, must remain an open question here. Supplying the 'correct' answers has been imbued with a large measure of social desirability, but this certainly does not exclude the possibility that a shadow aetiology may have continued to exist, one in which homosexuality *tout court* is the successor of prostitution and promiscuity.[40] Be that as it may, the fact that such views have to date been consigned to the shadows is a telling comment on the climate of opinion. They can scarcely be brought out in broad daylight.

While the increasing range of the debate on venereal disease has attenuated the influence of traditional moral attitudes, that is not to say that judgementalism has altogether vanished. If we are to understand how today's centres of moral authority and prevailing codes of behaviour have become established, we must look at another development that has resulted from the past few decades' expansion of the welfare state – the rise of *experts' regimes*. As collective facilities expanded, so too did the groups of professionals and semi-professionals involved in providing them. These groups succeeded, as De Swaan has noted, 'not only in forming close links with the state apparatus but also in establishing their "regimes" over increasing sections of the population, which accordingly became their clientele'.[41] The resulting ascendancy of the medical regime has already been discussed, but other experts – teachers and educationists, aid workers and lawyers – were likewise able to expand their field of operation considerably. These experts' regimes in turn helped to foster the extension of collectivization as well as influencing public attitudes in the welfare state. As people were increasingly drawn into these regimes, often in a casual way, they became more appreciative of what they had to offer: health, knowledge, self-knowledge and an assured income. Of these, it is the first – the increased value that people attach to their health – that is most important here.[42] Of course, this trend has been reinforced by the same changes that have boosted the authority of medical opinion – improved standards of living and associated higher life expectancy. Faced with the genuine prospect of a long life, it is more worthwhile than ever before to live in accordance with the precepts of medical science. So the expansion of medical knowledge itself has been accompanied by a considerable growth in the public's confidence in it.

All this makes it entirely logical that medical voices should have gradually drowned out the rest of the narrators' chorus in the debate on venereal disease – the second important development. Not that this dominance was established without a fight, however; some people did seize on AIDS to breathe new life into the outworn dogmas of traditional moralism. In the Netherlands, efforts to stir a moralist revival failed almost completely. Even in England and the United States, both of which witnessed far more of a struggle about interpretations of AIDS, the medical profession with its strictly medical definitions has prevailed. Basically, medical science has become the main foundation on which present-day morality concerning sexual relationships between consenting adults is based. It defines the limits of what is permissible and what is not – what is hazardous and what is safe. Everyone can fill in the space between these limits as he or she sees fit.

This development has greatly affected reactions to venereal disease. Medical dominance has shifted the focus of attention from the character of the perpetrator to that of the victim. Whereas in the past the debate largely concentrated on characters seen as miscreants – those held responsible for infecting 'innocent' third parties – medical ascendancy has meant that the main characters are now almost exclusively the 'victims', this time defined as the main groups of patients. Narrators who would prefer to cast present-day 'perpetrator' characters – bisexuals or mothers addicted to drugs – in the starring role, or single out gay men as the guilty parties, find themselves opposed by a medical stronghold that systematically divests every perpetrator of his or her human form. Only the germs remain; under the influence of medical science, the character of the

241

perpetrator has shrunk to a virus. It is because of this position, and the widespread support for it in society, that the medical profession has formed a 'thin white line' – by analogy with the 'thin blue line' used to refer to a police cordon – around gay men and other persons involved in the epidemic, to protect them from orchestrated hysteria and stigmatization.[43]

Increased confidence in medical science has thus made the debate on venereal disease less susceptible to moralistic interpretation in the traditional sense. In today's context, old moral standards and ideas about responsibility and guilt have lost their value and significance. Sexual practices are no longer judged in accordance with moral criteria; certain acts are simply defined as 'more hazardous' than others. As Michael Pollak puts it,

> Almost all the 'acceptable compromises' arrived at in the individual management of the risk of infection have in common their pragmatic nature. After all, whether they have to do with reducing the number of partners or using condoms, such changes in behaviour are seldom justified in moral terms. Furthermore, the biological risk that is attached to sexual practices is seldom translated into the sublimation of sexual desire in alternative activities: instead, it tends to produce a search for a course that will provide satisfaction with reduced risks.[44]

The moralistic attitudes that once dominated the fight against venereal disease have given way to a new moral position, informed by medical opinion, which has established a less repressive, though not always less compelling, regime of health-related precepts. The modern descendants of the late 19th-century midnight mission, who patrol the red light district, do so not out of any moral convictions or with the intention of dissuading men with a clear aim in mind from visiting a house of ill repute. Today's missionaries have a more pragmatic objective. They aim to make as many potential clients as possible aware of the need for condoms, which they provide free of charge when they go campaigning.[45]

The ascendancy of medical opinion does not automatically mean that medical practitioners are the main narrators. On the contrary, what it means is rather that other groups increasingly wield medical arguments or allow themselves to be swayed by them, in the same way that doctors once used the religious and moral terms that determined the debate in the past. These days, as we have seen, narrators are increasingly characters as well. Patient groups (organizations representing gay men or haemophiliacs) or people protecting their interests (in the case of drug-users and prostitutes) have acquired a voice alongside that of medical practitioners, but in general their views coincide, because a purely medical definition of AIDS is in the interests of all concerned. The most striking feature of the current debate is the prominent role of gay men. They, more than any other category of characters in history, have become organized, have ensured that they are represented in policy-making bodies, have set their stamp on the debate, have seen to it that their own people are well informed, and have themselves helped to create a practical and emotional support network for AIDS patients. The medical establishment engages in serious consultations with them. It may not be a marriage of true minds, this bond between doctors and gay men, but it can at least be characterized as a marriage of convenience.[46] Both parties benefit from maintaining good relations; medics because of their views on the workings of subcultures, namely the belief that the gay scene must be prevented at all costs from 'going underground', and the gay community because it needs the protection it is afforded by the medical profession, and wants to retain its influence in policy-making.

When one party wants to go further than the other, the strongest, but most conservative, partner has sometimes had to give way. For instance, pressure exerted by gay organizations has telescoped the procedure for trying out new drugs, and ensured the importation and distribution of alternative remedies outside the ordinary channels.[47] While autonomous campaigns of this kind may cause irritation, they do not truly undermine the authority of medical science. On the contrary, they underscore the primacy of the medical solution. The mammoth research drive and the fervent desire for effective drugs among HIV-positive individuals and AIDS patients, while entirely understandable, are nevertheless striking when one recalls the lukewarm reception that the medical establishment gave Salvarsan, and even penicillin, and the need for coercive measures, even after the Second World War, to ensure that uncooperative patients underwent or completed their treatment!

When the two sides of this coalition fail to agree, for instance in the case of unsolicited testing or large-scale epidemiological research, they can each present their case to a third party, made up of lawyers and ethicists. These latter groups sometimes intervene without being asked, however, much to the annoyance of medics, as their emphasis is largely on protecting the rights of patients when they see these as under threat from the introduction of medical examinations and their consequences. It is hence these lawyers and ethicists – far more than traditional sources of moral authority – that have now become the medical profession's chief adversaries.[48] They watch over the unintentional results of measures under consideration. In so doing, they do not set out to undermine the weight of medical opinion, but merely oppose any initiatives that could make the disease into more than a biomedical phenomenon. In their scheme of priorities, the right to self-determination and the protection of privacy rank higher than the accumulation of medical or epidemiological knowledge.

The most conspicuous feature of this configuration, of course, is the key role played by AIDS patients and associated high-risk groups. This brings us to the realm of narrators and characters, the third area in which a clear trend has become visible. In the current debate, it is no longer a simple matter to fit the relationship between the diverse groups into the familiar scheme of narrators and characters. Here, even more than in the case of herpes, the traditional cast – with medical practitioners as narrators and patients playing the characters – is no longer applicable. There has been so much crossing of frontiers, with the explicit involvement of homosexual medical practitioners on the one hand, and the substantial emancipation of patient groups on the other, that both roles have become blurred: some 'narrators' count themselves among the characters, and 'characters' increasingly make their views known. The gap between what could once be seen as two opposite poles has thus all but closed.

The stronger power position of characters in the debate on venereal disease reflects certain wider-ranging developments, which – once again – accompanied the expansion of the welfare state: one was the weakening of social contrasts, and the other was the rise of a large number of interest groups, representing an equally large number of minorities. The levelling influence of the welfare state enabled previously powerless groups to protect their interests more effectively. In the case of AIDS, gay men were in the middle of a successful process of liberation, and there were numerous organizations that could, and did, help fight the epidemic. The involvement of such organizations was not sought from outside; on the contrary, they were themselves the initiators, along with a vanguard of progressive medics, urging the government to take action and raising people's consciousness both in and beyond their own circles. Not only gay rights groups were involved; haemophiliacs, drug addicts and prostitutes also had groups watching over their interests, and soon after the first signs of crisis they joined the debate and continued to play an active role.

The resultant merging of narrators and characters reinforced the effect of the trends already mentioned – the scaling-up of operations and growth in authority of the medical profession. Now that those afflicted were also the people proposing solutions, there was little scope for moralists. Anyone joining in today's debate is obliged to take far more account of the groups affected than in the past. An outsider can expect to be rebuked for any observation that is taken amiss. The current debate on venereal disease in the Netherlands is characterized by a conspicuous and concerted rejection of moralizing, a fear of even being suspected of having expressed a moral judgement concerning other people's actions. Let us once again follow the present-day midnight missionaries on their intrepid expeditions into the red light districts of nine large towns. Although their doling out of free condoms in itself contrasts sharply with the moralist intervention of their 19th-century predecessors, their presence – despite their purely pragmatic intentions – was still capable of being misunderstood by the target group. One solution to this problem was to involve the people at risk – prostitutes and their clients. Given their expertise, based on their own experience, it was argued that

> they could make a significant contribution to developing information provisions. They would also be very suitable for deployment in the campaign itself. The distribution of condoms by members of the target group itself would be unlikely to provoke any opposition. No one would be wary of their adopting a moralizing or didactic tone.[49]

The open moralism that was once so much taken for granted simply does not work any more. At best, it arouses a defensive response, and at worst it is counter-productive – at any rate, that is what is generally believed.[50] Perhaps it never worked at all, but it once set the tone all the same. It is almost impossible to reconcile the present-day balance of power between the various groups involved in the problem of venereal disease with the accusatory tone of judgementalism.

The erosion of the traditional us-and-them polarization between narrators and characters also comes out in the resistance to the custom of casting certain individuals in the role of characters. These days many people have an aversion to identifying characters, or 'high-risk groups' in the current jargon, and a fear of stigmatization that was entirely alien to previous generations. For instance, in Chapter I of the future scenario report *AIDS in Nederland tot 2000* we read:

> The concept of a 'high-risk group' may unintentionally and wrongly create the impression that homosexuality or hard drug use in themselves carry the risk of infection with AIDS. Whenever possible, we shall speak of sub-epidemics, groups of patients, men with homosexual contacts etc. In some cases, however, the concept of a 'high-risk group', in the neutral epidemiological sense of the term, will be unavoidable.[51]

Never had the debate on venereal disease known such a cautious use of words. The link between the danger of contracting a venereal infection and specific, silent and anonymous characters was indeed one of the few certainties that one could cling to. But the increased faith in medical science reduced the need for social divisions of this kind, and with the changed social structure in which the debate was conducted, the way in which 'perpetrator characters' had been treated in the past was increasingly experienced as distasteful. We have already seen several consequences of this growing revulsion for the traditional presentation of the problem of VD: the present-day classification of patients on the basis of the route of infection, the removal of the perpetrator character from the debate, and the link between risks and sexual techniques rather than between the danger of infection and specific sections of the population. The habit that 'venereal entrepreneurs' had of bringing the subject to the attention of the general public by stressing that the generally 'innocent' victims of venereal infection were now found everywhere (which meant, in the past, in all social classes) was strengthened by this reversal of attitudes. At the same time, it underwent a fundamental change. The present-day variant of this approach is based not only on considerations of strategy but also on conscious idealism. Despite the fact that the AIDS epidemic quite clearly strikes at certain specific sections of the population, a definite effort has been made to ensure that AIDS is not seen as a problem of specific groups, which are marginal anyway, but as a disease that anyone could get and is therefore of relevance to the whole of society.[52] The general message propagated by AIDS prevention workers is attuned to this, and at the same time specific information campaigns aimed at the heterosexual population or certain parts of it – young people, migrants and holiday-makers – have been incorporated into the official prevention policy since 1987.

The revival of moralist intervention in sexual matters, which was so feared with the advent of AIDS, did not materialize in the Netherlands. The increased scale of activities, the new faith in medical science and the lessening of the gap in power between narrators and characters immunized the debate on venereal disease, as it were, against any such development. Ideas about sex, and controls on sexual behaviour, have been changed by the advent of AIDS, but they have not reverted to the old patterns. It is time to take stock of these changes.

Venereal disease and controls on sexual behaviour

The history of venereal diseases is in many ways bound up with the history of sexuality. The link is not just the obvious one of causation, but also has a more indirect component: dominant views on sexuality help determine society's response to the presence of venereal diseases and the danger of contracting them. Historical changes in these responses therefore tell us about developments in the history of sexuality, and in particular about the ways in which society tries to regulate it. While medicine was virtually helpless in the face of venereal disease, and the watchword was prevention – as was the case for much of the past hundred years, with the exception of the period from about 1950 to 1980 – the fight against VD focused mainly on the control of sexual relations, from the sheer lack of any alternative. Whether the terrifying aspects of infection were publicized deliberately as a deterrent, or information was supplied in a more matter-of-fact way; whether venereal diseases were seen primarily as a sin, or first and foremost as a disease; at each stage, reducing the risk of infection meant placing certain constraints on sexuality. So it is worth looking at the ways in which VD prevention workers have gone about this. Elias, once again, provides a convenient theoretical framework for this analysis.

Elias's theory of civilization dwells on the transition, in his terms, from *Fremdzwang* to *Selbstzwang* – from external constraints to self-restraint – that characterizes the civilization process as he describes it. Elias argues that as society is gradually woven into a vast mesh of connected lives, and social groups vie for ascendancy, people's behaviour and their emotional lives necessarily become less erratic. People learn to temper their impulses and passions, come to take more account of others, and look more to the future.

As this process unfolds, social precepts and prohibitions are internalized. Gradually, relations between people become less dependent on external constraints and more a question of individual conscience.[53] In Elias's work, the development briefly summarized here relates to European civilization from the late middle ages up to the 19th century. Whether the process continued during the 20th century, and in particular after the Second World War, became the subject of controversy in the 1970s, and remains a contentious issue today.[54] Should the slackening in codes of conduct since the war be seen as a continuation of this process, or rather as a reversal of it? Have the controls on people's behaviour and feelings multiplied, becoming more complex and sophisticated, or actually decreased?

When we apply Elias's theory of civilization to the history of sexual regulation in the fight against venereal disease, we soon encounter similar problems of interpretation. One way in which AIDS prevention to date has differed from previous episodes in the history of VD control is the heavy, and exclusive, emphasis placed on individual responsibility. The containment of the epidemic depends on individual, freely elected changes in sexual behaviour, or surrounding the use of drugs. Here I am focusing on the first of these two areas. This emphasis on people's individual responsibility and their ability to control their own sexual behaviour is scarcely a new element in the fight against venereal disease. Self-control has always figured in the debate – sometimes because nothing else was available, and sometimes as an obligatory extra, but often it has been the main objective, a lofty ideal pursued by moral reformers.

Yet today's insistence on self-control is in two ways a new departure. Firstly, the definition of self-control is itself gradually changing. It once meant sexual abstinence both before and outside marriage, a norm that was reinforced, but not created, by the danger of contracting VD. The self-control on which current AIDS prevention is so heavily reliant is remote from this form of abstinence; the danger of infection is its only *raison d'être*. Nowadays, people – and gay men in particular – are expected to refrain from high-risk activity; they are counselled to use condoms or to take other set precautions to ensure safe sex. This approach is clearly based on the workings of what we may call 'self-restraint imposed by external constraints', with the external constraints consisting both of the existence of the disease and of the social configuration that has evolved around it: alongside the dread of contracting a fatal infection, the relationship between the various groups involved in the AIDS epidemic has generated a good deal of social pressure, particularly on the gay community, to behave responsibly and to keep to the rules of safe sex.

Does compliance with these rules point to a finely tuned and highly developed level of self-control, one that can only be mustered by those who have attained supreme mastery over their sexual impulses and desires? Or is it rather a bare minimum, as people can scarcely be expected, since the liberalizing and de-civilizing process of the past few decades, to control their sexual urges? According to the latter view it is only when compelled to do so by dramatic external constraints that people are prepared to consider making strictly essential adjustments to their behaviour, and have enough will-power to keep to them. It is hard enough to resolve this divergence in interpretation, let alone to ascertain whether the factual level of self-control has increased or decreased over the years. A plausible case can be made for the proposition that life in the modern welfare state has made people in general less erratic in their behaviour, more focused on the future and less inclined to take risks.[55] But whether, when faced by the presence of a deadly venereal disease, they display *more* self-control – as opposed to a different form – than their predecessors, is simply impossible to determine.

The second way in which today's emphasis on self-control differs from previous efforts is the absence of supplementary coercive measures. In the past, although many saw self-control as an ideal to be pursued, wherever possible external measures were introduced to back it up: these included regulated prostitution, a ban on brothels and coercive regulations during and shortly after the Second World War. In contrast, none of the measures that might have been introduced in the attempt to contain AIDS – the closure of saunas and other meeting-places for anonymous sex – have been implemented in the Netherlands. What current trends make clear is therefore not so much whether people are better or worse at controlling their sexual impulses, but rather that there has been an increase in public confidence in self-control.

It is too soon to tell whether this confidence is well-founded. 15% of those responding to questionnaires conducted over the past few years state that they have changed their sexual behaviour under the influence of AIDS.[56] The use of condoms is the change most commonly reported. Condom sales figures reveal a 20% rise in 1988, to about 25 million a year, after which the figures gradually returned to their previous level.[57] Another way in which we can try to determine whether people have structurally changed their behaviour is by plotting the incidence of other venereal diseases. Among heterosexuals the statistics show no clear pattern, offering at best shaky evidence for the proposition that the advent of AIDS has led to any noteworthy change of behaviour.[58] Viewing the figures generated by questionnaires and epidemiological studies as a whole, it would appear fair to conclude that virtually everyone knows of the protection afforded by condoms, that many people plan to use them in the future, and that a small minority actually does so.[59]

The discrepancy between intention and practice probably reflects another incongruity, namely that between information campaigns stressing that everyone is at risk, and everyday experience, which quite fails to support this. In the Netherlands, AIDS has in fact remained largely a problem of specific groups. Where epidemiology is concerned, the changes of behaviour and the ability to exert self-control within these groups are therefore more interesting than they are within the largely heterosexual general population. In this connection, initial reports were very hopeful: studies conducted among gay men in Amsterdam revealed that a large majority had changed their sexual behaviour within a short space of time.[60] But perseverance proved to be essential, and around 1990 a new increase in the number of infections within the Amsterdam cohort gave rise to suspicions that many gays were becoming more lax in observing safe-sex rules, or that the changes in behaviour that they had adopted were inadequate.[61] The increased incidence of other venereal diseases (syphilis and anal gonorrhoea) among gay men in Amsterdam seemed to confirm these suspicions; nor did research into the use of condoms in this group present a reassuring picture.[62] International comparisons likewise tend to dampen the original mood of optimism. These reveal that Dutch policy on prevention among gay men has achieved poorer results, in the proportional increase in numbers of gay male AIDS patients, than those achieved in Germany and England, and far poorer than those in Switzerland and the Scandinavian countries.[63]

Although the explicit, matter-of-fact information that is distributed to the public takes little account of it, the rational control of sexual behaviour that is called for in this matter is a complicated business, one that dramatically affects the lives of those concerned and that is scarcely compatible with some of the needs and desires that are pursued in sexual relations.[64] Despite these difficulties, which tend to be glossed over, and despite the recent 'regression', the course adopted, one based on individual responsibility, has nevertheless yielded striking results in the group of gay men, a group that is reasonably well integrated into society. On the basis of theoretical considerations, it is questionable whether this also applies to groups that are less well organized and integrated – drug-users, for instance.[65] Given the ties that exist between drug addicts and the various care facilities available to them, the starting-point in the Netherlands is relatively favourable. But few changes in the sexual behaviour of drug addicts have been noted. Although the vast majority of addicted prostitutes state that they use condoms in their work, in their private sexual relationships they – like other hard drug-users – shun condoms almost completely.[66]

Self-restraint thus remains a shaky and intractable instrument to depend on. But the amount of information that is available in the realm of safe (or unsafe) sex is in itself an indication that confidence in self-restraint is prudently 'covered' by a fairly extensive monitoring system. An army of AIDS researchers studies attentively the behaviour of high-risk groups from a distance, and through a variety of channels. A far less elaborate, though by no means negligible, network watches over heterosexual activity. The surveillance that has thus grown up is far from comprehensive, but more inclusive than earlier forms of registration and external control. Traditional forms of surveillance – compulsory registration of new cases and tracing sources – have made way for a far-flung complex of cohort studies, surveys, questionnaires on behaviour and opinions, specified statistics on the incidence of venereal diseases, and a whole spectrum of isolated studies. Together, they make up the safety gauge of the policy that has been pursued.

Conclusion

In the course of this discussion of the Dutch response to the AIDS epidemic, several of the historical lines that run through the various chapters of this book have been mapped out. Now the moment has come to gather them together, to look at the constants and the variables in the history of venereal disease and the fight against it. The Introduction posed three questions: how have public responses to the problem of venereal disease changed in the course of time, what is the social function of peaks of concern, and what does a historical comparison of various stages in the venereal debate teach us?

First, the fluctuations in concern about the problem of venereal disease. Why has the subject commanded more public interest at some times than at others? These swings cannot be explained either theoretically or empirically in terms of contemporaneous or recent fluctuations in the prevalence of VD itself or of the danger posed by it. This is obviously not to say that matters such as incidence and the availability of a cure play no role. But while such factors help determine the threat posed by the presence of venereal diseases, they are not, it appears, decisive in determining the dynamics of the venereal debate. The advent of a *new* venereal disease, AIDS, did of course have an impact on the debate, but in this connection too, neither the intensity nor the nature of the current debate on venereal disease can be fully accounted for by the virulence of AIDS.

The previous chapters have described several periods during which the ever-present concern about venereal diseases swelled into a wave of public alarm or even panic. At such times, the debate acquired an unusual intensity, and otherwise disparate groups found themselves broadly agreeing on the diagnosis of the problem and the way it should be tackled. Unlikely alliances of this kind were far more in evidence at the end of the 19th century and shortly after the Second World War, both peak periods of concern, than at other times. The advent of AIDS triggered a third wave of public alarm, from the mid-1980s onwards.

The distinction between narrators and characters has proved very helpful in clarifying these fluctuations in concern. As we have seen, the changing relations between these categories could be explained, in the past, in terms of certain parameters: different social classes, men versus women, and doctors versus patients. It was changes in these more fundamental oppositions in society, in the first place, that generated the dynamics of the venereal debate. The emancipation of workers and women formed a significant backdrop to the late 19th-century struggle against prostitution and venereal disease, the economic power secured by girls between the wars provoked a reaction from middle-class men that simmered for a long time before finally boiling over immediately after the Second World War; and as for the current debate, here the emancipation of various groups of patients has played a crucial role.

The three sets of parameters have not always been prominent at the same time. During the period spanned by this book, class distinctions have gradually lost their relevance, and in today's debate they scarcely figure at all. To a lesser extent, one might say the same of the opposition between the sexes, as is clear from the herpes scare. Throughout the period studied, men and women can be found playing the respective roles of narrators and characters at various times, but the fierce battle of the sexes that was fought over the issue of venereal disease at the end of the 19th century is difficult to imagine now. The third opposition, that between doctor and patient, has become the dominant one since the Second World War. In the AIDS debate too, these two groups are very much in the foreground. This altered landscape in part explains the diminishing social resonance of the problem of venereal disease during the period under study. With narrators and characters gradually becoming defined as doctors and patients, much of the rich symbolism with which venereal disease was once imbued has been eroded.

The second question concerned the social function fulfilled by peaks of intensity in the venereal debate. This cannot be fully understood without first recalling the metaphorical nature of venereal disease. The struggle against VD has always had a wider frame of reference, although the decrease in social resonance already noted has resulted in the ulterior motives that were once trumpeted abroad vanishing discreetly into the wings. Spokespersons in the debate have been impelled by a variety of driving forces: by the determination to improve society or fight injustice, or sometimes, perhaps, simply by the urge to attack the views espoused by their foes. For speaking out on VD is one way of expressing views about society. This is the first social function of VD scares.

The second has to do with society's regulation of sexuality. Many authors have pointed out that sporadic attempted routs of venereal disease have played a role in controlling sexuality and preserving order in society.[67] Some believe that such subsidiary effects are created quite deliberately, for instance by inflating the statistics on incidence, exaggerating the danger of infection and placing added emphasis on the most terrifying aspects of venereal disease.[68] On the other hand, Foucault and his followers have identified subtler forms of control.[69] They do not view sex as having been the object of repression or liberation; their reading is that since the 18th century the aim has been to ensure that sexuality is discussed in all openness, to listen to, record and disseminate whatever is said about it. From this point of view, sexuality is monitored and controlled not through prohibitions, repression or deterrent strategies, but through the constant production of authentic discourse.

Although the restraining influence of the VD debate, and indeed of all concern with venereal diseases, whether moral or medical, has probably been pursued less deliberately than exponents of the first of these two approaches would have us believe, and has had less of an effect than the second school maintains, its existence is undeniable. Each chapter of the venereal chronicle we have followed in this book fulfilled some function in the social regulation of sexual relations. Whether intentionally imposed or subtly and unpremeditatedly interwoven in the plot, each narrative conveyed an edifying message. Of course, for a long time a venereal infection was intimately bound up in the public mind with moral and social degradation. But even when this link gradually weakened in significance, and health risks instead moved to the foreground, the message was much the same.

If we survey the venereal debate over a hundred years or more, it is clear that the way in which sexual regulation has figured as a deliberate aim in the fight against venereal disease has greatly changed in the course of time. The main change is the growing confidence in people's ability to achieve self-control, with coercive measures and other external modes of control gradually making way for freely elected behavioural adjustments and the assumption of personal responsibility. This is the first development that emerges from a historical comparison of various phases in the venereal debate. There are three others.

First, the range of the debate has expanded enormously. This increase of scale reflects public awareness of the existence of a larger and denser network of sexual relations among people and of the related external effects. This is clearly expressed in the succession of dominant epidemiological models: the wheel was superseded by the chain, which in time yielded to the network. Taken as a series, these three visualizations of ideas exhibit an ascending range and degree of complexity. And as each model was replaced by a more large-scale conceptualization, the main factor *within* the model – the key factor in the aetiology of VD – changed as well. Within the wheel, VD infections were inextricably bound up with prostitution, the chain model focused on promiscuity, and in sexual networks the main vehicle of transmission consists of specific sexual acts.

Second, the medical establishment has become by far the most authoritative voice in the chorus of narrators. We have already noted that narrators representing a particular social class or one of the sexes have become less significant in the course of time. But besides achieving dominance, medical opinion has changed in character; medical pronouncements have a much larger sociological content than in the past. The new views that were expressed on the causal relationship between promiscuity and venereal disease in the 1960s and the theory of behavioural change that achieved wide currency in medical circles with the advent of AIDS are striking instances of the incorporation of sociological ideas into medical thought.

Third, the gap between narrators and characters has all but closed. In the latter half of the 19th century, an impenetrable wall stood between them, and the debate – or what we can glean of it – was conducted exclusively on one side of it. In the 1930s and 1940s, narrators were more inclined to refer to developments in a world that was visible to them and close at hand, although this closer proximity did not generate any exchange of ideas worthy of the name. After the Second World War, characters acquired a voice of their own for the first time in history, and the traditional divide started to crumble. Today's narrators are often speaking of their own experiences; today's characters join in the debate and respond to what others say.

Each one of these developments – the increase of scale, the increased authority of the medical establishment and the sociological input into its views, and the character's procurement of an influential voice – has reinforced the others. The combined effect is a debate on venereal disease that, compared to the past, is more anonymous, less focused on particular individuals and groups, and less susceptible to the traditional influence of those who have a moral or religious axe to grind.

Notes

1. See Pollak 1988:125-6. For an extremely detailed account of the beginning of the epidemic in the United States and of all the controversies it spawned, see the well-known AIDS chronicle of Shilts [1987].

2. For details of this controversy, see Heilbron & Goudsmit 1986; Shilts [1987]; Grmek [1989], Chapters VI and VII. After the isolation of a related virus, researchers started speaking of HIV-1 and HIV-2, the latter occurring mainly in Africa. In the Netherlands, AIDS is caused by HIV-1, and the term 'HIV' is always understood to refer to HIV-1.

3. A more differentiated analysis is called for. Not all sexual acts pose the same risk, as will be known. Anal sex carries by far the greatest risk of infection, particularly for the passive partner. During vaginal heterosexual intercourse, the risk of infection is far lower, and likewise asymmetrical: the risk of a woman contracting the disease from a single act of unprotected vaginal intercourse with a male HIV carrier is higher than the obverse, and has been estimated as 0.14%, although certain circumstances, such as the presence of other sexually transmitted diseases, may increase this probability dramatically (see *Aids in Nederland tot 2000*:55-6). Iatrogenic transmission in blood has declined sharply since the early 1980s: in the Netherlands, the risk of infection through blood products administered to haemophiliacs or in transfusions is now virtually negligible. The most frequent type of infection in blood occurs through needle-sharing by intravenous drug-users. Mother–child infection occurs during pregnancy or shortly after birth, the risk of infection in this case being approximately 30%. All in all, HIV has a pattern of

transmission strongly resembling that of hepatitis B, although the former is considerably less infectious.

The status of HIV in the aetiology of AIDS is still the subject of controversy. The most extreme position is that propagated by American virologist Peter Duesberg, who holds that HIV is a harmless virus unrelated to the development of AIDS. Duesberg has pitted himself against virtually the entire medical profession, which regards HIV as at least a necessary condition for the development of AIDS. On the question of whether it is also a sufficient condition, however, opinions are more varied. Some experts, including the French researcher Luc Montagnier, who first isolated the virus, believe that other factors – including many that are still unknown – also play a role. In this chapter I shall follow the vast majority of medical experts in assuming that HIV, whether or not aided by other factors, is the cause of AIDS.

4. See *Bibliotheek- en documentatiegids AIDS*. Amsterdam: National AIDS Committee 1991.

5. For the interested reader, however, it may be useful to mention a few of the most outstanding contributions. As far as I have been able to ascertain, the work of the French sociologist Michael Pollak and that of Mirko Grmek, a historian of medicine and biology, are among the best foreign studies with an international perspective. Also of interest are the anthologies edited by Fee & Fox (1988 and 1992) and (partly overlapping with these volumes) special issues of several journals; see *Aids: the public context of an epidemic* (1986); *In time of plague* (1988); *Living with aids* (1989). *Fumento* (1990) is also thought-provoking. The Dutch literature is dealt with in the following note.

6. A concise survey of AIDS in the Netherlands, which gives a historical account as well as looking forward, is given in *Aids in Nederland tot 2000*, published in 1992. There are also several volumes containing articles on policy-related issues, epidemiological, social, economic and ethical aspects of AIDS in the Netherlands; see e.g. Danner & Lange 1986; Vuysje & Coutinho 1989; Ravenschlag, De Wachter & Zwart 1990. For a brief account of the main findings of the ongoing cohort studies among gay men and drug-users respectively, see *The Amsterdam cohort study of HIV infection and AIDS in homosexual men. A summary of the results* (1984-1992) and *The Amsterdam cohort study of HIV infection and AIDS among drug-users. A summary of the results* (1985-1992). Both were published by Amsterdam University Press in 1992.

7. The term 'iatrogenesis' was coined and elaborated in Illich 1975.

8. For an overview of these recent developments in virology and microbiology, see Grmek [1989]: Chapter 5.

9. Grmek [1989]: Chapters 9–12. His argument is based largely on the epidemiological pattern of AIDS – the epidemic spread from several different places – as well as on old medical files and preserved blood samples in which HIV antibodies have been found. Grmek believes that HIV had already existed for centuries in various parts of the world, sporadically manifesting itself in small outbreaks, which were visible only as fluctuations of morbidity and mortality as a result of other diseases and were therefore scarcely perceptible as a specific phenomenon. The present AIDS epidemic began in the USA and Africa independently; in the second phase, the disease spread in the rest of the world largely from America. The much-publicized theory that the AIDS virus originated in Africa is therefore false, at least as far as HIV-1 is concerned, which is the issue here. HIV-2 is a related virus from a different strain which did originate in Africa, probably from monkeys.

10. See Grmek [1989]: Chapter 14.

11. See the article by Smit & Rosendaal, in Vuysje & Coutinho 1989:47-66. In the Netherlands, 17% of haemophilia patients became infected. In Germany and France, which used products imported from the United States, the corresponding percentage is about 60% (51).

12. See McNeill 1976:155 ff.

13. Grmek [1989]:161.

14. See *Aids in Nederland tot 2000*:48; see also Appendix 2. These figures, along with those given in the rest of the chapter, derive from the records of the Chief Health Inspectorate. It is not compulsory to register cases of AIDS, but anonymous AIDS diagnoses are voluntarily passed on – sometimes rather late – to the Inspectorate. The figures I give here were not known precisely in the years that they concern. Late registrations meant that the statistics constantly needed updating, sometimes up to two or three years later.

15. H. Houweling *et al.*, 'Epidemiologie van aids en hiv-infecties in Nederland; huidige situatie en prognose voor de periode 1987–1990', *NTvG* 131 (1987):818-24.

16. Knowing the number of HIV-positive individuals is of course extremely important for predicting the likely course of the AIDS epidemic. Divergent forecasts exist in this area. One highly attractive prediction, not only because of its optimistic conclusions but also because of its simple formula and clear calculations, is the prognosis based on Farr's Law. This law, dating from 1840, is based on the simple principle that the beginning and end of an epidemic are symmetrical. When applied to the AIDS epidemic in the

Netherlands, Farr's Law predicted that the peak would be reached in
1990–1991. After this, a decline would set in, eventually tailing off at
a low endemic level. Where the United States was concerned, Farr's
Law predicted that the epidemic would peak in or around 1989. See
J.P. Vandenbroucke, 'Het toekomstige verloop van de aids-epidemie
in Nederland volgens de wet van Farr', *NTvG* 134 (1990):2479-82.
On the US, see also Fumento 1990:311-19. For other, less optimistic
estimates, see *Aids in Nederland tot 2000*: Chapter 6; H.P.A. van de
Water *et al.*, 'Schatting van het aantal hiv-seropositieven in
Nederland; implicaties voor het toekomstig verloop van de aids-
epidemie', *NTvG* 134 (1990):2482-86; J.C. Jager et al., 'Prognose
aangaande hiv-infectie en aids-epidemie in Nederland op basis van
wiskundige analyse', *idem*:2486-91.

17. The accusation of sluggishness was directed at various government
departments, not at the medical profession. For the US, see on this
point Shilts [1987]; for the Netherlands, see Groeneveld, in Vuysje &
Coutinho 1989. Commenting on this accusation, it is fair to say that
when viewed in a historical perspective, the government's response
can be labelled extremely fast and effective.

18. See *Sociaal en Cultureel Rapport 1988*:28-29; De Vroome *et al.* 1990.
The findings of regular tests among the general public likewise point
to an extremely high level of knowledge.

19. See Voortgangsnotitie Aidsbeleid, proceedings of the Lower House
1991–1992, 19218, no. 48:58. This sum obviously does not include
all AIDS-related expenditure. Other ministries help fund specific
projects; municipal authorities subsidize local initiatives and facilities;
and private individuals, the public health service and medical
insurances together meet the costs of testing and a major share of the
costs of medical treatment.

20. Schnabel 1989b:18-19.

21. See De Vries 1992:1-7.

22. Schnabel 1989b:29.

23. Becker [1963]:157.

24. Sontag 1989:86-7. Sontag's remarks concern the situation in the
United States, where the AIDS epidemic is more extensive, the
reactions to it more hysterical, and the worst-case scenarios more
extreme and doom-laden than in the Netherlands; nevertheless, the
US also has a circuit of professionals with interests to protect, and the
mechanisms of competition described here can be applied equally
well to that country.

25. See Duyves 1986; Goudsblom 1987; Schnabel 1989b; De Vroome *et
al.* 1990:268; *Aids in Nederland tot 2000* 1992, Chapter 4.

26. See Het Nederlandse aidsbeleid, Fact Sheet V-3-N 1992, Rijswijk: Ministry of Welfare, Health and Culture.

27. This is not only the conclusion reached by certain commentators (Van Wijngaarden in Vuysje & Coutinho 1989:36-8, *Aids in Nederland tot 2000* 1992:102), but is also apparent from opinion polls conducted by the Social and Cultural Planning Office. These opinion polls show that the social acceptance of homosexuals continued to increase between 1980 and 1991. See *Sociaal en Cultureel Rapport*, Rijswijk: Sociaal Cultureel Planbureau 1992:465. A similar picture emerges from a survey of the articles that appeared in numerous Dutch popular magazines between 1982 and 1989: the information supplied is correct and the tone of the articles is 'down-to-earth, open, and non-judgemental, though not without a sense of drama and sensationalism. Stigmatization ... is almost completely absent from the articles'. Nor does this magazine survey turn up any articles urging the introduction of more restrictive measures *vis-à-vis* AIDS patients or individuals or groups known to be at increased risk from AIDS. See Drent, Reinking & Van den Boom 1992:24.

28. On the successful progress of gay liberation, see Tielman 1982, esp. Chapters 12 and 13; Van Stolk 1991, Chapter 2.

29. See the articles by IJssel and Duyvendak, respectively, in Costera Meijer, Duyvendak & Van Kerkhof 1991:48-56.

30. See *Adviesnota Album Amsterdam*, Amsterdam 1992:9, 21.

31. Goudsblom 1987:209-10.

32. See Veenker, in Vuysje & Coutinho 1989:67-87; Van den Boom, Schnabel & Reinking 1991; *Aids in Nederland tot 2000* 1992:101-2.

33. De Swaan 1988.

34. De Swaan 1988. For the consequences of the post-war expansion of the welfare state described here see 223 ff.

35. De Swaan 1988:10.

36. See Klovdahl 1985; Straver & Van Stolk 1988; *Aids in Nederland tot 2000* 1992:5-6,95-7.

37. See Pollak 1987:331.

38. See e.g. De Vroome *et al.* 1990:268; *Aids in Nederland tot 2000* 1992:5-6.

39. See Coutinho 1989:24, who goes on to remark that this message does not correspond to reality.

40. Montefiore (1992) discusses the problem, albeit in a somewhat irritatingly breezy tone, that people – in this case, American youth – questioned in the AIDS era about their sexual behaviour are more likely to say what they ought to do than what they actually do.

41. De Swaan 1988:226.

42. Opinion polls confirm this. When people were asked shortly after the
Second World War 'What does happiness mean to you?' the answer
'good health' came third, with 26% choosing it. In first place was 'a
good standard of living, money' (35%) and second came 'a good
marriage, family life' (29%) (see Blom 1981:142). In 1966
questionnaires issued by the Socio-Cultural Planning Office tackled a
similar theme. In answer to the question of what people considered
most important, the answers 'good health' and 'a good married life'
tied for first place, with each being chosen by 35% of respondents.
After this came 'strong religious faith', which 15% saw as the most
important thing in life. Between 1966 and 1991 the numbers opting
for 'good health' increased from 35% to 60%. During this same
period, the answer 'a good married life' dropped from 35% to 14%.
'Strong religious faith' likewise lost ground: 15% gave this answer in
1966 as against 5% in 1991. See *Sociaal en Cultureel Rapport*, The
Hague, Socio-Cultural Planning Office 1992:438. The authors
conclude: 'The view that good health is the most important thing in
life appears to have achieved a dominant position in the pattern of
values' (*idem*:421-2). See also Rolies (ed.) 1988.
43. My thanks are due to Abram de Swaan, who first used this image.
44. Pollak 1988:70.
45. S. Biersteker, in Van Gelder & H. ten Hoeve, '"Er gebeurt vanavond
iets speciaals in deze buurt". Verslag van de experimentele
condoomuitdeelactie aan prostituanten', *SOA-bulletin* 10 (1989) 5:7-8.
46. See Pollak 1987:331.
47. See Van den Boom, Schnabel & Reinking 1991:4-5.
48. See H. Vuysje, 'Het evenwicht tussen medici en ethici is duidelijk
zoek' (interview with R. Coutinho), *NRC Handelsblad*, 1-4-1989, Z-
supplement:3; J.P. Vandenbroucke, 'Medische ethiek en
gezondheidsrecht; hinderpalen voor de verdere toename van kennis
in de geneeskunde?', *NTvG* 134 (1990):5-6; Kimsma, in
Ravenschlag, De Wachter & Zwart 1990:57-74.
49. S. Biersteker, in van Gelder & H. ten Hoeve, '"Er gebeurt vanavond
iets speciaals in deze buurt": Verslag van de experimentele
condoomuitdeelactie aan prostituanten', *SOA-bulletin* 10 (1989), 5:7.
50. See Dallas's assessment of the prevention message that was
propagated for gay men until a few years ago, in which men were
advised against practising anal sex, and warned that those who still
insisted on practising this form of sex should use condoms. 'This
advice had several undesirable side-effects', Dallas points out. Firstly,
it could lead someone to conclude that condoms are apparently not
completely safe after all, so it does not matter so much if you

occasionally do without one. Moreover, the message could itself be interpreted as moralistic. For an external advisory body to warn against having anal sex may provoke resistance that will block changes of behaviour (I'm not having that taken away from me). Dallas 1990:83-4; for the anticipated negative effects of a moralistic approach, see also Veenker, in Vuysje & Coutinho 1989:80.
Aids in Nederland tot 2000 1992:5-6.
See Van den Boom, Schnabel & Reinking 1991. The authors regard the gay rights movement as the motor behind the successful effort to conceptualize AIDS as a problem that concerns everyone instead of one that is of sole relevance to certain marginal sections of society.
See Elias [1939], vol. II.
For this debate, see *Amsterdams Sociologisch Tijdschrift*: Brinkgreve & Korzec, *AST* 3 (1976), no.1:17-32; Wouters, *AST* 3 (1976), no.3:336-60; Brinkgreve & Korzec, *AST* 3 (1976):361-4; Benjo Maso, *AST* 5 (1978), no.2:258-83; Paul ten Have, *AST* 5 (1978), no.4:713-43; Benjo Maso, *AST* 7 (1980), no.3:222-57; Paul Kapteyn, *AST* 7 (1980), no.4:467-86; Benjo Maso, *AST* 7 (1980), no.4:487-500. See also Kapteyn 1980; Wouters 1990.
This theory is expounded in De Swaan 1988, esp. 246-52.
Van Zessen & Sandfort 1991:175-6. De Vroome *et al.* (1990:272) reveal that the proportion of persons stating that they have changed their behaviour because of the risk of contracting AIDS has since increased (i.e. between April 1987 and October 1988) to 17%. The average of the various assessments that have been made is about 12%. The percentage for persons who have a variety of sexual partners is much higher, at about 47%.
These figures relate to the turnover of the London Rubber Company (Durex), which has 93% of the market. See *Aids in Nederland tot 2000* 1992:70; 'Nederland is nog geen condoomland' (interview with LRC's director of marketing J.H.A.J. Jacobs), *De Tijd* 27-7-1990:44-5. The Netherlands lags behind other countries in the use of condoms.
See J.S.A. Fennema *et al.*, 'Het vóórkomen van seksueel overdraagbare aandoeningen bij de bezoekers van twee geslachtsziektenpoliklinieken in Amsterdam 1981-1987', *NTvG* 133 (1989):886-90; Mooij 1990:139-41.
This may be inferred from De Vroome *et al.* 1990:273-4.
See J.S.A. Fennema *et al.*, 'Het vóórkomen van seksueel overdraagbare aandoeningen bij de bezoekers van twee geslachtsziektenpoliklinieken in Amsterdam, 1981-1987', *NTvG* 133 (1989):886-90; L. Wigersma, H.A. Lemette & E.H. Hochheimer, 'Hulpvragen inzake geslachtsziekten en aids in de weekendpolikliniek

voor homoseksuele mannen: ontwikkelingen 1983-1987', *NTvG* 133 (1989):1033-5; Van Griensven 1989.

61. Dallas 1990; J.A.R. van den Hoek, G.J.P. van Griensven & R.A. Coutinho, 'Aanwijzingen voor toename van onveilig seksueel gedrag bij homoseksuele mannen in Amsterdam', *NTvG* 134 (1990):1229-30; J.B.F. de Wit *et al.*, 'Stijging van de incidentie van hiv-infectie, het gevolg van een toename in onveilig seksueel gedrag? Bevindingen in een cohort homoseksuele mannen in Amsterdam', *Tijdschrift voor Sociale Gezondheidszorg* 69 (1991), no. 1:26-30.

62. On the increased incidence of other venereal diseases among gay men, see *Jaarverslag Geslachtsziektenbestrijding GG en GD Amsterdam over de jaren 1989–1991*; on the use of condoms among gay men, see Duyvendak & Koopmans 1991.

63. See Duyvendak & Koopmans 1991; Pollak 1991. Duyvendak and Koopmans explain the difference between Switzerland and the Netherlands in the effects of AIDS prevention among gay men – despite certain similarities such as a strong gay movement and a rapid response to the advent of AIDS – by pointing to the different content of the prevention message issued to gay men in the two countries. In Switzerland the message was clear from the outset: condoms were essential. In the Netherlands the initial advice was to refrain from anal sex, with the added advice: 'if you do it anyway, do it with a condom'. The authors maintain that this ambiguous message, alongside the climate of reassurance that prevails in Dutch society concerning AIDS (panic must be avoided at all costs), may have impaired the effectiveness of Dutch prevention policy.

64. See Van Kerkhof 1990.

65. See Schnabel 1989b:30; Douglas & Calvez 1990.

66. Van den Hoek 1990; *Aids in Nederland tot 2000* 1992:64-6.

67. The most detailed discussion of this point of view may be found in Brandt 1987.

68. See Van Ussel [1968]; Corbin 1981.

69. See Foucault [1976]; Armstrong 1983.

Bibliography

Adler, Alfred, Syphilidophobie. In: *Praxis und Theorie der Individualpsychologie. Vorträge zur Einführung in die Psychotherapie für Ärzte, Psychologen und Lehrer.* München: J.F. Bergmann, 1924, 108-14.

Agreement (The) of Brussels (1924), respecting facilities to be given to merchant seamen for the treatment of venereal diseases. Geneva: World Health Organization, 1958 (Technical report series no.150).

AIDS in Nederland tot 2000. Epidemiologische, sociaal-culturele en economische scenario-analyse. Houten/Zaventem: Bohn Stafleu Van Loghum, 1992.

AIDS: The public context of an epidemic. *The Milbank Quarterly*, vol. 64 (1986), suppl.1.

Akkerman, Tjitske & Siep Stuurman (eds.), *De zondige riviera van het katholicisme. Een lokale studie over feminisme en ontzuiling, 1950–1975.* Amsterdam: SUA, 1985.

Ali Cohen, L., et al., *Handboek der openbare gezondheidsregeling en der geneeskungeneeskundige politie, met het oog op de behoeften en de wetgeving in Nederland.* Groningen: J.B. Wolters, 1872 (2 vols.)

Altman, Dennis, *AIDS in the mind of America. The social, political, and psychological impact of a new epidemic.* New York: Anchor Press, 1987.

Antonovsky, Aaron, Social class, life expectancy and overall mortality. *The Millbank Memorial Fund Quarterly*, vol.XLV (1967), nr.2, p.31-73.

Armstrong, David, *Political anatomy of the body. Medical knowledge in Britain in the twentieth century.* Cambridge etc.: Cambridge University Press, 1983.

Bakker, Gerard, Geneeskundig onderzoek voor het huwelijk, van geneeskundig en christelijk-zedelijk standpunt beschouwd. *Stemmen des Tijds*, 14 (1925), nr.1, p.392-409; nr.II, p.50-67.

Bäumler, Ernst, *Amors vergifteter Pfeil. Kulturgeschichte einer verschwiegenen Krankheit.* Hamburg: Hoffmann und Campe, 1976.

Becker, Howard S., *Outsiders. Studies in the sociology of deviance.* New York: The Free Press, 1966 [1963].

263

Bibliography

Beelaerts van Blokland-Kneppelhout & A. van Hogendorp, *Gedenkboek 1884–1909. Vijfentwintig jaren arbeids van den Nederlandschen Vrouwenbond tot verhooging van het zedelijk bewustzijn.* Groningen: Römelingh & Co., 1909.

Bekker, B.V., Verslag lues enquête 1959. *GHI Bulletin,* April 1960, 2-9.

Belt, Henk van den, De zonden der vaderen. Syfilis in wetenschap en literatuur omstreeks 1900. *Wetenschap & Samenleving,* 40 (1988), nr.1, 33-40.

Berdenis van Berlekom, J.J. & Ch. Bles, *Geneeskundig onderzoek vóór het huwelijk.* Baarn: Hollandia, 1914 (Pro en Contra, serie IX, no.4).

Bergh, W. van den, *De strijd tegen de prostitutie in Nederland. Geschiedkundig overzicht, gevolgd door een overzicht der «verordeningen en voorschriften betreffende de publieke vrouwen en huizen van ontucht» in Nederland bestaande, en daaromtrent uitgebracht advies van een medicus, verslag eener commissie van enquête en resolutiën van het congres te Genève.* 's-Gravenhage: W.A. Beschoor, 1879.

Berkel, Dymphie van, *Moederschap tussen zielzorg en psychohygiëne. Katholieke deskundigen over voortplanting en opvoeding, 1945–1970.* Assen: Van Gorcum, 1990.

Berkman, Lisa F., Physical health and the social environment: a social epidemiological perspective. In: Leon Eisenberg & Arthur Kleinman (eds), *The relevance of social science for medicine.* Dordrecht/Boston/London: Reidel Publishing Company, 1981, 51-75.

Bervoets, Liesbeth, Het ontstaan van het sociaal werk als resultaat van een gelukkige coïncidentie. De articulatie van een vrouwelijke professionaliteit in het sociaal werk rond de eeuwwisseling. *Tijdschrift voor Vrouwenstudies,* 9 (1988), nr.34, 157-73.

Best, Joel, Rhetoric in claims-making: constructing the missing children problem. *Social Problems,* 34 (1987), 101-21.

Bestrijding (de) van de thans heerschende epidemie van geslachtsziekten. Verhandelingen van het instituut voor praeventieve geneeskunde. Leiden: Stenfert Kroese, z.j. [1946].

Bie, Tineke de & Wantje Fritschy, De 'wereld' van Reveilvrouwen, hun liefdadige activiteiten en het ontstaan van het feminisme in Nederland. In: *De eerste feministische golf. Zesde Jaarboek voor Vrouwengeschiedenis.* Nijmegen: SUN, 1985, 30-58.

Bijkerk, H., Luesenquête 1963. *GHI Bulletin,* juni 1966, 3-40.

Bijkerk, H., *Het vóórkomen van geslachtsziekten in Nederland, 1967.* 's-Gravenhage: Staatsdrukkerij, 1969 (2 vols.).

Bijkerk, H., Epidemiologie. In: E. Stolz & D. Suurmond (eds.), *Seksueel overdraagbare aandoeningen.* Alphen aan den Rijn/Brussel: Stafleu, 1982, 27-41.

Bland, Lucy, 'Guardians of the race' or 'Vampires upon the nation's health'?
    Female sexuality and its regulation in early twentieth-century Britain.
    In: Elizabeth Whitelegg et al. (eds.), *The changing experience of
    women*. Oxford: Basil Blackwell, 1989 [1982], 373-88.
Bland, Lucy, 'Cleansing the portals of life': the venereal disease campaign in
    the early twentieth century. In: M. Langan & B. Schwarz (eds.),
    Crises in the British state, 1880–1930. London etc.: Hutchinson,
    1985, 192-208.
Blok, Els, *Loonarbeid van vrouwen in Nederland, 1945–1955*. Nijmegen:
    SUN, 1978.
Blok, Els, *Uit de schaduw van de mannen. Vrouwenverzet 1930–1940*.
    Amsterdam: Feministische Uitgeverij Sara, 1985.
Blok, Josine, et al. (eds.), *Vrouwen, kiesrecht en arbeid in Nederland,
    1889–1919*. Groningen: Stichting ter bevordering van de Studie der
    Geschiedenis in Nederland, 1978.
Blom, J.C.H., Jaren van tucht en ascese. Enige beschouwingen over de
    stemming in Herrijzend Nederland. In: P.W. Klein & G.N. van der
    Plaat (ed.), *Herrijzend Nederland. Opstellen over Nederland in de
    periode 1945–1950*. 's-Gravenhage: Martinus Nijhoff, 1981, 125-58.
Boom, Frans van den, Paul Schnabel & Dick Reinking, AIDS als bedreiging
    en uitdaging voor de homobeweging. *Tijdschrift voor Gezondheid en
    Politiek*, 9 (1991), nr.5, 2-5.
Bottema, C.W., *Het venereologisch archief der marine. Beschouwingen over
    den invloed der toegepaste therapie op de gevolgen der syphilis*. Den
    Helder: N.V. Drukkerij v/h C. de Boer, 1931.
Boudier-Bakker, Ina, *De klop op de deur. Amsterdamsche familie-roman*.
    Amsterdam: Van Kampen, 1930.
Brandt, Allan M., *No magic bullet. A social history of venereal disease in the
    United States since 1880*. New York/Oxford: Oxford University Press,
    1987.
Breukelen, Joh.H. van, *Alcoholisme, tuberculose en syphilis. De ouders
    verantwoordelijk voor het lijden der kinderen*. Baarn: Hollandia, 1911
    (Uit Zenuw- en Zieleleven. Uitkomsten van psychologisch
    onderzoek, serie I, no.9).
Brieux, E., *De beschadigden. Toneelstuk in drie bedrijven*. Vertaald door Titia
    van der Tuuk. Amsterdam: W. Versluys, 1902 [1901].
Brugmans, I.J., *De arbeidende klasse in Nederland in de 19e eeuw
    (1813–1870)*. Utrecht/Antwerpen: Het Spectrum, 1967 [1925].
Bruijn, Jan de, *Geschiedenis van de abortus in Nederland. Een analyse van
    opvattingen en discussies, 1600–1979*. Amsterdam: Van Gennep, 1979.
Brusse, M.J., *Rotterdamsche zedeprenten*. Rotterdam: W.L. & J.Brusse's
    Uitgeversmaatschappij, 1921.

Bibliography

Bryder, Linda, *Below the magic mountain. A social history of tuberculosis in twentieth-century Britain.* Oxford: Clarendon Press, 1988.

Butler, Josephine E., *The voice of one crying in the wilderness.* London, 1913 [1875].

Caljé, P.A.J. & J.C. den Hollander, *De nieuwste geschiedenis. Vanaf 1870 tot heden.* Utrecht: Het Spectrum, 1990.

Cassel, Jay, *The secret plague. Venereal disease in Canada, 1838–1939.* Toronto/Buffalo/London: University of Toronto Press, 1987.

Centrale Gezondheidsraad, *Bestrijding der geslachtsziekten.* z., 1919.

Chanfleury van IJsselstein, J.L., *Het toezicht op de prostitutie uit een hygiënisch oogpunt beschouwd.* Amsterdam: Van Rossen, 1889.

Clark, E. Gurney & Niels Danbolt, The Oslo Study of the natural course of untreated syphilis. An epidemiologic investigation based on a re-study of the Boeck-Bruusgaard material. *Medical Clinics of North America,* 48 (1964), nr.3, 613-23.

Clurman, Harold, *Ibsen.* New York: Da Capo Press, 1989 [1977].

Conrad, Peter & Joseph W. Schneider, *Deviance and medicalization, from badness to sickness.* St. Louis: Mosby, 1980.

Corbin, Alain, *Les filles de noce. Misère sexuelle et prostitution (19e siècle).* Paris: Flammarion, 1982 [1978].

Corbin, Alain, L'hérédosyphilis ou l'impossible rédemption. Contribution à l'histoire de l'hérédité morbide. *Romantisme. Revue du dix-neuvième siècle,* 11 (1981), nr.31, 131-49.

Costera Meijer, Irene, Jan Willem Duyvendak & Marty P.N. van Kerkhof, *Over normaal gesproken. Hedendaagse homopolitiek.* Amsterdam: Schorer, 1991.

Coutinho, R.A., *Sexually transmitted diseases among homosexual men. Studies on epidemiology and prevention.* Amsterdam: Rodopi, 1984.

Coutinho, Roel, *Van pokken, syfilis en AIDS. Geschiedenis van de infectiebestrijding door de eeuwen heen.* Inaugurele rede, Amsterdam, 1989.

Daalen, Rineke van, Het begin van de Amsterdamse 'zuigelingenzorg': medicalisering en verstatelijking. *Amsterdams Sociologisch Tijdschrift,* 8 (1981), nr.3, 461-98.

Daalen, Rineke van, Tot behoud van de gezondheid. Leefregels en een sociaal programma op wetenschappelijke basis. *Amsterdams Sociologisch Tijdschrift,* 17 (1990), nr.1, 47-73.

Dallas, Michael. *Onveilige seks bij homomannen. Een verkennend onderzoek naar omvang en achtergronden.* Publikatiereeks Homostudies Utrecht, deel 17, 1990.

Danner, S.A. & J.M.A. Lange (eds.), AIDS. *Ziekte, patiënt en samenleving.* Utrecht: Wetenschappelijke Uitgeverij Bunge, 1986.

Deinse, F.J.H. van, *Het vraagstuk der venerische ziekten bij de marine.* Academisch proefschrift, RUL, 1918.

Dekker, Rudolf, De Middernachtzending, een buitenparlementaire actiegroe In: S. Faber et al., *Criminaliteit in de negentiende eeuw.* Hilversum: Uitgeverij Verloren, 1989, 109-13 (Hollandse Studiën 22).

Dercksen, Adrianne & Loes Verplanke, *Geschiedenis van de onmaatschappelijkheidsbestrijding in Nederland, 1914–1970.* Academisch Proefschrift, RUU, 1987.

Derks, Marjet, Steps, shimmies en de wulpsche tango. Dansvermaak in het interbellum. *Spiegel Historiael,* 26 (1991), nr.9, 388-96.

Deyssel, L. van [K.J.L. Alberdingk Thijm], *Een liefde.* Amsterdam: Bert Bakker, 1976 [1887].

Dongen, A.W.H. van, *Register van onmaatschappelijkheidsonderzoek, 1945–1966.* Amsterdam: Noord-Hollandsche Uitgevers Maatschappij, 1968.

Donzelot, Jacques, *The policing of families.* New York: Pantheon Books, 1979 [1977].

Doorn, Jac.A.A. van, *De proletarische achterhoede. Een sociologische critiek.* Meppel: Boom, 1954.

Douglas, Mary & Marcel Calvez, The self as risk taker: a cultural theory of contagion in relation to AIDS. *The Sociological Review,* 38 (1990), 445-64.

Dowling, Harry F., Comparisons and contrasts between the early arsphenamine and early antibiotic periods. *Bulletin of the History of Medicine,* 47 (1973), 236-49.

Dowling, Harry F., *Fighting Infection. Conquests of the twentieth century.* Cambridge, Massachusetts/London: Harvard University Press, 1977.

Drent, Jasper, Dick Reinking & Frans van den Boom, AIDS-berichtgeving in populaire tijdschriften. *Tijdschrift voor Seksuologie,* 16 (1992), nr.1, 17-26.

Drenth, Annemieke van, Het massa-meisje. *Comenius* 17, 5 (1985), nr.1, 7-30.

Drenth, Annemieke van & Aty Pilon, Tussen gloeilamp en transistor. Meisjes in de electronische industrie, 1940–1960. *Amsterdams Sociologisch Tijdschrift,* 16 (1989), nr.1, 39-62.

Drenth, Annemieke van, *De zorg om het Philipsmeisje. Fabrieksmeisjes in de elektrotechnische industrie in Eindhoven (1900–1960).* Zutphen: Walburg Pers, 1991.

Dubos, René, *Mirage of health. Utopias, progress and biological change.* New York etc.: Harper & Row, 1979 [1959].

Duyvendak, J.W. & R. Koopmans, Weerstand bieden aan AIDS; de invloed van de homobeweging op de AIDS-preventie. *Beleid en Maatschappij,* 18 (1991), nr.5, 237-45.

Duyves, Mattias, Sloopbedrijf onder de hamer. Vijf jaar AIDS-bestrijding, een tussenbalans. *Homologie*, 6 (1986), nr.4, 22-5.

Elias, Norbert, *The civilizing process*. New York: Pantheon Books, 1982 [1939] (2 vols.).

Elias, Norbert, *What is sociology?* London: Hutchinson, 1978 [1970].

Evans, Richard J., *The feminists. Women's emancipation movements in Europe, America and Australasia 1840–1920*. London/Sydney: Croom Helm, 1977.

Everard, Myriam, De woede van Wilhelmina Drucker. *Lover*, 19 (1992), nr.4, 234-6.

Festen, H., *125 Jaar geneeskunst en maatschappij. Geschiedenis van de Koninklijke Nederlandsche Maatschappij tot bevordering der Geneeskunst*. z., 1974.

Fleck, L., *Genesis and development of a scientific fact*. Chicago: University of Chicago Press, 1981 [1935].

Flegel, Kenneth M., Changing concepts of the nosology of gonorrhea and syphilis. *Bulletin of the History of Medicine*, 48 (1974), 571-88.

Foucault, Michel, *Discipline and punish: the birth of the prison*. London: Allen Lane, 1977 [1975].

Foucault, Michel, *The history of sexuality*. Vol. 1. New York: Pantheon Books, 1978 [1976].

Fournier, Alfred, *Syphilis en huwelijk*. Vertaald door dr. H. Boshouwers. Amsterdam: Scheltema & Holkema, 1905 [1880].

Fox, Daniel M. & Elizabeth Fee (eds.), *AIDS. The burdens of history*. Berkeley/Los Angeles/London: University of California Press, 1988.

Fox, Daniel M. & Elizabeth Fee (eds.), *AIDS. The making of a chronic disease*. Berkeley/Los Angeles/Oxford: University of California Press, 1992.

Frenken, Jos (ed.), *Seksuologie. Een interdisciplinaire benadering*. Deventer: Van Loghum Slaterus, 1980.

Frenken, Jos, Seksuele moeilijkheden in Nederland. Een overzicht. *Maandblad Geestelijke Volksgezondheid*, 42 (1987), nr.1, 3-18.

Fumento, Michael, *The myth of heterosexual AIDS. How a tragedy has been distorted by the media and partisan politics*. New York: Basic Books, 1990.

Galtier-Boissière, *Oorzaken, gevolgen en behandeling der syphilitische ziekte*. Amsterdam: A. van Klaveren, z.j. [1906].

Gastelaars, Marja, *Een geregeld leven. Sociologie en sociale politiek in Nederland 1925–1968*. Amsterdam: SUA, 1985.

Gerritsen, C.V., *Eenige bezwaren tegen het reglementeeren der prostitutie*. Amersfoort: Slothouwer, 1882.

Geschiedenis van het moderne Nederland. Politieke, economische en sociale ontwikkelingen. Houten: De Haan, 1988.

Bibliography

Glucksmann, Miriam, *Women assemble. Women workers and the new industries in inter-war Britain.* London/New York: Routledge, 1990.

Goudsblom, J., Openbare gezondheidszorg en het civilisatieproces. In: *De sociologie van Norbert Elias.* Amsterdam: Meulenhoff, 1987, 183-210.

Graaf, A. de, Het wezensverschil tusschen man en vrouw [1923]. In: *Feest en strijd. Uit de geschriften van mr. A. de Graaf, 1867–1937.* Amsterdam: H.J. Paris, 1937, 274-83.

Graaf, A. de, De bestrijding van de geslachtsziekten. In: *De Volkenbond en de strijd tegen de onzedelijkheid.* Zeist: Ruys' Uitgevers Mij., 1929, 89-113.

Greidanus, S., *Geneeskundig onderzoek vóór het huwelijk, een zedelijke verplichting. Tuberculose, syphilis, alcoholisme, krankzinnigheid.* Baarn: Hollandia, 1904.

Greiling, Walter, *Paul Ehrlich. Zijn leven en werk.* Leiden: Stafleu, 1955.

Griensven, G.J.P. van, *Epidemiology and prevention of HIV infection among homosexual men.* Academisch proefschrift, UvA, 1989.

Grinten, Tom van der, *De vorming van de ambulante geestelijke gezondheidszorg. Een historisch beleidsonderzoek.* Baarn: Ambo, 1987.

Grmek, Mirko D., *History of AIDS: emergence and origin of a modern pandemic.* Princeton: Princeton University Press, 1990 [1989].

Gusfield, J.R., *The culture of public problems. Drinking-driving and the symbolic order.* Chicago/London: University of Chicago Press, 1981.

Haan, Francisca de, *Sekse op kantoor. Over vrouwelijkheid, mannelijkheid en macht, Nederland 1860–1940.* Hilversum: Verloren, 1992.

Haan, Tjarda de, '*De beteugeling van een volksziekte', of de bestrijding der geslachtsziekten in Amsterdam van 1919 tot 1926.* Amsterdam, 1991 (ongepubliceerde scriptie).

Habermas, Jürgen, *Legitimationsprobleme im Spätkapitalismus.* Frankfurt: Suhrkamp Verlag, 1973.

Handelingen van het nationaal congres tegen de prostitutie. 's-Gravenhage: W.A. Beschoor, 1889.

Haustein, H., Statistik der Geschlechtskrankheiten. *Handbuch der Haut- und Geschlechtskrankheiten,* XXII (1927), 238-1018.

Heertje, H., Het ateliermeisje van Amsterdam. *Mensch en Maatschappij,* 10 (1934), 39-55.

Heilbron, Johan & Jaap Goudsmit, De ontdekking van het AIDS-virus. Over weerstanden en wedijver in een prioriteitsgeschil. *De Gids,* 149 (1986), nr.1, 3-14.

Hekma, Gert, *Homoseksualiteit, een medische reputatie. De uitdoktering van de homoseksueel in negentiende-eeuws Nederland.* Amsterdam: SUA, 1987.

Bibliography

Helwegen, F. A., *Opvattingen over geslachtsziekten in de eerste helft van de negentiende eeuw*. Scripta Tironum: Nijmeegse medisch-historische scriptiereeks no.11. Instituut voor Geschiedenis der Geneeskunde, KUN, 1987.

Hermanides, S. R., *Reglementeering der prostitutie, hygiënisch gerechtvaardigd? Openbare brief aan prof. dr. G. van Overbeek de Meyer*. 's-Gravenhage: W. A. Beschoor, 1883.

Hermans, E. H., *Nieuwe wegen bij de bestrijding van geslachtsziekten*. Zwolle: erven J. J. Tijl, z.j. [1934].

Hermans, E. H., *Ten voeten uit. Mens en dokter*. Leiden: Stafleu & Zoon, 1976.

Herzlich, Claudine & Janine Pierret, *Illness and self in society*. Baltimore/London: The Johns Hopkins University Press, 1987 [1984].

Hijmans, A., *Oorzaak en bestrijding van zedeloosheid onder de tegenwoordige jeugd*. Zutphen: Ruys' Uitg. Mij.,1934.

Hilgartner, Stephen & Charles L. Bosk, The rise and fall of social problems: A public arenas model. *American Journal of Sociology*, 94 (1988), nr.1, 53-78.

Hirschfeld, Magnus & Andreas Gaspar (Hrsg.), *Sittengeschichte des Ersten Weltkrieges*. Hanau: Müller & Kiepenheuer, z.j. [1929].

Hoek, Anneke van den, *Epidemiology of hiv infection among drug users in Amsterdam*. Amsterdam: Rodopi, 1990 (Academisch proefschrift, UvA).

Hoog, P. H. van der, *De bestrijding der geslachtsziekten*. Academisch Proefschrift, RUL, 1922.

Hoog, P. H. van der, *De bestrijding der geslachtsziekten in Nederland*. Santpoort: C.A. Mees, z.j. [1930].

Houwaart, E. S., *De hygiënisten. Artsen, staat en volksgezondheid in Nederland, 1840–1890*. Groningen: Historische Uitgeverij Groningen, 1991.

Huitzing, A.M.I., Prostituées en hun klanten in de negentiende eeuw: een literatuuroverzicht. *Tijdschrift voor Sociale Geschiedenis*, 7 (1981), nr.3, 223-46.

Huitzing, An, *Betaalde liefde. Prostituées in Nederland 1850–1900*. Bergen: Octavo, 1983.

Hulsmeyer, C., *Staatsbordeelen. Practische oplossing der prostitutie-kwestie. Dringende voorstellen aan besturen, geneesheren, staatslieden en publiek*. 's-Gravenhage: Volksuitgaven-Bureau, z.j. [1893].

Ibsen, Henrik, *Ghosts and other plays*. Harmondsworth: Penguin, 1984 [1881].

Idsoe, O. & T. Guthe, The rise and fall of the treponematoses. Ecological aspects and international trends in venereal syphilis. *British Journal of Venereal Diseases*, 43 (1967), 227-43.

Illich, Ivan, *Medical Nemesis. The expropriation of health*. London: Calder & Boyars, 1975.

Bibliography

In time of plague. The history and social consequences of lethal epidemic disease. *Social Research,* vol. 55 (1988), nr.3.

Jacobs, Aletta H., Over het geslachtsleven. *Minerva. Algemeen Nederlandsch Studenten-Weekblad,* 27 (1902), nr.6, 71-3.

Jacobs, Aletta H., *Herinneringen.* Nijmegen: SUN, 1985 [1924].

Jones, James H., *Bad blood. The Tuskegee syphilis experiment.* New York: The Free Press, 1981.

Kaam, Ben van, *Parade der mannenbroeders. Protestants leven in Nederland, 1918–1938.* Wageningen: Zomer & Keuning, 1964.

Kam, B.J., *Meretrix en medicus. Een onderzoek naar de invloed van de geneeskundige visitatie op handel en wandel van Zwolse publieke vrouwen tussen 1876 en 1900.* Zwolle: Geert Groote, 1983 (Academisch proefschrift, KUN).

Kapteyn, Paul, *Taboe, macht en moraal in Nederland.* Amsterdam: Arbeiderspers, 1980.

Kass, Edward H., Infectious diseases and social change. *Journal of Infectious Diseases,* 123 (1971), nr.1, 110-14.

Kerkhof, Marty P.N. van, Voorbij het risico wenkt de extase. *Homologie,* 12 (1990), nr.3, 8-13.

Kern, Stephen, *Anatomy and destiny. A cultural history of the human body.* Indianapolis/New York: The Bobbs-Merrill Company, 1975.

Keyser, Marja, *Komt dat zien! De Amsterdamse kermis in de negentiende eeuw.* Amsterdam: B.M. Israel, Rotterdam: Ad. Donker, 1976.

Kleijngeld, A.M.P., *Gemobiliseerde militairen in Tilburg tijdens de Eerste Wereldoorlog.* Tilburg: Stichting Zuidelijk Historisch Contact, 1983 (Bijdragen tot de geschiedenis van het zuiden van Nederland, LVII).

Klerck-Van Hogendorp, [Marianne], *Een woord aan de vrouwen van Nederland.* 's-Gravenhage: W.A. Beschoor, 1883/1884.

Klöters, Jaques, *100 Jaar amusement in Nederland.* 's-Gravenhage: Staatsuitgeverij, 1987.

Klovdahl, Alden S., Social networks and the spread of infectious diseases: the AIDS example. *Social Science and Medicine,* 21 (1985), nr.11, 1203-16.

Kluit, M. Elisabeth, *Het protestantse Réveil in Nederland en daarbuiten, 1815–1865.* Amsterdam: Paris, 1970.

Kooy, G. A., *Seksualiteit, huwelijk en gezin in Nederland. Ontwikkelingen en vooruitzichten.* Deventer: Van Loghum Slaterus, 1975.

Kooy, G.A., Ontwikkelingen met betrekking tot de intieme levenssfeer. In: *Nederland na 1945. Beschouwingen over ontwikkeling en beleid.* Deventer: Van Loghum Slaterus, 1980, 40-62.

Lammerts van Bueren, J., Sexueele gevaren en zedelijke kracht. In: J. van der Spek (ed.), *Het zedelijkheidsvraagstuk.* Rotterdam: J.M. Bredée's Uitg.Mij., z.j. [1931].

Bibliography

Leenaars, P.E.M., G.H. de Weert-Van Oene & A.J.P. Schrijvers, *Circuitkeuze van SOA-patiënten*. Vakgroep Algemene Gezondheidszorg en Epidemiologie, RUU, 1989.

Leeuwen, Th. M. van, *De invloed der nieuwe onderzoekingen op de therapie der syphilis. Eenige opmerkingen voor den medicus practicus*. Utrecht: H. de Vroede, 1911.

Leeuwen, Th.M., Geneeskundig onderzoek voor het huwelijk. *Waarheid en Vrede. Evangelisch Tijdschrift voor de Protestantsche Kerken*, 61 (1924), 790-808.

Lewandowski, Herbert & P.J. van Dranen, *Beschavings- en zedengeschiedenis van Nederland*. Amsterdam: Uitgevers-maatschappij Enum, 1933.

Liagre Böhl, Herman de, De Nederlandse pers over de omgang van vrouwen met Canadezen in de zomer van 1945. *De Gids*, 148 (1985), nr.3/4, 243-56.

Liagre Böhl, Herman de, Zedeloosheidsbestrijding in 1945. Een motor van wederopbouw. In: Hansje Galesloot & Margreet Schrevel (eds.), *In fatsoen hersteld. Zedelijkheid en wederopbouw na de oorlog*. Amsterdam: SUA, z.j. [1987], 15-28.

Liagre Böhl, Herman de & Guus Meershoek, *De bevrijding van Amsterdam. Een strijd om macht en moraal*. Zwolle: Uitgeverij Waanders, 1989.

Liagre Böhl, Herman de, Jan Nekkers & Laurens Slot (eds.), *Nederland industrialiseert! Politieke en ideologiese strijd rondom het naoorlogse industrialisatiebeleid 1945–1955*. Nijmegen: SUN, 1981.

Lieburg, M.J. van, De syfilitische patiënt in de geschiedenis van het Nederlandse ziekenhuiswezen vóór 1900. *Tijdschrift voor Sociale Geschiedenis*, 8 (1982), 156-79.

Lieburg, M.J. van, *Van zeemanshospitaal tot havenziekenhuis. De geschiedenis van de Stichting Havenziekenhuis en Instituut voor Tropische Ziekten te Rotterdam*. Rotterdam: Erasmus Publishing, 1992.

Lieshout, Peter van, Veertig jaar geestelijke volksgezondheid. Een analyse van het MGv. *Maandblad Geestelijke Volksgezondheid*, 40 (1985), nr.12, 1243-74.

Living with AIDS, I en II. *Daedalus*, vol.118 (1989), nr.2 en 3.

Mansholt, W. H. & E. A. Keuchenius, *Reglementeering der prostitutie*. Baarn: Hollandia, 1906 (Pro en Contra, serie II no.4).

McKeown, Thomas, *The modern rise of population*. London: Edward Arnold, 1976a.

McKeown, Thomas, *The role of medicine. Dream, mirage or nemesis?* London: The Nuffield Provincial Hospitals Trust, 1976b.

McNeill, William H., *Plagues and peoples*. New York: Anchor Press/Doubleday, 1976.

Bibliography

Meer, Pieter van der, Vergelding. In: *Het geheime. Vreemde verhalen.* Rotterdam: Meindert Boogaerdt, 1906, 43-142.

Meyerowitz, Joanne J., *Women adrift. Independent wage earners in Chicago, 1880–1930.* Chicago/London: University of Chicago Press, 1991 [1988].

Michielse, H.C.M., *Welzijn en discipline. Van tuchthuis tot psychotherapie: strategieën en technologieën in het sociaal beheer.* Meppel/Amsterdam: Boom, 1989.

Miltenburg, H.M.Th.M. *et al., Gonorroe in Nederland (en enkele beschouwingen over andere soa). Verslag van een telefonische enquête onder behandelaars naar het voorkomen van gonorroe in Nederland.* Utrecht: SOA-Stichting, 1988.

Mol, Annemarie & Peter van Lieshout, *Ziek is het woord niet. Medicalisering, normalisering en de veranderende taal van huisartsgeneeskunde en geestelijke gezondheidszorg, 1945–1985.* Nijmegen: SUN, 1989.

Montefiore, Simon Sebag, Love, lies and fear in the plague years. *Psychology Today,* 25 (1992), nr.5, 30-5.

Mooij, Annet, De ziektes van de revolutie. Geslachtsziektes in Nederland vanaf de jaren zestig. In: Gert Hekma et al. (eds), *Het verlies van de onschuld. Seksualiteit in Nederland.* Groningen: Wolters Noordhoff, 1990, 121-50. (ook: *Amsterdams Sociologisch Tijdschrift,* 17 (1990), nr.2).

Morée, Marjolein & Marjan Schwegman, *Vrouwenarbeid in Nederland, 1870–1940.* Rijswijk: Elmar BV, 1981.

Mort, Frank, *Dangerous sexualities. Medico-moral politics in England since 1830.* London/New York: Routledge & Kegan Paul, 1987.

Mounier, G.J.D., *Onderzoek naar de beteekenis van de statistiek der venerische en syphilitische ziekten bij de landmacht in het Koninkrijk der Nederlanden.* 's-Gravenhage: W.A. Beschoor, 1889.

Muller, L., *Over bestrijding van geslachtsziekten. Sociaal-geneeskundige beschouwingen op grond van de ervaringen te Rotterdam.* Amsterdam: H.J. Paris, 1939.

Munster, J.N. van, *Met zegen bekroond. Grepen uit de geschiedenis van veertig jaren der Nederlandsche Middernachtzending-vereeniging.* Amsterdam: Bureau Ned. Middernachtzending-vereeniging, z.j.

Munster, J.N. van, *In een duistere wereld. Grepen uit het werk der Nederlandsche Middernachtzending.* Utrecht: F. Wentzel & Co., 1901.

Nabrink, Gé, *Seksuele hervorming in Nederland. Achtergronden en geschiedenis van de Nieuw-Malthusiaanse Bond (NMB) en de Nederlandse Vereniging voor Seksuele Hervorming (NVSH), 1881–1971.* Nijmegen: SUN, 1978.

Bibliography

Nathanson, Constance A., Illness and the feminine role: a theoretical
review. *Social Science and Medicine*, 9 (1975), 57-62.

Nationale Vrouwenraad van Nederland, *Bespreking van het Prostitutie-
vraagstuk op de Openbare Vergadering te Rotterdam van 2 April 1902*,
door mejonkvrouw W. van Hogendorp, dr. Aletrino, mevrouw
M.W.H. Rutgers-Hoitsema, mr. A. de Graaf & mevr. dr. Aletta H.
Jacobs. Rotterdam: J.M. Bredee, 1902.

Nijhoff, G.C., *De noodzakelijkheid van geneeskundig onderzoek vóór het
huwelijk*. Rotterdam: Brusse, 1908.

Noordam, D. J., Een gezond lichaam of een reine geest. Kruistochten tegen
onzedelijkheid in Leiden. *Jaarboekje voor geschiedenis en oudheidkunde
van Leiden en omstreken*, deel 84, 1992, 150-81 (Leids Jaarboekje
1992).

Noordegraaf, Leo & Gerrit Valk, *De gave Gods. De pest in Holland vanaf de
late middeleeuwen*. Bergen: Octavo, 1988.

Noordman, Jan, *Om de kwaliteit van het nageslacht. Eugenetica in Nederland,
1900–1950*. Nijmegen: SUN, 1989.

Nye, Robert A., *Crime, madness and politics in modern France. The medical
concept of national decline*. Princeton: Princeton University Press, 1984.

Overbeek de Meijer, G. van, *Geneeskundig toezicht op de prostitutie opnieuw
verdedigd*. Amsterdam: F. van Rossen, 1883.

Peiss, Kathy, 'Charity girls' and city pleasures: historical notes on working-
class sexuality, 1880–1920. In: Ann Snitow, Christine Stansell &
Sharon Thompson (eds), *Desire. The politics of sexuality*. London:
Virago Press, 1984.

Peiss, Kathy, *Cheap amusements. Working women and leisure in turn-of-the-
century New York*. Philadelphia: Temple University Press, 1986.

Pfohl, Stephen J., The 'discovery' of child abuse. *Social Problems*, 24 (1977),
310-23.

Pierson, H., *Gewettigde ontucht*. Arnhem: J.W. & C.F. Swaan, 1878.

Pivar, David J., *Purity crusade. Sexual morality and social control,
1868–1900*. London: Greenwood Press, 1973.

Pollak, Michael, AIDS: Risikomanagement unter widersprüchlichen
Zwängen. Reaktionen und Verhaltensänderungen unter
französischen Homosexuellen. *Journal für Sozialforschung*, 27
(1987), nr.3/4, 329-45.

Pollak, Michael, *Les homosexuels et le sida. Sociologie d'une Épidémie*. Paris:
Métailié, 1988.

Pollak, Michael, *Assessing AIDS prevention. AIDS prevention for men having
sex with men. Final report*. Lausanne: Institut universitaire de
médicine sociale et préventive, 1991 (Cahiers de recherche et de
documentation).

Poortstra, Jacob, Jeugd en zedelijkheid na de oorlog. Quid leges sine moribus. In: Hansje Galesloot & Margreet Schrevel (eds.), *In fatsoen hersteld. Zedelijkheid en wederopbouw na de oorlog.* Amsterdam: SUA, z.j. [1987], 29-46.

Poppel, Frans van, Marriage as a farewell to youth: regional and social differentiation in the age at marriage in the nineteenth-century Netherlands. *Paedagogica Historica,* XXIX (1993), nr. 1, 93-123.

Posthumus-Van der Goot, W.H. & Anna de Waal (eds), *Van moeder op dochter. De maatschappelijke positie van de vrouw in Nederland vanaf de Franse tijd.* Nijmegen: SUN, 1977 [1968].

Praag, Ph. van, *Het bevolkingsvraagstuk in Nederland. Ontwikkelingen van standpunten en opvattingen, 1918–1940.* Deventer: Van Loghum Slaterus, 1976.

Prakken, J.R., *Leerboek der geslachtsziekten.* Amsterdam: Scheltema en Holkema, 1948.

Prakken, J.R., Hygiënisten en moralisten bij de geslachtsziektenbestrijding in de negentiende eeuw. *NTvG* 117 (1973), 1042-9.

Proksch, J.K., *Die Litteratur über die venerischen Krankheiten, von den ersten Schriften über Syphilis aus dem Ende des fünfzehnten Jahrhunderts bis zum Jahre 1889.* Bonn: Hanstein, 1889–1891 (3 vols.).

Prostitutie-kwestie, De. Amsterdam: Vereeniging Opbeuring, z.j. (2 vols.).

Quétel, Claude, *History of syphilis.* Cambridge: Polity Press, 1990 [1986].

Raamplan voor de positie van de soa stichting in een gecoördineerde soa-bestrijding. Utrecht: SOA-Stichting, 1987.

Rapport der commissie tot onderzoek naar de te nemen maatregelen ten opzichte van de bestrijding van syphilis en gonorrhoe, ingesteld bij besluit van de 58ste algemeene vergadering, gehouden 6, 7, en 8 juli 1908 te Rotterdam. *NTvG* 55 (1911), IB, 1709-1808.

Rapport der regeerings-commissie inzake het dansvraagstuk. 's-Gravenhage: Rijksuitgeverij, 1931.

Rapport van de commissie tot onderzoek naar den omvang en den aard der hier bestaande prostitutie, 1897. Gemeente Archief Amsterdam, inv.nr. 5136.

Ravenschlag, I., M.A.M. de Wachter & H.A.E. Zwart (eds.), *AIDS. Instellingen, individu, samenleving.* Baarn: Ambo, 1990.

Rebmann, Petra, Syfilis 1834–1850: de geboorte van een epidemie. *Belgisch Tijdschrift voor Nieuwste Geschiedenis / Revue Belge d'Histoire Contemporaine,* XXII (1991), nr.3/4, 569-623.

Regt, Ali de, Ontoelaatbare gezinnen: over het ontstaan van onmaatschappelijkheid. *Amsterdams Sociologisch Tijdschrift,* 7 (1981), nr.4, 385-432.

Regt, Ali de, *Arbeidersgezinnen en beschavingsarbeid. Ontwikkelingen in Nederland 1870–1940; een historisch-sociologische studie.* Amsterdam/Meppel: Boom, 1985 [1984].

Bibliography

Regt, Ali de, Onmaatschappelijke gezinnen: over het verdwijnen van een categorie. In: J.W. de Beus & J.A.A. van Doorn (eds.), *De geconstrueerde samenleving. Vormen en gevolgen van classificerend beleid.* Meppel/Amsterdam: Boom, 1986, 133-54.

Regt, Ali de, "Het eeuwige kostgeldprobleem". *Amsterdams Sociologisch Tijdschrift,* 16 (1990), nr.4, 27-49.

Rénon, Louis, *De drie volksziekten. Geslachtsziekten, alcoholisme, tuberculose.* Vertaald door M. Kamerling. Amsterdam: F. van Rossen, 1906 [1904].

Ribbius Peletier, E., De jonge vrouw, die na het verlaten der lagere school in het beroepsleven treedt. *Congresverslag het gezin,* Nederlandsche Vereeniging voor Geestelijke Volksgezondheid, 1937, 38-57.

Robinson, Paul, *The modernization of sex. Havelock Ellis, Alfred Kinsey, William Masters and Virginia Johnson.* New York: Cornell University Press, 1989 [1976].

Rodway, Margaret & Marianne Wright (eds.), *Decade of the plague: The sociopsychological ramifications of STD.* New York/London: Harrington Park Press, 1988.

Rolies, Jan (ed.), *De gezonde burger. Gezondheid als norm.* Nijmegen: SUN, 1988.

Röling, H.Q., Sacralisering en trivialisering. Van seksualiteit in verlichtings- en reformpedagogiek. In: Gert Hekma, Dorelies Kraakman & Willem Melching (eds), *Grensgeschillen in de seks. Bijdragen tot een culturele geschiedenis van de seksualiteit.* Amsterdam: Rodopi, 1990, 117-27.

Röling, H.Q., Permanente seksuele revolutie in Nederland? *Spiegel Historiael,* 26 (1991), nr.9, 376-80.

Romein, Jan, *Op het breukvlak van twee eeuwen.* Amsterdam: Querido, 1976 [1967].

Romein-Verschoor, Annie, *Vrouwenspiegel. Een literair-sociologische studie over de Nederlandse romanschrijfster na 1880.* Nijmegen: SUN, 1977 [1935].

Rooy, P. de, *Werklozenzorg en werkloosheidsbestrijding, 1917–1940. Landelijk en Amsterdams beleid.* Amsterdam: Van Gennep, 1979.

Rooy, P. de, Vetkuifje waarheen? Jongeren in Nederland in de jaren vijftig en zestig. In: *Wederopbouw, welvaart en onrust.* Houten: De Haan, 1986, 119-46.

Rooy, Piet de, Jugendpolitik in den Niederlanden 1945–1955. In: Horst Lademacher & Jac Bosmans (Hrsg.), *Tradition und Neugestaltung. Zu Fragen des Wiederaufbaus in Deutschland und den Niederlanden in der frühen Nachkriegszeit.* Münster: Verlag Regensberg, 1991, 233-49.

Rooy, Piet de, "Dat de evenaar noch naar links, noch naar rechts doorzwikke". De confessionelen en de moderne natie. In: Uwe Becker (ed.), *Nederlandse politiek in historisch en vergelijkend perspectief.* Amsterdam: Het Spinhuis, 1992, 39-60.

Rosebury, Theodor, *Microbes and morals. The strange story of venereal disease.* London: Secker & Warburg, 1971.

Rosenberg, Charles E., *The cholera years. The United States in 1832, 1849 and 1866.* Chicago/London: The University of Chicago Press, 1962.

Rutgers, J., Skizzen aus Holland. *Zeitschrift für Bekämpfung der Geschlechtskrankheiten,* 5 (1906), 343-459.

Rutgers, J., *Is de prostitutie een noodzakelijk kwaad?* Baarn: Hollandia, 1914 (Levensvragen Serie VII, no.4).

Saal, C.D., *Hoe leeft en denkt onze jeugd. Resultaten van een in 1946–1947 gehouden enquête.* 's-Gravenhage: Boekencentrum, 1950.

Savornin Lohman, W.H. de, *De verhouding van den staat tot de prostitutie.* Groningen: J.B. Wolters, 1881.

Schnabel, Paul, Seksualiteit in de welvaartsstaat. *Sociologische Gids,* XX (1973), nr.3, 189-206.

Schnabel, Paul, De ethische emancipatie van de seksualiteit. *Civis Mundi,* 17 (1978), 133-40.

Schnabel, Paul, Seksualiteit, sociologisch gezien. In: Jos Frenken (ed.), *Seksuologie. Een interdisciplinaire benadering.* Deventer: Van Loghum Slaterus, 1980, 13-35.

Schnabel, Paul, Een veranderende kijk op seksualiteit. *Tijdschrift voor Seksuologie,* 13 (1989a), 208-18.

Schnabel, P., De diepten van een epidemie. Over de maatschappelijke gevolgen van AIDS. In: Atti Noordhof-De Vries (ed.), *AIDS. Een nieuwe verantwoordelijkheid voor gezondheidszorg en onderwijs.* Amsterdam/Lisse: Swets & Zeitlinger, 1989b, 15-33.

Schnabel, Paul, Het verlies van de seksuele onschuld. In: Gert Hekma et al. (eds.), *Het verlies van de onschuld. Seksualiteit in Nederland.* Groningen: Wolters-Noordhoff, 1990, 11-50 (ook: *Amsterdams Sociologisch Tijdschrift,* 17 (1990), nr.2).

Schneider, Joseph W. & John I. Kitsuse (eds), *Studies in the sociology of social problems.* Norwood: Ablex, 1984.

Schoemaker-Frentzen, M., *Mogen wij zwijgen?* Leiden: A.W. Sijthoff, z.j. [1913].

Schoon, Lidy, *Een trage ontsluiting. Vrouwengeneeskunde politiek doorgelicht.* Boskoop: Macula, 1985.

Schoonheid, P.H., *De geslachtsziekten. (Haar ontstaan, verschijnselen en bestrijding).* Baarn: Hollandia, 1917.

Schram, P.L., *Hendrik Pierson. Een hoofdstuk uit de geschiedenis van de inwendige zending.* Kampen: J.H. Kok, 1968.

Schultetus Aeneae, B.W., *De Syphilis der onschuldigen. Een warm pleidooi voor moeders en kinderen toegelicht door eene statistiek.* 's-Gravenhage: Cremer & Co., 1889.

Schwegman, Marjan, Tussen traditie en moderniteit: de Nederlandse vrouw tijdens het interbellum. In: A. Jespers & B. Koevoets (eds.), *Bericht uit 1929. Het veelzijdig gezicht van de Nederlandse samenleving ten tijde van de oprichting van het PTT Museum.* 's-Gravenhage: Stichting het Nederlandse PTT Museum, 1989a, 32-45.

Schwegman, Marjan, Een zaak die alle vrouwen raakt? De prostitutiekwestie opnieuw bekeken. In: *Het raadsel vrouwengeschiedenis. Tiende Jaarboek voor Vrouwegeschiedenis.* Nijmegen: SUN, 1989b, 75-95.

Scott, James C., *Weapons of the weak. Everyday forms of peasant resistance.* New Haven: Yale University Press, 1985.

Scott, James C., *Domination and the arts of resistance: hidden transcripts.* New Haven/London: Yale University Press, 1990.

Scott, Joan Wallach, *Gender and the politics of history.* New York: Columbia University Press, 1988.

Searle, G.R., *The quest for national efficiency. A study in British politics and political thought.* Oxford: Basil Blackwell, 1971.

Selhorst, S.B., Prostitution et maladies vénériennes dans les Pays-Bas. In: Dubois-Havenith, *Conférence internationale pour la prophylaxie de la syphilis et des maladies vénériennes: enquêtes sur l'état de la prostitution et la fréquence de la syphilis et des maladies vénériennes dans les différents pays.* Bruxelles: H.Lamartin, 1899.

Sevenhuijsen, Selma L., *De orde van het vadersche Politieke debatten over ongehuwd moederschap, afstamming en het huwelijk in Nederland 1870–1900.* Amsterdam: Stichting beheer IISG, 1987.

Shilts, Randy, *And the band played on. Politics, people and the AIDS epidemic.* Penguin Books, 1988 [1987].

Sickenga, F.N., *Korte geschiedenis van de tuberculosebestrijding in Nederland, 1900–1960.* 's-Gravenhage: Koninklijke Nederlandse Centrale Vereniging tot Bestrijding van Tuberculose, 1980.

Sijmons, Diet, *"De prostitutie-quaestie", 1878–1911.* Doctoraalscriptie RUU, 1976.

Slobbe, J.F. van, *Bijdrage tot de geschiedenis en de bestrijding der prostitutie te Amsterdam.* Amsterdam: Scheltema & Holkema, 1937.

Smit, C., *Nederland in de Eerste Wereldoorlog (1899–1919).* Groningen: Wolters Noordhoff, 1971-1973 (3 vols.).

Sontag, Susan, *Illness as metaphor.* Harmondsworth: Penguin Books, 1987 [1978].

Sontag, Susan, *AIDS and its metaphors.* New York: Farrar, Straus and Giroux, 1989.

Spector, Malcolm & John I. Kitsuse, Social problems: a re-formulation. *Social Problems*, 21 (1973), 145-59.

Spencer, Herbert, *The study of sociology*. New York: D. Appleton and Company, 1889 [1873].

Spink, Wesley W., *Infectious diseases. Prevention and treatment in the nineteenth and twentieth centuries*. Minneapolis: University of Minnesota Press, 1978.

Splinter, Leony van der, *Dertig jaar streven naar rein leven. De Rein Leven Beweging in Nederland (1901–1931)*. Doctoraalscriptie Geschiedenis, RUL, 1986.

Standing, Hilary, 'Sickness is a woman's business?': reflections on the attribution of illness. In: Lynda Birke *et al.* (eds), *Alice through the microscope. The power of science over women's lives*. London: Virago, 1980, 124-38.

Steenbergen, E.P. van, *De directe bestrijding der syphilis in de Universiteitskliniek voor huid- en geslachtsziekten te Utrecht in de jaren 1940–1945*. Academisch Proefschrift, RUU, 1950.

Stemvers, F.A., Geslachtsziektenbestrijding 1850–1880. *Tijdschrift voor de Geschiedenis der Geneeskunde, Natuurwetenschappen, Wiskunde en Techniek*, 4 (1981), nr.1, 1-24.

Stemvers, F.A., Prostitutie, prostituées en geneeskunde in Nederland, 1850–1900. *Spiegel Historiael*, 18 (1983), 316-23.

Stemvers, F.A., *Meisjes van plezier. De geschiedenis van de prostitutie in Nederland*. Weesp: Fabula-Van Dishoeck, 1985.

Stolk, Bram van, *Eigenwaarde als groepsbelang. Sociologische studies naar de dynamiek van zefwaardering*. Houten/Zaventem: Bohn Stafleu Van Loghum, 1991.

Stolz, E. & D. Suurmond (eds), *Seksueel overdraagbare aandoeningen*. Alphen aan den Rijn/Brussel: Stafleu, 1982.

Straver, Cees & Bram van Stolk, De kans op verbreiding van AIDS onder de Nederlandse bevolking. *Maandblad Geestelijke Volksgezondheid*, 43 (1988), nr.4, 379-93.

Stuurman, Siep, *Verzuiling, kapitalisme en patriarchaat. Aspecten van de ontwikkeling van de moderne staat in Nederland*. Nijmegen: SUN, 1983.

Swaan, Abram de, Lust en last, 1,2 en 3. In: *Het lied van de kosmopoliet*. Amsterdam: Meulenhoff, 1987, 19-29.

Swaan, Abram de, *In care of the state. Health care, education and welfare in Europe and the USA in the modern era*. Cambridge: Polity Press, 1988.

Swaan, Abram de, *The management of normality. Critical essays in health and welfare*. London/New York: Routledge, 1990.

Syme, S. Leonard & Lisa F. Berkman, Social class, susceptibility and sickness. *Journal of Epidemiology*, vol.104 (1976), 1-8.

Bibliography

Temkin, O., On the history of 'morality and syphilis' [1927]. In: *The double face of Janus, and other essays in the history of medicine.* Baltimore/London: The Johns Hopkins University Press, 1977, 472-84.

Tielman, Rob, *Homoseksualiteit in Nederland. Studie van een emancipatiebeweging.* Amsterdam/Meppel: Boom, 1982.

Tielman, Rob & Frits van Griensven, Sociaal-wetenschappelijk AIDS-onderzoek. *Sociologische Gids,* XXXII (1985), nr.5/6, 416-30.

Tuuk, Titia van der, *Mensch of voorwerp?* Arnhem: Arnhemsche Uitgevers-Maatschappij, 1898.

Tuuk, Titia van der, *De vrouw in haar seksueele leven. Een physiologisch-maatschappelijke studie met geneeskundige en hygiënische wenken.* Almelo: W. Hilarius, 1915.

Ussel, J.M.W. van, *Geschiedenis van het seksuele probleem.* Meppel/Amsterdam: Boom, 1982 [1968].

Valk, J.W. van der, *Bijdrage tot de kennis van de geschiedenis der syphilis in ons land.* Academisch Proefschrift, UvA, 1910.

Velde, Henk te, *Gemeenschapszin en plichtsbesef. Liberalisme en nationalisme in Nederland, 1870–1918.* 's-Gravenhage: Sdu Uitgeverij, 1992.

Velle, Karel, De syfiliskwestie in België in de 19de en het begin van de 20ste eeuw. *Tijdschrift voor Sociale Wetenschappen,* 32 (1987), 331-63.

Verbreiding (de) van de geslachtsziekten en hare gevolgen. Uitgegeven door de Nederlandsche Vereeniging tot Bestrijding der Geslachtsziekten. Zeist: J. Ploegsma, 1921.

Verdoorn, J.A., *Volksgezondheid en sociale ontwikkeling. Beschouwingen over het gezondheidswezen te Amsterdam in de 19e eeuw.* Utrecht/Antwerpen: Het Spectrum, 1965.

Verdoorn, J.A., *Arts en oorlog. Medische en sociale zorg voor oorlogsslachtoffers in de geschiedenis van Europa. Inleiding in de medische polemologie.* Amsterdam: Stichting Uitgeverij Lynx, 1972 (2 vols.).

Vergeer, Charles, *Toen werden schoot en boezem lekkernij. Erotiek van de Tachtigers.* Amsterdam: Thomas Rap, 1990.

Verkaik, Jan Paul, *Gewrichten en tijdsgewrichten. Ontwikkelingen in de Nederlandse reumabestrijding, 1905–1990.* Amsterdam: Historisch Seminarium van de UvA, 1991 (Amsterdamse Historische Reeks, nr.20).

Versluys-Poelman, A.W.L., Onderlinge Vrouwenbescherming. *Minerva, Algemeen Nederlandsch Studenten-Weekblad,* 27 (1902), nr.4, 41-3.

Vigarello, Georges, *Le propre et le sale. L'hygiéne du corps depuis le Moyen Age.* Paris: Editions du Seuil, 1985.

Vinks, P.A., *Gegevens over syphilis, uit de universiteitskliniek voor huid- en geslachtsziekten te Utrecht in de jaren 1940 t/m 1950.* Academisch Proefschrift, RUU, 1954.

Vliet, Ron van der, De opkomst van het seksuele moratorium. In: Gert Hekma et al. (eds), *Het verlies van de onschuld. Seksualiteit in Nederland.* Groningen: Wolters-Noordhoff, 1990, 51-68 (ook: *Amsterdams Sociologisch Tijdschrift,* 17 (1990), nr.2).

Vluchten voor de groote oorlog. Belgen in Nederland, 1914–1918. Amsterdam: De Bataafsche Leeuw, 1988.

Voorhoeve, H.C., *De jacht op de bleke microbe. De geschiedenis van de syphilis.* Amsterdam: Amsterdamsche Boek- en Courantmaatschappij, 1951.

Vries, Geert de, *Nederland verandert. Sociale problemen in de jaren tachtig en negentig.* Amsterdam: Het Spinhuis, 1992.

Vroome, E.M.M. de, *et al.*, AIDS in the Netherlands: the effects of several years of campaigning. *International Journal of STD & AIDS,* 1 (1990), 268-75.

Vuysje, Herman & Roel Coutinho (eds.), *Dilemma's rondom AIDS.* Amsterdam/Lisse: Swets & Zeitlinger, 1989.

Wain, Harry, *A history of preventive medicine.* Springfield/Illinois: Charles C. Thomas, 1970.

Walkowitz, Judith R., *Prostitution and victorian society. Women, class, and the state.* Cambridge etc.: Cambridge University Press, 1989 [1980].

Watney, Simon, *Policing desire. Pornography, AIDS and the media.* London: Methuen, 1987.

Waugh, Michael, STDs in the modern world. *Venereology,* 3 (1990), nr.4, 104-6.

Wederopbouw, welvaart en onrust. Nederland in de jaren vijftig en zestig. Houten: De Haan, 1986.

Weeks, Jeffrey, *Sex, politics and society. The regulation of sexuality since 1800.* London/New York: Longman, 1981.

Weeks, Jeffrey, *Sexuality and its discontents. Meanings, myths and modern sexualities.* London/Melbourne/Henley: Routledge & Kegan Paul, 1985.

Westland, Cora [C.M.E. Wisboom Verstegen-Kautzmann], *Levenswond.* Leiden: Sijthoff, z.j. [1913].

Westland, Cora [C.M.E. Wisboom Verstegen-Kautzmann], *Eugéne Brieux.* 's-Gravenhage: C.L.G. Veldt, 1915.

Wibaut-Berdenis van Berlekom, M. & L. Nathans, *Geslachtelijke voorlichting.* Baarn: Hollandia, 1909 (Pro en Contra, serie V, no.3).

Wiebes, P.E., *Geslachtsziektenbestrijding in Nederland. Historische ontwikkeling van curatieve en niet-curatieve functies en het belang van drempelvrije voorzieningen.* WVC-literatuurrapport nr.32, 1986.

Wijmans, L.L., *Beeld en betekenis van het maatschappelijke midden. Oude en nieuwe middengroepen 1850 tot heden.* Amsterdam: Van Gennep, 1987.

Bibliography

Wijnaendts Francken, C.J., *Wenschelijk huwelijksverbod*. Haarlem: Tjeenk
  Willink, 1901.
Wijnaendts Francken, C.J., *Het vraagstuk der sexueele voorlichting*.
  Groningen/Den Haag: Wolters, 1920.
Wootton, Barbara, *Social science and social pathology*. London: George Allen
  & Unwin Ltd., 1959.
Wouters, Cas, *Van minnen en sterven. Informalisering van omgangsvormen
  rond seks en dood*. Amsterdam: Bert Bakker, 1990.
Wright Mills, C., *The sociological imagination*. London/Oxford/New York:
  Oxford University Press, 1977 [1959].
Zessen, Gertjan van & Theo Sandfort (eds.), *Seksualiteit in Nederland.
  Seksueel gedrag, risico en preventie van AIDS*. Amsterdam/Lisse: Swets
  & Zeitlinger, 1991.

Journals [*]

Geneeskundige Bladen uit Kliniek en Laboratorium voor de Praktijk
  (1894–1964)
Geneeskundige Courant voor het Koninkrijk der Nederlanden (1860–1912)
Maandblad voor de Geestelijke Volksgezondheid (1946–1970)
Marineblad (1886/87–1977)
Medisch Contact (1947–1989)
Medisch Weekblad voor Noord en Zuid Nederland (1894/95–1924/25)
Militair Geneeskundig Tijdschrift (1897–1919 en 1935–1940)
Nederlands Militair Geneeskundig Tijdschrift (1947–1957)
Nederlands Tijdschrift voor Geneeskunde (*NTvG*) (1856–1990)
Sexueele Hygiëne (SH) (1921–1949)
Sexueel Overdraagbare Aandoeningen (SOA), later: *SOA-Bulletin*
  (1979–1990)
Tijdschrift voor Sociale Hygiëne (1899–1933)
Tijdschrift voor Sociale Geneeskunde (1923–1970)

---

[*]   References to articles and reports appearing in these journals are
       given in the notes. With a few exceptions these are not included in
       the bibliography.

Appendices

Appendix 1

Annual figures of new patients with primary or secondary syphilis or gonorrhoea as registered by the VD advice centres, 1940–1980.

Year	Syphilis				Gonorrhoea			
	M	F	T	%[1]	M	F	T	%
1940	125	80	205	6	593	557	1150	17
1941	229	152	381	11	797	763	1560	24
1942	324	313	637	18	1083	1280	2363	36
1943	745	705	1450	41	1775	2379	4154	63
1944	717	878	1595	45	1329	1386	2715	41
1945	679	928	1607	45	1439	1899	3338	51
1946	1458	1791	3249	91	3342	3173	6515	99
1947	1569	2011	3580	100	3803	2770	6573	100
1948	1275	1065	2340	65	2383	1480	3863	59
1949	1130	724	1854	52	1890	1100	2990	45
1950	1280	369	1649	46	1170	599	1769	27
1951	714	375	1089	30	1158	593	1751	27
1952	168	181	349	10	674	395	1069	16
1953	129	123	252	7	862	409	1271	19
1954	113	73	186	5	772	402	1174	18
1955	112	53	165	5	959	410	1369	21
1956	83	37	120	3	1013	364	1377	21
1957	70	42	112	3	881	327	1208	18
1958	72	35	107	3	867	287	1154	18
1959	52	15	67	2	788	283	1071	16
1960	79	19	98	3	931	288	1219	19

continues on next page

Source: Bijkerk 1969, vol. II:33 (1940–1967) and the Chief Health Inspectorate (1968–1980)

[1] Annual totals expressed as percentages of the total number of patients (=100%) in 1947

[2] Number of patients whose sex was not recorded

Appendix 1 (cont'd)

1961–1980

Year	Syphilis				Gonorrhoea			
	M	F	T	%[1]	M	F	T	%
1961	102	33	135	4	1030	288	1318	20
1962	162	41	203	6	1014	314	1328	20
1963	214	53	267	7	950	346	1296	20
1964	244	49	293	8	878	284	1162	18
1965	241	40	281	8	1071	359	1430	22
1966	146	44	190	5	1194	371	1565	24
1967	168	29	197	6	1386	435	1821	28
1968	117	20	137	4	1356	393	1749	27
1969	185	30	215	6	1549	752	2301	35
1970	223	25	248	7	2424	1035	3459	53
1971	260	19	279	8	2957	1350	4307	66
1972	272	59	331	9	2950	1753	4734	72 (31)[2]
1973	220	31	253	7	2035	984	3027	46 (10)
1974	382	76	458	13	3544	1730	5274	80
1975	363	68	431	12	3704	1453	5157	78
1976	453	99	586	16	2886	1424	4424	67 (148)
1977	509	87	596	17	5147	2575	7722	118
1978	723	187	910	25	4859	2457	7316	111
1979	890	230	1120	31	5940	2878	8818	134
1980	792	190	982	27	5865	2680	8545	130

Source: Bijkerk 1969, vol. II:33 (1940–1967) and the Chief Health Inspectorate (1968–1980)

[1] Annual totals expressed as percentages of the total number of patients (=100%) in 1947

[2] Number of patients whose sex was not recorded

Appendix II

Numbers of cases of primary or secondary syphilis, gonorrhoea or AIDS as supplied by the Chief Health Inspectorate, with the figures per 100,000 inhabitants given in parentheses.

Year	Syphilis		Gonorrhoea		AIDS
1976	691	(5.0)	7336	(53.3)	
1977	767	(5.5)	9005	(65.0)	
1978	999	(7.2)	9613	(69.2)	
1979	1196	(8.5)	11051	(78.8)	
1980	1169	(8.3)	12264	(87.0)	
1981	998	(7.0)	14855	(104.6)	
1982	1026	(7.2)	13425	(94.0)	5
1983	913	(6.4)	13199	(92.1)	19
1984	938	(6.5)	14400	(100.0)	31
1985	584	(4.0)	12451	(86.1)	64
1986	540	(3.7)	9841	(67.1)	136
1987	388	(2.7)	5636	(38.6)	239
1988	394	(2.7)	3347	(22.8)	321
1989	539	(3.6)	3024	(20.4)	387
1990	499	(3.4)	3669	(24.6)	410

Source: Chief Health Inspectorate

Index

Index

B

Barnhoorn, J.A.J. *155-6*
Bavaria *25*
Becker, Howard *230-1*
Belgian refugees *114*
Bergen op Zoom *23*
Bilderdijk, Willem *38*
bismuth *85, 143, 146*
Blaschko, Alfred *27*
blood banks *223-4*
Blooker, C.J.F. *52-3*
Böhl, Herman de Liagre *152-3*
Bonaparte, Napoleon *22*
Boudier-Bakker, Ina: *De Klop op der Deur 1-4, 135*
Bouman, A. *147, 154, 156, 164*
Brandt, Allan *203*
  No Magic Bullet 10-12, 13
Brielle *23*
Brieux, Eugène: *Les Avariés (Damaged Goods) 49-50, 93*
Bromberg, R. *106*
brothels
  abolitionists and *39*
  demise of *58-60*
  regulation of *21, 22, 23, 24-5, 33, 43, 52-4*
  sexual perversity in *53-4, 58*
Brusse, M.J. *129-30, 133*
Butler, Josephine *37, 45*

C

calomel ointment *103, 105*
Canada *12*
  armed forces of *149-50, 152*
cancer *8*
  cervical *201, 205*
case-finding/case-holding *138, 139*
Cassel, Jay: *The Secret Plague 12*
Catholics *38, 41, 43, 61, 129, 130, 135*
cervical cancer *201, 205*

chancroid *25, 27, 112, 128, 190*
  'syphilisation' *28-9*
Chanfleury van IJsselstein, J.L. *40-1*
children
  as innocent victims *44-5*
  see also infants/neonates
chlamydia *188-9, 190*
cholera *8-9, 24, 112*
Christian political parties *61-2, 66*
class, social *see* social class
Clean Living Society *56*
clinics *80-3, 112, 113*
collective provisions *237-9*
Committee for Moral Recovery *147, 154*
Committee for the Promotion of Medical Examinations before Marriage *96*
condoms *103, 104, 105-6, 107, 145, 183*
  in AIDS era *105-6, 242, 245, 249-50, 251*
contagion, theories of *23-4*
contagion médiate 47
contraception *43, 62, 93, 194, 195*
  see also condoms
Corbin, Alain *48, 57-60*
  Les Filles de Noce 22
Cosmopolitan 206-7
Credé, Karl *46-7*
cytomegalovirus *189, 199*

D

da Costa, Isaac *38*
dancing *130-1, 133-4, 136*
de Graaf, Andrew *88, 89, 142, 163*
de Mooij, P. *104-5*
de Regt, Ali *63, 158*
de Savornin Lohman, A.F. *41*
de Swaan, Abram *8, 196, 197, 237-8, 240*
  theory of medicalization *35-6*

287

sociological approach to *6-9*
see also venereal disease(s)
information *93-5*
  advice centres *89-90, 113, 138-9, 140, 151, 179, 191*
  safe sex *250-1*
  sex education *94-5, 99-100, 154, 156, 164*
Institute of Preventive Medicine *148*
interdependency: in society *237-9*
international relations *65-6, 185, 190*
  maritime trade *112-13*

J

Jacobs, Aletta *48-9, 55, 93-4*
Janet, Jules *30*
Japan *104*

K

Kampen *23*
Kaposi's sarcoma *220, 221*
Keuchenius, E.A. *54*
Keuchenius, L.W.C. *41*
Klerck-Van Hogendorp, Dowager Marianne *39, 56-7*
Knoop, Jeanne *99-100*
Kruisinga, State Secretary *191*
Kuypers, J. *125*

L

labour camps *160-1*
lawyers *243-4*
leprosy *224*
Liberals *31-2, 41, 61-2, 66-7, 101*
Limburg *179*
living standards *6-7, 62-3*
  see also sanitation
lymphogranuloma inguinale *112*

M

Maandblad voor de Geestelijke 154
McKeown, Thomas *6*
McNeill, William *202*
  Plagues and Peoples 5-6, 189, 224
malaria treatment *85-6*
Mansholt, W.H. *54-5*
marriage
  female employment and *132*
  medical examination prior to *95-7, 99*
  prostitution and *33, 44-5, 49-51, 53-4, 58, 59*
  sexual perversity outside *53-4*
  syphilis and *19-20*
  timing of *58, 59*
measles *10*
media coverage: of herpes debate *198-9, 200-1, 204-5, 206-7*
medical examination
  before marriage *95-7, 99*
  of prostitutes *21, 24-5, 31, 37, 40-1, 42, 47, 51*
medical profession *87, 90, 97-8, 167*
  AIDS professionals *229-33*
  moral authority of *195-8, 240-6, 254*
  and prophylaxis *107-8*
  and prostitution regulation *34-7, 40-1, 42*
  and sex education *95*
  and sexual abstinence *54-5*
  and social workers *140-1*
  and syphilis treatments *83, 84-5*
  see also medical examination; treatment
medicalization, theory of *35-6*
men *98, 166-7*
  AIDS debate and *235-6*
  functional democratization and *63-5, 66-7*